Planning, Implementing, and Evaluating Health Promotion Programs

A Primer

THIRD EDITION

James F. McKenzie

Ball State University

Jan L. Smeltzer

Allyn and Bacon

Boston • London • Toronto • Sydney • Tokyo • Singapore

Publisher: *Joseph E. Burns*
Editorial Assistants: *Tanja Eise, Annemarie Kennedy*
Marketing Manager: *Richard Muhr*
Editorial-Production Administrator: *Annette Joseph*
Editorial-Production Coordinator: *Susan Freese*
Editorial-Production Service: *Lynda Griffiths*
Electronic Composition: *Omegatype Typography, Inc.*
Manufacturing Buyer: *Julie McNeill*
Cover Administrator: *Linda Knowles*

Copyright © 2001, 1997, 1993 by Allyn & Bacon
A Pearson Education Company
160 Gould Street
Needham Heights, MA 02494

Internet: www.abacon.com

Between the time website information is gathered and then published, it is not unusual for some sites to have closed. Also, the transcription of URLs can result in unintended typographical errors. The publisher would appreciate being notified of any problems with URLs so that they may be corrected in subsequent editions. Thank you.

Library of Congress Cataloging-in-Publication Data

McKenzie, James F.
     Planning, implementing, and evaluating health promotion programs: a primer / James
  F. McKenzie, Jan L. Smeltzer.—3rd ed.
       p. ; cm.
     Includes bibliographical references and indexes.
     ISBN 0–205–31915–7
     1. Health promotion—Planning. 2. Health promotion—Evaluation. I. Smeltzer, Jan L.
  II. Title
     [DNLM: 1. Health Promotion. 2. Health Education. 3. Health Planning. WA 525
  M4785p 2000]
  RA427.8 .M39 2000
  613'.068—dc21

                                                                                    00-030578

Printed in the United States of America

10 9 8 7 6 5 4 3   RRDV   05 04 03 02 01

This book is dedicated to five special people—
Bonnie, Anne, Greg, Hilary, and Mike—

and to our teachers and mentors—
Marshall H. Becker (deceased), Mary K. Beyrer,
Norren M. Clark, Nancy Kinney, Terry W. Parsons,
Irwin M. Rosenstock, and Yuzuru J. Takeshita

Contents

Preface

This book is written for students who are enrolled in their first professional course in health promotion program development. It is designed to help them understand and develop the skills necessary to carry out program development regardless of the setting. The book is unique among the health program–planning textbooks on the market in that it provides readers with both theoretical and practical information. A straightforward, step-by-step format is used to make concepts clear and the full process of health promotion programming understandable. This book also provides, under a single cover, material on all three areas of program development: planning, implementing, and evaluating.

Learning Aids

Each chapter of the book includes chapter objectives, a list of key terms, presentation of content, chapter summary, review questions, activities, and web activities. In addition, many of the key concepts are further explained with information presented in figures, tables, and the appendixes.

Chapter Objectives. The chapter objectives identify the content and skills that should be mastered after reading the chapter, answering the end-of-chapter questions, and completing both sets of activities. Most of the objectives are written using the cognitive and psychomotor (behavior) educational domains. For most effective use of the objectives, we suggest that they be reviewed before reading the chapter. This will help readers focus on the major points in each chapter and will facilitate answering the questions and completing the activities at the end.

Key Terms. Key terms are introduced in each chapter of the textbook and are important to the understanding of the chapter. The terms are presented in a list at the beginning of each chapter and then are printed in boldface at the appropriate points within the chapter. Again, as with the chapter objectives, we suggest that readers skim the list before reading the chapter. Then as the chapter is read, particular attention should be paid to the definition of each term.

Presentation of Content. Although each chapter in this book could be expanded—in some cases, entire books have been written on topics we have covered in a chapter or less—we believe that each chapter contains the necessary information to help readers understand and develop many of the skills required to be a successful health promotion program planner, implementor, and evaluator.

Chapter Summary.   At the end of each chapter, readers will find a one- or two-paragraph review of the major concepts contained in the chapter.

Review Questions.   The purpose of the questions at the end of each chapter is to provide readers with some feedback regarding their mastery of the content. We have endeavored to ask questions that would reinforce the chapter objectives and key terms presented in each chapter.

Activities.   Each chapter also includes several activities that will allow readers to put their new knowledge and skills to use. The activities are presented in several different formats for the sake of variety and to appeal to the different learning styles of readers. It should be noted that, depending on the ones selected for completion, the activities in one chapter can build on those in a previous chapter and lead to the final product of a completely developed health promotion program.

Web Activities.   The final portion of each chapter consists of several activities based on the World Wide Web. These activities allow readers to explore a number of different websites that are available to support program planning, implementation, and evaluation efforts.

New to This Edition

In revising this textbook, we incorporated as many suggestions from reviewers, colleagues, and former students as possible. In addition to updating material throughout the text, the following points reflect the major changes in this new edition:

- Chapter 1 has been expanded to include information about how the Framework for Competency-Based Health Education has been revised to include competencies for advanced-level health practitioners.
- Chapter 2 on planning models has been reorganized with the addition of the MATCH (Multilevel Approach to Community Health), CDCynergy, and SMART (Social Marketing Assessment and Response) planning models. Also, the most recent updates to the PRECEDE-PROCEED model are included.
- Chapter 4 has been expanded to include strategies on using the World Wide Web to assist in the needs assessment process. In addition, the needs assessment process has been broadened to allow for ease of application.
- Chapter 7 on theories and models used for interventions has been expanded with additional information about the transtheoretical model.
- Chapter 8 on interventions has been restructured to place greater emphasis on communication intervention activities.

- Chapter 9 has been extended by adding the concept of community building to the discussion of community organizing.
- The information presented on social marketing in Chapter 11 has been expanded.
- Chapter 14 has been reorganized with the addition of the Framework for Program Evaluation from the Centers for Disease Control and Prevention.
- Throughout the textbook, new applications of and references to planning programs in multicultural settings have been included.
- At the end of each chapter, World Wide Web activities have been added to support the readers in their program-planning efforts.

Readers will find this book easy to understand and use. We are confident that if the chapters are carefully read and an honest effort is put into completing the activities and web activities, readers will gain the essential knowledge and skills for program planning, implementation, and evaluation.

Acknowledgments

A project of this nature could not have been completed without the assistance and understanding of many individuals. First, we thank all our past and present students, who have had to put up with our "working drafts" of the manuscript.

Second, we are grateful to those professionals who took the time and effort to review and comment on various editions of this book. For the first edition, they included Vicki Keanz, Eastern Kentucky University; Susan Cross Lipnickey, Miami University; Fred Pearson, Ricks College; Kerry Redican, Virginia Tech; John Sciacca, Northern Arizona University; and William K. Spath, Montana Tech. For the second edition, reviewers included Gordon James, Weber State; John Sciacca, Northern Arizona University; and Mark Wilson, University of Georgia. For this third edition, the reviewers included Joanna Hayden, William Paterson University; Raffy Luquis, Southern Connecticut State University; Teresa Shattuck, University of Maryland; Thomas Syre, James Madison University; and Esther Weekes, Texas Women's University.

Third, we thank our friends for providing valuable feedback on all three editions of this book: Robert J. Yonker, Ph.D., Professor Emeritus in the Department of Educational Foundations and Inquiry, Bowling Green State University; Lawrence W. Green, Dr.P.H., Distinguished Service Fellow/Visiting Scientist, Office on Smoking and Health, National Center for Chronic Disease Prevention and Health Promotion, Centers for Disease Control and Prevention; Bruce Simons-Morton, Ed.D., M.P.H., Chief, Prevention Research Branch, National Institute of Child Health and Human Development, National Institutes of Health; and Jerome E. Kotecki, H.S.D., Associate Professor, Department of Physiology and Health Science, Ball State University.

Fourth, we thank Brad Neiger, Ph.D., C.H.E.S., Associate Professor, Health Science Department, Brigham Young University, for writing the largest portion of Chapter 2 and for his organization of the whole chapter.

Fifth, we appreciate the work of Allyn and Bacon employees Joe Burns, series editor for health and physical education, and his assistants Tanja Eise and Annemarie Kennedy. We also appreciate the careful work of freelancers Susan Freese and Lynda Griffiths.

Finally, we express our deepest appreciation to our families for their support, encouragement, and understanding of the time that writing takes away from our family activities.

J. F. M.
J. L. S.

1

Health Education, Health Promotion, Health Educators, and Program Development

After reading this chapter and answering the questions at the end, you should be able to:

- Explain the relationship between good health behavior, health education, and health promotion.
- Write your own definition of health education.
- Explain the role of the health educator as defined by the Role Delineation Project.
- Explain how the Framework for Competency-Based Health Education is used by colleges and universities, the National Commission for Health Education Credentialing, Inc. (NCHEC), the National Council for the Accreditation of Teacher Education (NCATE), and the SOPHE/AAHE Baccalaureate Program Approval Committee (SABPAC).
- Explain how the Framework has been expanded for advanced-level health practitioners.
- Identify the assumptions upon which health education is based.
- Name the generic components for developing a program.

Key Terms

advanced-level practitioners
entry-level health educator
health behavior

health education
health educator
health promotion

health promotion and
    disease prevention
Role Delineation Project

In looking back over the twentieth century, we can see that much progress was made in the health and life expectancy of Americans: "People are living longer than previously and with greater freedom from the threat of disease" (Breslow, 1999, p. 1031). Since 1900, we have seen a sharp drop in infant mortality (Hoyert, Kochanek, & Murphy, 1999); the eradication of smallpox; the elimination of polio-myelitis in the Americas; the control of measles, rubella, tetanus, diphtheria, Hae-mophilus influenzae type b, and other infectious diseases; better family planning (CDC, 1999d), and an increase of 29.2 years in the average life span of a person in the United States (Hoyert, Kochanek, & Murphy, 1999). Over this same time, we have witnessed disease prevention change "from focusing on reducing environmental exposures over which the individual had little control, such as providing potable water, to emphasizing behaviors such as avoiding use of tobacco, fatty foods, and a sedentary lifestyle" (Breslow, 1999, p. 1030). In fact, in the latter part of the twenti-eth century, it was reported that better control of behavioral risk factors alone—such as lack of exercise, poor diet, use of tobacco and drugs, and alcohol abuse—could prevent between 40 and 70% of all premature deaths, one-third of all acute disabilities, and two-thirds of chronic disabilities (USDHHS, 1990b).

Though the focus on good health, wellness, and **health behavior** (those behav-iors that impact a person's health) seem commonplace in our lives today, it was not until the last fourth of the twentieth century that health promotion was recognized for its potential to help control injury and disease and to promote health.

> Most scholars, policymakers, and practitioners in health promotion would pick 1974 as the turning point that marks the beginning of health promotion as a signif-icant component of national health policy in the twentieth century. That year Canada published its landmark policy statement, *A New Perspective on the Health of Canadians* (Lalonde, 1974). In the United States, Congress passed PL 94-317, the Health Information and Health Promotion Act, which created the Office of Health Information and Health Promotion, later renamed the Office of Disease Prevention and Health Promotion. (Green, 1999, p. 69)

This led the way for the U.S. government's publication *Healthy People: The Surgeon General's Report on Health Promotion and Disease Prevention* (*Healthy People*, 1979). This document brought together much of what was known about the relationship of personal behavior and health status. The document also presented a "personal re-sponsibility" model that provided Americans with a prescription for reducing their health risks and increasing their chances for good health.

It may not have been the content of *Healthy People* that made the publication so significant, because several publications written before it provided a similar message. Rather, *Healthy People* was important because it summarized the research available up to that point, presented it in a very readable format, and made the in-formation available to the general public. *Healthy People* was then followed by the release of the first set of health goals and objectives for the nation, titled *Promoting Health/Preventing Disease: Objectives for the Nation* (USDHHS, 1980). These goals and objectives, now in their third generation, have defined the nation's health agenda and guided its health policy since their inception. And, in part, they have kept the importance of good health visible to all Americans.

This focus on good health has given many people in the United States a desire to do something about their health. This desire, in turn, has created a greater need for good health information that can be easily understood by the average person. One need only look at the current best-seller list, read the daily newspaper, observe the health advertisements delivered via the mass media, or consider the increase in the number of health-promoting facilities (not illness or sickness facilities) to verify the interest that American consumers have in health. Because of the increased interest in health, health professionals are now faced with providing the public with the health information they want and need.

Health Education and Health Promotion

In the simplest terms, **health education** is the process of educating people about health. However, two more formal definitions of health education have been frequently cited in the literature. The first comes from the Joint Committee on Health Education Terminology report (1991, p. 103). The committee defined the health education process as the "continuum of learning which enables people, as individuals and as members of social structures, to voluntarily make decisions, modify behaviors, and change social conditions in ways which are health enhancing." The second definition was proposed by Green and Kreuter (1999), who defined health education as

> any combination of learning experiences designed to facilitate voluntary actions conducive to health. *Combination* emphasizes the importance of matching the multiple determinants of behavior with multiple learning experiences or educational interventions. *Designed* distinguishes health education from incidental learning experiences as a systematically planned activity. *Facilitate* means predispose, enable, and reinforce. *Voluntary* means without coercion and with full understanding and acceptance of the purposes of the action. *Actions* means behavioral steps taken by an individual, group, or community to achieve an intended health effect or to build their capacity for health. (p. 27)

Another term that is closely related to health education, and sometimes incorrectly used in its place, is **health promotion.** *Health promotion* is a broader term than *health education.* One of the early definitions of this term stated that health promotion was "any combination of health education and related organizational, political and economic interventions designed to facilitate behavioral and environmental adaptations that will improve or protect health" (USDHHS, 1980, p. 1). A more recent definition of health promotion was offered by Green and Kreuter (1999): Health promotion is "the combination of educational and ecological supports for actions and conditions of living conducive to health." In this definition "*combination* again refers to the necessity of matching multiple determinants of health with multiple interventions or sources of support" (p. 27). *Educational* refers to health education as defined by Green and Kreuter (Green & Kreuter, 1999). "*Ecological* refers to the social, political, economic, organizational, policy, regulatory, and other environmental circumstances interacting with behavior in affecting health" (Green & Kreuter, 1999, p. 27).

A third definition of health promotion was provided in the Joint Committee on Health Education Terminology report (1991, p. 102). The committee defined **health promotion and disease prevention** as "the aggregate of all purposeful activities designed to improve personal and public health through a combination of strategies, including the competent implementation of behavioral change strategies, health education, health protection measures, risk factor detection, health enhancement and health maintenance." To help us to further understand and operationalize the terms *health promotion* and *disease prevention*, Breslow (1999) has stated, "Each person has a certain degree of health that may be expressed as a place in a spectrum. From that perspective, promoting health must focus on enhancing people's capacities for living. That means moving them toward the health end of the spectrum, just as prevention is aimed at avoiding disease that can move people toward the opposite of the spectrum" (p. 1031). According to all three of these definitions of health promotion, health education is an important component of health promotion and firmly implanted in it (see Figure 1.1). "Without health education, health promotion would be a manipulative social engineering enterprise" (Green & Kreuter, 1999, p. 19).

The effectiveness of health promotion programs can vary greatly. However, the success of a program can usually be linked to the planning that takes place before implementation of the program. Programs that have undergone a thorough

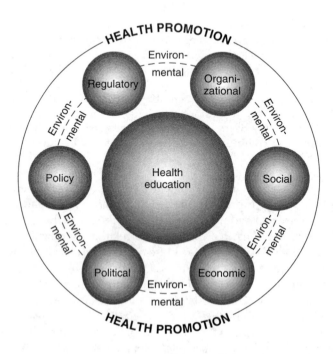

FIGURE 1.1 *Relationships of Health Education and Health Promotion*

planning process are usually the most successful. As the old saying goes, "If you fail to plan, your plan will fail."

Health Educators

The role of the **health educator** in the United States has evolved over time based on the need to provide people with educational interventions to enhance their health. The earliest signs of the role of the health educator appeared in the mid-1800s with school hygiene education, which was closely associated with physical activity. By the early 1900s, the need for health education spread to the public health arena, but it was the writers, journalists, social workers, and visiting nurses who were doing the educating—not health educators as we know them today (Deeds, 1992). As we gained more knowledge about the relationship between health, disease, and health behavior, it was obvious that the writers, journalists, social workers, visiting nurses, and primary caregivers—mainly physicians, dentists, other independent practitioners, and nurses—were unable to provide the needed health education. The combination of the heavy workload of the primary caregivers, the lack of formal training in the process of educating others, and the need for education at all levels of prevention (see Figure 1.2) created a need for health educators.

Today, health educators can be found working in a variety of settings, including schools (K–12, colleges, and universities), community health agencies (governmental and nongovernmental), worksites (business, industry, and other work settings), and medical settings (clinics, hospitals, and managed care organizations).

Though the need for health educators grew out of the need to provide the appropriate educational interventions, the role has expanded over the years such that health educators are now involved in all aspects of health promotion. As the role of health educators has grown, there has been a movement by those in the discipline to clearly define their role so that people inside and outside the discipline would have a better understanding of what the health educator does. In 1978, the **Role Delineation Project** was begun (National Task Force [on the Preparation and Practice of Health Educators, Inc.], 1985). Through a comprehensive process, this project yielded a generic role for the **entry-level health educator**—that is, responsibilities for health educators taking their first job regardless of their work setting. In more recent years, the list of responsibilities has become known as "A Competency-Based Framework for Professional Development of Certified Health Education Specialists," or just simply the Framework (NCHEC, 1996). This Framework comprises seven major areas of responsibility and several different competencies and subcompetencies, which further delineate the responsibilities. The seven major areas of responsibility identified through the Role Delineation Project and still in use today include:

1. Assessing individual and community needs for health education.
2. Planning effective health education programs.
3. Implementing health education programs.
4. Evaluating the effectiveness of health education programs.

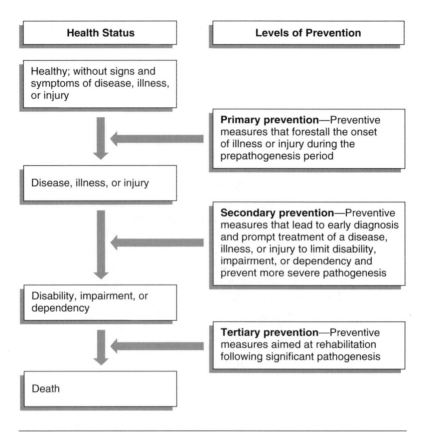

FIGURE 1.2   *Levels of Prevention*

Source: Adapted from Pickett and Hanlon (1990).

5. Coordinating provision of health education services.
6. Acting as a resource person in health education.
7. Communicating health and health education needs, concerns, and resources (National Task Force, 1985, pp. 15–16).

In reviewing the seven areas of responsibility, it is obvious that four of the seven are directly related to program planning, implementation, and evaluation and that the other three could be associated with programming, depending on the type of program being planned. In effect, these responsibilities distinguish health educators from other professionals who try to provide health education experiences.

The importance of the defined role of the health educator is becoming greater as the profession of health education continues to mature. This is exhibited by its use in several major professional activities. First, the Framework has provided a guide for all colleges and universities to use when designing and revising their curricula in health education. Second, the Framework was used by the National Commission for Health Education Credentialing, Inc. (NCHEC) to develop the core criteria for the examination that is used to certify individuals as health educators (Certified Health Education Specialist, or CHES).

> In 1990 the first group of individuals received the CHES credential through successful completion of a criterion-referenced examination, based on the Framework. This nationwide testing program was a landmark event in the profession. As of October 1998, over 5,000 individuals are active CHES, the CHES examination is given twice a year and some employers are requiring/preferring the CHES credential in job announcements. (AAHE, NCHEC, & SOPHE, 1999, p. 5)

Third, the Framework is used by program accrediting and approval bodies to review college and university academic programs in health education. The National Council for the Accreditation of Teacher Education (NCATE) uses the Framework to review and accredit teacher preparation programs in health education at institutions of higher education. Also, a joint committee of the Society for Public Health Education, Inc. (SOPHE) and the American Association for Health Education, known as the SOPHE/AAHE Baccalaureate Program Approval Committee (SABPAC), uses the Framework to review and approve undergraduate health education programs via a self-study and external reviewers.

The use of the Framework by the profession to guide academic curricula, provide the core criteria for the health education specialist examination, and form the basis of program approval processes (AAHE, NCHEC, & SOPHE, 1999) has done much to advance the health education profession. "In 1998 the U.S. Department of Commerce and Labor formally acknowledged 'health educator' as a distinct occupation. Such recognition was justified, based to a large extent, on the ability of the profession to specify its unique skills" (AAHE, NCHEC, & SOPHE, 1999, p. 9).

Prior to the recognition of "health educator" as a singular occupational classification code by the U.S. Department of Commerce and Labor, the initial responsibilities of the health educator that had served the profession so well were beginning to show their age and did not express the responsibilities and competencies of a health educator with an advanced degree in the field. As early as 1992, a Joint Committee for Graduate Standards was established by the Association for the Advancement of Health Education (now known as the American Association for Health Education (AAHE)) and the Society for Public Health Education (SOPHE) to help define the role of an advanced practitioner. Over the course of the next few years, the joint committee, with the help of many professionals, completed its work and submitted its final report and graduate competencies to the boards of AAHE and SOPHE. Both boards accepted the report in 1996. Then, in July 1997, the National Commission for Health Education Credentialing's (NCHEC) Board of Commissioners endorsed the competencies (AAHE, NCHEC, & SOPHE, 1999). In March 1998, the Competencies Update Project (CUP) was initiated by NCHEC to reverify the entry-level competencies to make sure they were up to date with current health education practice and to further delineate and verify the advanced-level competencies derived from the joint committee report, "A Competency-Based Framework for Graduate-Level Health Educators" (AAHE, NCHEC, & SOPHE, 1999). At the time of the writing of this book, it appears that three new responsibilities for **advanced-level practitioners** will be added to the seven that were already in place for the entry-level health educators. The three added responsibilities are:

8. Applying appropriate research principles and techniques to health education.
9. Administering health education programs.
10. Advancing the profession of health education.

In addition to the new areas of responsibility, several new competencies and subcompetencies reflecting advanced-level practitioner skills were to be incorporated into the existing entry-level Framework (AAHE, NCHEC, & SOPHE, 1999). At the time of this writing, the completion date for CUP had not been determined. For more information about the development of the project, contact the NCHEC. (*Note:* Its website address is noted at the end of the chapter in Activities on the Web.)

Assumptions of Health Promotion

So far, we have discussed the need for health, what health education and health promotion are, and the role health educators play in delivering successful health promotion programs. We have not yet discussed the assumptions that underlie health promotion—all the things that must be in place before the whole process of health promotion begins. In the mid-1980s, Bates and Winder (1984) outlined what they saw as four critical assumptions of health education. Their list has been modified by the authors by adding several items and referring to them as "assumptions of health promotion." This expanded list of assumptions is critical to understanding what we can expect from health promotion programs. Health promotion is by no means the sole answer to the nation's health care problem or, for that matter, the sole means of getting the smoker to stop smoking or the nonexerciser to exercise. Health promotion is an important part of the health care system, but it does have limitations. Here are the assumptions:

1. Health status can be changed.
2. Disease occurrence theories and principles can be understood (Bates & Winder, 1984).
3. Appropriate prevention strategies can be developed to deal with the identified health problems (Bates & Winder, 1984).
4. An individual's health is affected by a variety of factors, not just lifestyle. Other factors include heredity, environment, and the health care system.
5. Changes in individual and societal health behaviors and lifestyles will affect an individual's health status positively (Bates & Winder, 1984).
6. "Individuals, families, small groups, and communities can be taught to assume responsibility for their health, which in turn changes their health behaviors and lifestyles" (Bates & Winder, 1984, p. 2).

7. Individual responsibility should not be viewed as victim blaming.
8. For health behavior change to be permanent, an individual must be motivated and ready to change.

The importance of these assumptions is made clearer if we refer to the definitions of health education presented earlier in the chapter. Implicit in those definitions was a goal of having the participants of health education programs voluntarily adopt actions conducive to health. To achieve such a goal, the assumptions must indeed be in place. We cannot expect people to adopt lifelong health-enhancing behavior if we force them into such change. Nor can we expect people to change their behavior just because they have been exposed to a health education program. Health behavior change is very complex, and health educators should not expect to change every person with whom they come in contact. However, the greatest chance for success will come to those who have the knowledge and skills to plan, implement, and evaluate appropriate programs.

Program Development

Since many of health educators' responsibilities are involved in some way with program planning, implementation, and evaluation, health educators need to become well versed in these processes. "Planning an effective program is more difficult than implementing it. Planning, implementing, and evaluating programs are all interrelated, but good planning skills are prerequisite to programs worthy of evaluation" (Breckon, Harvey, & Lancaster, 1998, p. 145). All three processes are very involved, and much time, effort, practice, and on-the-job training are required to do them well. Even the most experienced health educators find program planning challenging because of the constant changes in settings, resources, and target populations.

Today, it is generally accepted that the process of health promotion program development can take many different forms. That is, there are many different ways of getting from point A to point B. However, all approaches usually center on a generic set of tasks that include:

1. Understanding the community and engaging the target population
2. Assessing the needs of the target population
3. Developing appropriate goals and objectives
4. Creating an intervention that considers the peculiarities of the setting
5. Implementing the intervention
6. Evaluating the results (see Figure 1.3)

The remaining chapters of this book present a process that health educators can use to plan, implement, and evaluate successful health promotion programs and will introduce you to the necessary knowledge and skills to carry out these tasks.

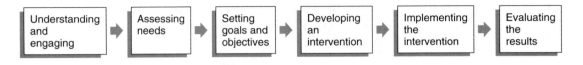

FIGURE 1.3 *A Generalized Model for Program Development*

Summary

The increased interest in personal health and the flood of new health information have created a need to provide quality health promotion programs. Individuals are seeking guidance to enable them to make sound decisions about behavior that would be conducive to their health. Those best prepared to help these people are health educators who have received appropriate training. Properly trained health educators are aware of the limitations of the discipline and understand the assumptions on which health promotion is based.

Questions

1. Explain the role *Healthy People* played in the relationship between the American people and health.

2. How is *health education* defined by the Joint Committee on Health Education Terminology (1991)?

3. What are the key phrases in the definition of health education presented by Green and Kreuter (1999)?

4. What is the relationship between health education and health promotion?

5. Why is there a need for health educators?

6. What is the Role Delineation Project?

7. How is the Framework for Competency-Based Health Education used by colleges and universities? By NCHEC? By NCATE? By SABPAC?

8. What are the seven major responsibilities of entry-level health educators? What are the additional three responsibilities for the advanced-level health educators?

9. What assumptions are critical to health promotion?

10. What are the components of the generalized model for program development?

Activities

1. Based on what you have read in this chapter and your knowledge of the profession of health education, write your own definitions for *health, health education, health promotion*, and *health promotion program*.

2. Write a response indicating what you see as the importance of each of the eight assumptions presented in the chapter. Write no more than one paragraph per assumption.

3. With your knowledge of health promotion, what other assumptions would you add to the list presented in this chapter? Provide a one-paragraph rationale for each.

4. If you have not already done so, go to the government documents section of the library on your campus and read *Healthy People: The Surgeon General's Report on Health Promotion and Disease Prevention* (*Healthy People*, 1979).

Activities on the Web

1. Visit the website for the National Commission on Health Education Credentialing, Inc. **<http://www.nchec.org/>** and answer the following questions:
   a. What is the next test date for the CHES examination?
   b. What publications does the NCHEC offer for those preparing for the examination?
   c. Who is eligible to take the CHES examination?
   d. What is the process one must complete to take the CHES examination?

2. Visit the website for the American Association for Health Education (AAHE) **<http://www.aahperd.org/aahe/aahe-main.html>** and answer the following questions:
   a. What is the mission of AAHE?
   b. What publications are available from AAHE?
   c. What is the purpose of the NCATE Review Committee?

3. Visit the website for the Society for Public Health Education (SOPHE) **<http://www.sophe.org>** and answer the following questions:
   a. What is the mission of SOPHE?
   b. What publications are available from SOPHE?
   c. Is there a chapter of SOPHE in your state? If so, what is it called and who is the president?
   d. What is the purpose of SABPAC?

2

Models for Health Education and Health Promotion Programming

After reading this chapter and answering the questions at the end, you should be able to:

- Explain the importance of using a model for planning a program.
- Identify the models commonly used in planning health education and health promotion programs and briefly explain each.
- Identify the major components of the planning models presented.
- Apply a planning model to a program you are planning.

Key Terms

administrative and policy
   assessment
behavioral and environmental
   assessment
CDCynergy or Cynergy
educational and ecological
   assessment
EMPOWER

enabling factors
epidemiological assessment
evaluation
formative research
health communication
impact evaluation
implementation
MATCH

outcome evaluation
PRECEDE-PROCEED
predisposing factors
process evaluation
reinforcing factors
social assessment
social marketing

As noted in Chapter 1, a major portion of the role of the health educator is associated with health promotion programming—planning, implementing, and evaluating health education programs. Good health promotion programs are not created by chance; they are the product of much effort and should be based on a systematic planning model. Models are the means by which structure and organization are given to the programming process. They provide planners with direction and supply a frame on which to build. Many different planning models have been developed, some of which are used more frequently than others. Although many of the models have common elements, those elements may have different labels. In fact, "the underlying principles that guide the development of the various models are similar; however, there are important differences in sequence, emphasis, and the conceptualization of the major components that make certain models more appealing than others to individual practitioners" (Simons-Morton, Greene, & Gottlieb, 1995, pp. 126–127). Also be aware that there are no perfect planning models. Planners may have to "adapt them to fit the needs of the planning situation and the cultural characteristics of the target group, setting, and health problem" (Kline & Huff, 1999, p. 109).

Most planners find occasions when they do not need to use a model in its entirety or when it is necessary to combine parts of different models to meet specific needs and situations. As Gilmore, Campbell, and Becker (1989, p. 13) have pointed out, "It may not be feasible for every programming effort to use all of the cited considerations at each stage, [but] they do provide prompters for planning committee, and administrative discussions."

The remainder of this chapter will present several different models that have been used by practitioners in planning health promotion programs. Four models, PRECEDE-PROCEED, MATCH, CDCynergy, and SMART, which have been used in a variety of settings, will be presented in detail. Others, which are not as widely known, will be briefly presented and referenced so you may explore them further.

PRECEDE-PROCEED

Currently, the best-known and most often used model for health promotion programming is the **PRECEDE-PROCEED** model. "PRECEDE is an acronym for *p*redisposing, *r*einforcing, and *e*nabling *c*onstructs in *e*ducational/*e*cological *d*iagnosis and *e*valuation" (Green & Kreuter, 1999, p. 34). "PROCEED stands for *p*olicy, *r*egulatory, and *o*rganizational *c*onstructs in *e*ducational and *e*nvironmental *d*evelopment" (Green & Kreuter, 1999, p. 34).

PRECEDE-PROCEED is a model with which all students should become very familiar. It is considered "the model" by most people in the health profession and has been the basis for many professional projects at the national level. PRECEDE-PROCEED is well received because it is theoretically grounded and comprehensive in nature; it combines a series of phases in the planning, implementation, and evaluation process.

PRECEDE-PROCEED was developed over the course of about 15 to 20 years. The Precede framework was conceived in the early 1970s (Green, 1974) and evolved as a planning model during the late 1970s (Green, 1975, 1976; Green, Levine, & Deeds, 1975; Green et al., 1978; Green et al., 1980). "The identification of priorities and the setting of objectives in the Precede phases provide the objectives and criteria for policy, implementation, and evaluation in the Proceed phases" (Green & Kreuter, 1999, p. 35).

The Proceed framework was developed in the 1980s (Green, 1979, 1980, 1981a, 1981b, 1982, 1983a, 1983b, 1984a, 1984b, 1984c, 1984d, 1986a, 1986b, 1986c, 1986d, 1986e, 1987a, 1987b; Green & Allen, 1980; Green & McAlister, 1984; Green, Mullen, & Friedman, 1986; Green, Wilson, & Lovato, 1986; Green, Wilson, & Bauer, 1983) and "is essentially an elaboration and extension of the administrative diagnosis step of PRECEDE, which was the final and least developed link in the PRECEDE framework" (Green & Kreuter, 1991, p. 25). It was influenced by the participation of Green and Kreuter in national policy initiatives and the development of community health promotion programs such as Planned Approach to Community Health (PATCH) (Green & Kreuter, 1992).

Though the basic components of the PRECEDE-PROCEED model have stayed the same over the years, the model has been revised and updated as the practice of health promotion has advanced. For example, as Precede was used in the 1980s, it became apparent that the model needed to be expanded and thus the addition of Proceed. One subtle change to the most recent presentation of the model (Green & Kreuter, 1999) was the dropping of the word *diagnosis* in the first five phases of the model and replacing it with *assessment*. Though Green and Kreuter still feel diagnosis to be the appropriate denotation, this change came as the result of many of the users of the model feeling uncomfortable with the term *diagnosis*, associating the model with clinical procedures. It also suggests that all assessments must start with or find a problem, which is not the case. As Green and Kreuter (1999) point out, in assets-based approaches to community assessment, planners build on the strengths of the community.

The Nine Phases of PRECEDE-PROCEED

As can be seen in Figure 2.1, PRECEDE-PROCEED is composed of nine phases or steps. At first glance, the model seems overly complicated, but on close examination, the continuous series of steps reveals a very logical sequence for health promotion programming. The underlying approach of this model is to begin by identifying the desired outcome, to determine what causes it, and finally to design an intervention aimed at reaching the desired outcome. In other words, PRECEDE-PROCEED begins with the final consequences and works backward to the causes. Once the causes are known, an intervention can be designed to deal with them.

Phase 1 in the model is called **social assessment** and seeks to subjectively define the quality of life (problems and priorities) of those in the target population. The designers of this model suggest that this is best accomplished by involving individuals in the target population in a self-study of their own needs and

PRECEDE

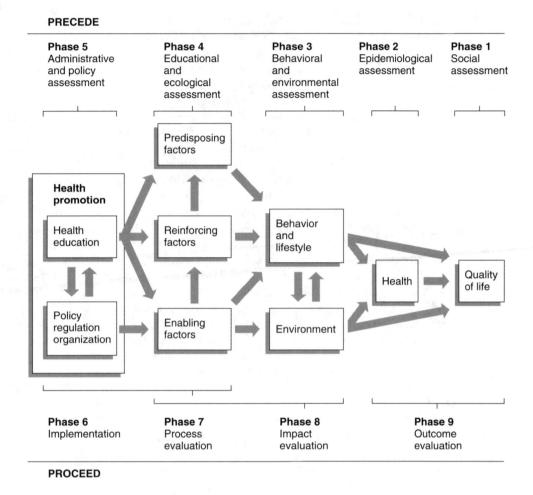

FIGURE 2.1 *The PRECEDE-PROCEED Model for Health Promotion Planning and Evaluation*

Source: From *Health Promotion Planning: An Educational and Ecological Approach, Third Edition* by Lawrence W. Green and Marshall W. Kreuter. Copyright © 1999 by Mayfield Publishing Company. Reprinted by permission of the publisher.

aspirations. Some of the social indicators of quality of life include absenteeism, alienation, crime, discrimination, happiness, illegitimacy, riots, self-esteem, unemployment, and welfare.

Phase 2, **epidemiological assessment,** is the step in which the planners use data to identify and rank the health goals or problems that may contribute to the needs identified in Phase 1. Those data might include disability, discomfort, fertility, fitness, morbidity, mortality, and physiological risk factors and their dimensions (distribution, duration, functional level, incidence, intensity, longevity, and prevalence). It is important to note that ranking the health problems in this phase is critical, because there are rarely, if ever, enough resources to deal with all or multiple problems. Also, this phase of the model is used to plan health programs. "A general community development program might apply this model to other problems or social goals identified in Phase 1, skipping Phase 2" (Green & Kreuter, 1999, p. 38).

Phase 3, **behavioral and environmental assessment,** involves determining and prioritizing the behavioral and environmental risk factors or risk conditions that might be linked to the health problems selected in Phase 2. Depending on health concerns noted in Phase 2, the behavioral factors could be the behavior or actions of individuals, groups, or communities. Behavioral indicators include such things as compliance, consumption patterns, coping, preventive actions, self-care, and utilization. These indicators can be expressed in the dimensions of frequency, persistence, promptness, quality, and range (Green & Kreuter, 1999). "Environmental factors are those determinants outside an individual that can be modified to support behavior, health, and quality of life" (Green & Kreuter, 1999, p. 40). Examples of environmental indicators include economic, physical, services, and social, and their dimensions (access, affordability, and equity) (Green & Kreuter, 1999). Note that in Figure 2.1, arrows connect both of the boxes in Phase 3 with Phases 1 and 2. The arrows from Phase 3 to Phase 1 represent the skipping of Phase 2 if the model is applied to something other than a health problem.

Once identified, the risk factors and/or risk conditions need to prioritized. This can be accomplished by first ranking the factors/conditions by importance and changeability and then using the 2 × 2 matrix presented in Figure 2.2.

	More important	**Less important**
More changeable	High priority for program focus (Quadrant 1)	Low priority except to demonstrate change for political purposes (Quadrant 3)
Less changeable	Priority for innovative program; evaluation crucial (Quadrant 2)	No program (Quadrant 4)

FIGURE 2.2 *Prioritization Matrix*

Source: From *Health Promotion Planning: An Educational and Ecological Approach, Third Edition* by Lawrence W. Green and Marshall W. Kreuter. Copyright © 1999 by Mayfield Publishing Company. Reprinted by permission of the publisher.

Phase 4, **educational and ecological assessment,** identifies and classifies the literally hundreds of factors that have the potential to influence a given behavior into three categories: predisposing, reinforcing, and enabling. **Predisposing factors** include knowledge and many affective traits such as a person's attitude, values, beliefs, and perceptions. These factors can facilitate or hinder a person's motivation to change and can be altered through *direct* communication. Barriers or vehicles created mainly by societal forces or systems make up **enabling factors,** which include access to health care facilities, availability of resources, referrals to appropriate providers, enactment of rules or laws, and the development of skills. "These factors thus include all those that *make possible* a change in behavior on in the environment that people want" (Green & Kreuter, 1999, p. 41). **Reinforcing factors** comprise the different types of feedback and rewards that those in the target population receive after behavior change, which may either encourage or discourage the continuation of the behavior. Reinforcing behaviors can be delivered by, but not limited to, family, friends, peers, teachers, self, and others who control rewards. "Social benefits—such as recognition; physical benefits such as convenience, comfort, relief of discomfort, or pain; tangible rewards such as economic benefits or avoidance of cost; imagined or vicarious rewards such as improved appearance, self-respect, or association with an admired person who demonstrates the behavior—all reinforce behavior" (Green & Kreuter, 1999, p. 171). As with the previous phases, planners must set priorities. The prioritized factors identified in this phase become the focus of the intervention that will be planned (Green & Kreuter, 1999).

Phase 5 consists of an **administrative and policy assessment,** in which planners determine if the capabilities and resources are available to develop and implement the program. It is between Phases 5 and 6 that PRECEDE (the assessment portion of the model) ends and PROCEED (implementation and evaluation) begins. However, there is not a clean break between the two phases; they really run together, and planners can move back and forth between them.

The four final phases of the model—Phases 6, 7, 8, and 9—make up the PROCEED portion. In Phase 6—**implementation**—with appropriate resources in hand, planners select the methods and strategies of the intervention and implementation begins. Phases 7, 8, and 9 focus on the **evaluation, process, impact,** and **outcome,** respectively, and are based on the earlier phases of the model, when objectives were outlined in the assessment process. Whether all three of these final phases are used depends on the evaluation requirements of the program. Obviously, the resources needed to conduct evaluations of impact (Phase 8) and outcome (Phase 9) are much greater than those needed to conduct process evaluation (Phase 7). (See Chapter 6 for a discussion on the relationship of objectives to evaluation.)

Applying PRECEDE-PROCEED

To assist you in understanding how PRECEDE-PROCEED is used, consider the following hypothetical example using a worksite setting. Remember Phase 1 of the model, social assessment, seeks to define the quality of life of the target population so that the desired outcomes can be identified. This is best done by including those in the target population. Thus, in a worksite, planners need to involve both the employer and the employees in the process of assessing the needs. So, having representation from the various groups within the target population (labor, management, clerical, etc.) on a planning committee, and letting this committee coordinate a self-study of the target population would be important. In a worksite setting, it would not be surprising to find such an assessment identifying that employers are concerned with economic outcomes of the company—turning a profit. Employees may also be concerned about economic outcomes—their own salary or wages—but also about working conditions. Social indicators that may reflect these desired outcomes include production rates; absenteeism for all reasons (use of personal days, vacation days, and sick days), aesthetics of the work environment, morale of the workers, lack of quality leisure time of the job, and little feeling of worth as an employee of this company.

In Phase 2 of the model, epidemiological assessment, planners use data to identify and rank health goals or problems that are associated with the economic concerns and working conditions that were uncovered in Phase 1. Therefore, planners would want to collect and analyze data that reflect the health status of the workforce. Such sources of data could include reviewing the reasons for the use of sick days, reviewing company safety records, providing health screenings for all employees so that physiological risk factors can be identified, and analyzing the health and disability insurance claims of the company. Once identified, planners need to rank those health concerns as they relate to the quality-of-life issues identified in Phase 1. Common occupational diseases and disorders that arise in work settings include musculoskeletal conditions (e.g., back injuries), dermatological conditions resulting from exposure to chemical or other agents, and lung diseases resulting from the inhalation of toxic substances (McKenzie, Pinger, & Kotecki, 1999). For the purpose of this example, let's assume that back injuries received the highest priority in the epidemiological assessment. Employees with back injuries have both an impact on the economic outcome of the company via lost productivity and on the quality of life of the employee who is off the job.

Having prioritized back injuries as the health concern, planners move to Phase 3, behavioral and environmental assessment. In this phase, they want to determine what risk factors or risk conditions contribute to the back injuries. Is lifting a big part of the employees' work? If so, are they using good lifting techniques? Are they lifting more weight than they should? Is the work environment conducive to the work the employees are asked to do? Is the work area set up in an ergonomically correct way? Have the workers been provided with appropriate back supports? Answers to these questions will provide the planners with the information they need to conduct the educational and ecological assessment, Phase 4.

The educational and ecological assessment may include (1) surveying the employees to find out what they know about lifting, (2) surveying the employer to find out what kind of training and equipment are provided for new employees and determining what policies are in place to reward injury-free work days, and (3) observing the workers to determine if they are using good lifting techniques.

From this assessment, it might be found that the workers know little about appropriate lifting techniques (predisposing factor), they have not been taught any skills for proper lifting, they have not been provided with back supports (enabling factors), and they are not rewarded for injury-free days (reinforcing factor). Thus, the planners decide that an appropriate health promotion intervention would be comprised of an education component to increase knowledge and skills, and the implementation of new corporate polices that require the use of back braces and financial bonuses for a certain number of injury-free work hours.

Through the administrative and policy assessment (Phase 5), planners must determine what organizational and administrative support and resources are available to carry out the health promotion intervention. Will the educational component of the intervention be conducted on company time, employee time, or a combination of the two? Can the educational component of the intervention be conducted by a current employee or will a consultant have to be hired? Are there financial resources to buy every employee a back brace or will braces have to be shared between workers on the different shifts?

Once the availability of program resources is determined, Phase 6, implementation, can begin. The evaluation components (Phases 7, 8, and 9) of this program will be based on the objectives that were created during assessment phases. As each of the objectives were written, it would be important to ensure that criteria (standards of acceptability) noted in each objective were clear. For example, in Phase 7 (process evaluation), the planners may be concerned with determining the availability of the educational component of the intervention for each employee. In Phase 8 (impact evaluation), the planners would be interested in evaluating changes in the behavior of the employees (e.g., proper lifting technique) and the work environment (e.g., availability of back braces for employees). As for outcome evaluation, Phase 9, the planners may be looking for a reduction in the incidence and prevalence of back injuries, or an increase in productivity.

Expert Methods for Planning and Organization within Everyone's Reach (EMPOWER)

Using the PRECEDE-PROCEED model to plan, implement, and evaluate a health promotion program requires that a certain level of knowledge, experience, and resources are available to planners. Unfortunately, this is not always the case. However, there is now a computer program, **EMPOWER,** developed by a group of health educators (Bob Gold, Larry Green, and Marshall Kreuter), that allows users to work through a decision matrix based on the PRECEDE-PROCEED model (Gilbert & Sawyer, 1995). This program is designed to help planners design community-based cancer prevention and control programs targeted to the health education needs of communities with diverse minority and other high-risk populations. The technology in the program is related to artificial intelligence and expert systems, and provides users with access to experts for help and advice, external databases, and other planning documents as they work through the planning and evaluation processes (Green et al., 1994; Gold, 1995). EMPOWER is available from Jones and Bartlett

Publishers, 40 Tall Pine Drive, Sudbury, MA, 01776 (telephone: 978/443–5000; email: info@jbpub.com; and website: **<www.jbpub.com>**).

MATCH

MATCH is an acronym for Multilevel Approach to Community Health. This planning model (see Figure 2.3) was developed in the late 1980s (Simons-Morton et al., 1988). Like the PRECEDE-PROCEED model, MATCH has also been been used in a variety settings, including in the development of several intervention handbooks created by the Centers for Disease Control and Prevention (Simons-Morton et al., 1995). MATCH is an ecological planning perspective that recognizes that intervention activities can and should be aimed at a variety of objectives and individuals (B. Simons-Morton, personal communication, October 10, 1999). This is represented in Figure 2.3 by the various levels of influence. The MATCH framework is recognized for emphasizing program implementation (Simons-Morton et al., 1995). "MATCH is designed to be applied when behavioral and environmental risk and protective factors for disease or injury are generally known and when general priorities for action have been determined, thus providing a convenient way to turn the corner from needs assessment and priority setting to the development of effective programs" (Simons-Morton et al., 1995, p. 155).

The Phases and Steps of MATCH

As can be seen in Figure 2.4, MATCH is comprised of five phases and several steps within each phase. Phase I of MATCH is *goals selection*. In this phase of MATCH, planners select health-status goals based on several different factors, including the prevalence of the health problem, the relative importance of the health problem, the changeability of the problem, and other considerations unique to the program. Also in this phase, planners need to select the high-priority target populations, identify the health behaviors most associated with the health-status goals in order to create health behavior goals, and identify the environmental factors—such as access, availability of resources, enabling practices, and barriers—so that environmental goals can be created (Simons-Morton et al., 1995).

In Phase II of MATCH, *intervention planning*, the planner "matches intervention objectives with the intervention targets and intervention actions" (Simons-Morton et al., 1995, p. 163). This begins with identifying the targets of the intervention actions (TIAs). TIAs are those individuals that exert influence or control over the personal or environmental conditions that are related to the target health and behavior goals (i.e., the level of society at which the intervention will be aimed). The levels include (1) individual level (e.g, persons in the target population); (2) interpersonal level (e.g., family members, coworkers, friends, teachers, and others close to those in the target population); (3) organizational level (e.g., a decision maker in an organization); (4) societal level (e.g., community leaders); and (5) governmental level. After identifying the TIAs, they are matched with the

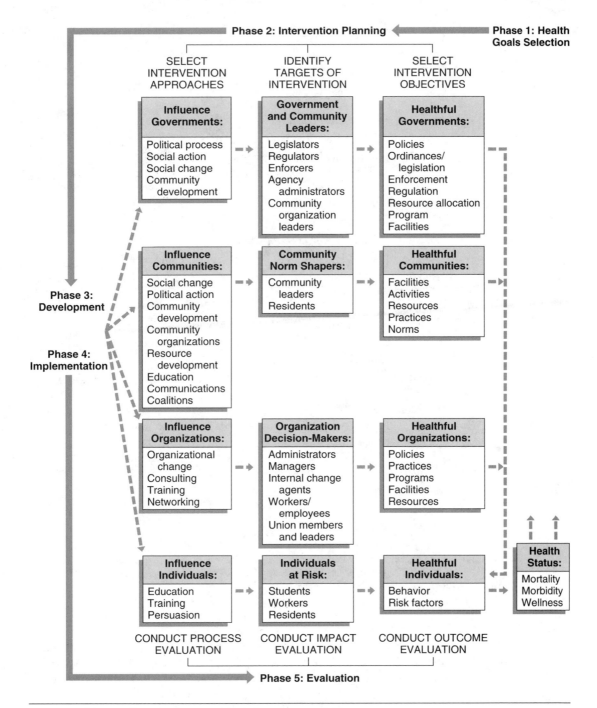

FIGURE 2.3   *MATCH: Multilevel Approach to Community Health*

Source: Reprinted by permission of Waveland Press, Inc. from B. G. Simons-Morton, W. H. Greene, and N. H. Gottlieb, *Introduction to Health Education and Health Promotion* (2nd ed.). Prospect Heights, IL: Waveland Press, Inc., 1995. All rights reserved.

FIGURE 2.4 *MATCH Phases and Steps*

Phase I: *Goals Selection*
    Step 1: Select health-status goals
    Step 2: Select high-priority target population(s)
    Step 3: Identify health behavior goals
    Step 4: Identify environmental factor goals

Phase II: *Intervention Planning*
    Step 1: Identify the targets of the intervention
    Step 2: Select intervention objectives
    Step 3: Identify mediators of the intervention objectives
    Step 4: Select intervention approaches

Phase III: *Program Development*
    Step 1: Create program units or components
    Step 2: Select or develop curricula and create intervention guides
    Step 3: Develop session plans
    Step 4: Create or acquire instructional materials, products, and resources

Phase IV: *Implementation Preparations*
    Step 1: Facilitate adoption, implementation, and maintenance
    Step 2: Select and train implementors

Phase V: *Evaluation*
    Step 1: Conduct process evaluation
    Step 2: Measure impact
    Step 3: Monitor outcomes

Source: Reprinted by permission of Waveland Press, Inc. from B. G. Simons-Morton, W. H. Greene, and N. H. Gottlieb, *Introduction to Health Education and Health Promotions* (2nd ed.). Prospect Heights, IL: Waveland Press, Inc., 1995. All rights reserved.

health behavioral and environmental factors identified in Phase I. Once this match is made, the planner selects an intervention action(s) to be used. Intervention actions commonly used by health educators include teaching, training, counseling, policy advocacy, consulting, community organization, social marketing, and social action. If the TIAs are individuals, planners need to consider those mediating factors causally associated with target behaviors, such as knowledge, attitudes, skills, experiences, and reinforcements (Simons-Morton et al., 1995).

    The third phase of MATCH is *program development* and begins with the creation of the program units or components. "Components are frequently organized according to target population subgroup (e.g., males, females, minority or age groups), objective (e.g., smoking, diet, physical activity), intervention target and level, setting and structural unit (e.g., classroom, food service, health services), or intervention approach or channel (e.g., interpersonal, media)" (Simons-Morton et al., 1995, p. 175). After the creation of the program components, planners either select from already developed curricula or develop their own guides. This would include the development of individual session or lesson plans, and the acquisition or creation of instructional materials, products, and resources (Simons-Morton et al., 1995).

In Phase IV, *implementation preparations,* planners prepare for implementation and conduct the interventions. To achieve effective implementation, planners must (1) develop a specific proposal and advocate for the adoption of change; (2) develop the need, readiness, and environmental supports for change; (3) provide evidence that the intervention works; (4) identify and select change agents and opinion leaders and sell them on the need for change; and (5) establish good working relationships with the decision makers (Simons-Morton et al., 1995). In addition, depending on who will implement the program, there may be a need select, train, support, and monitor those who do the implementation (Simons-Morton et al., 1995).

Phase V of MATCH is **evaluation.** Like the PRECEDE-PROCEED model, MATCH's evaluation also includes process, impact, and outcome components. "Process evaluation is concerned with the utility of the implementation plan and procedures, the extent and quality of implementation, and the effects of implementation on immediate learning outcomes" (Simons-Morton et al., 1995, p. 183). Impact evaluation is concerned with measuring the targeted mediators (usually knowledge, attitudes, and practices), health behaviors, and environmental factors (Simons-Morton et al., 1995). Outcome evaluation is typically focused on health behaviors but may also monitor long-term maintenance of changes in behavior or environmental factors. However, because of the time it takes for some outcomes to develop, there are often occasions in health promotion program development when there is not enough time or resources to do outcome evaluation (Simons-Morton et al., 1995).

Applying MATCH

To help you understand the phases and steps of MATCH, consider this implementation example. As you read through this example, it will help if you refer to a diagram of the model in Figure 2.3. As is common when using MATCH, let's assume that the needs assessment is complete and that heart disease is the focus of the program we are planning. The behavioral risk factors that are apparent are lack of exercise and poor eating habits, and the environmental risk factors we are concerned with are the lack of exercise facilities in the community and meals served in the school lunch program. See Table 2.1 for a presentation of the program focus.

We begin our planning with goals selection (Phase I). Based on the epidemiological data available to us, it is obvious that heart disease is the number-one

TABLE 2.1   *Behavioral and Environmental Risk Factors for MATCH Example*

Health Problem	Behavioral Risk Factors	Environmental Risk Factors
Heart disease	1. Lack of exercise 2. Poor eating habits	1. Lack of exercise facilities 2. School lunch program

killer in our community and that the heart disease death rate is much greater than the national average. We also know that several of the behaviors associated with the disease are changeable. Therefore, our health-status goal will be to reduce the prevalence of heart disease. We have decided to target elementary school children for the program because they are accessible, they possess a number of the behavior risks, and the school administration is interested in seeing such a program in the school. The health behavior goals chosen will be to decrease sedentary lifestyle and to improve eating habits. These were chosen because of their prevalence in the children, their association with heart disease, and their changeability. Environmental goals will focus on available exercise facilities, the school's curriculum with regard to physical activity and nutrition, and school policies that can influence physical activity and eating habits.

For Phase II, intervention planning, we need to identify the levels of society at which we plan to intervene, what our intervention objectives will be, what mediators with which we will be concerned, and what intervention approaches we will take (see Table 2.2). It is decided that we will intervene at the (1) individual level, with the fifth- and sixth-graders, to influence their exercise and eating behaviors with an educational approach aimed at knowledge, attitudes, skills, and behaviors; (2) organizational level, with the members of the board of education, school administrators, teachers, and school cafeteria workers, to change the physical education and nutrition curricula and policies related to the creation of school lunch menus via organization change and training approaches; and (3) governmental level, with the city parks and recreation division, to lobby for enhanced resources by better equipping the recreational areas within the city.

Phase III, program development, will focus on several program components, including (1) the training of teachers for classroom instruction for the fifth and sixth-graders in physical activity and nutrition, (2) the training of cafeteria workers to create healthier school lunches, and (3) lobbying the city parks and recreation board for better equipped parks. The training for the teachers will include the selection or development of a curriculum, scheduled in-service sessions, and the acquisition of the materials to support the curriculum development. A similar approach will be taken with the cafeteria workers by conducting in-service sessions aimed at planning and preparing nutritious meals. In preparation for the lobbying, policy advocacy, and interest-group pressure of city council and the parks and recreation board, sessions will need to be planned with appropriate resources to training advocates in political action techniques.

TABLE 2.2   *MATCH Phase II—Objectives, Mediators, Intervention Approaches by Societal Level*

Step 1 *Targets of the Intervention*	Step 2 *Objectives*	Step 3 *Mediators*	Step 4 *Intervention Approaches*
Individual Students • 5th-graders • 6th-graders	Health behaviors • Exercise • Eating habits	Knowledge Attitudes Skills Behavior	Educational • Teaching • Positive reinforcement
Organizational Board of education School administrators Teachers School cafeteria workers	Programs Practices Policies Resources	Knowledge Attitudes Skills Behavior	*Organizational Change* • Curricula change • School lunch menu policy • In-service training
Governmental City council City parks and recreation board City parks and recreation workers	Programs Practices Policies Resources	Knowledge Attitudes Skills Behavior	*Political Action* • Lobbying • Policy advocacy • Interest-group pressure

With the program components in place, Phase IV, implementation preparations, can begin. Planners will next facilitate the adoption, implementation, and maintenance of their program components by preparing those impacted by the program for change. This will mean selling them on the need for change. This can be done by showing those who are affected the possible consequences of no change, that many of the opinion leaders in the community support the change, and that similar programs have been successful in other communities. Of course, with implementation, planners will need to select and, if necessary, train the implementors so they can conduct the in-service sessions for the teachers and cafeteria workers, and prepare those who will be lobbying the city parks and recreation board.

Finally, the planners will need to plan for program evaluation (Phase V). Process evaluation will examine the success of the implementation of the various program components. How was the quality of the in-service sessions? What was good about them? How could they be improved? What were the immediate learning outcomes for the teachers, cafeteria workers, and those learning lobbying skills? What was the quality of the curriculum offered for the fifth- and sixth-graders? How did the implementation go with the school lunches using the new menu? The impact evaluation will measure the the knowledge, attitudes, and health practices of the fifth- and sixth-graders with regard to physical activity and nutrition. It will also include an examination of changes that may have occurred at the city parks. Since the health goal of the program was to reduce the prevalence of heart disease in the community and aimed at students in grades 5 and 6, the resources would not be available to track these students for a long period of time. Thus, outcome evaluation would not be conducted.

Consumer-Based Planning

PRECEDE-PROCEED and MATCH are examples of time-honored models that have been used successfully in many health promotion settings. It is fitting and important for health educators to understand and be able to apply these models. More recently, there has been some different planning models that have shown promise for many health promotion applications. The focus of these newer planning models is consumer based. Though the other planning models presented in this chapter (referred to by some as *practitioner-driven models*) use data from the consumer (target population) in the planning process, in *consumer-based planning*, all program decisions are based on consumer input and made with consumers in mind. In other words, consumer-based planning, includes consumers throughout the entire planning process. Data are collected to target an appropriate population segment, to understand the wants, needs, and preferences of the targeted population, then to continually test all aspects of intervention and communication strategies. There is mounting evidence to suggest that this planning approach is more effective than practitioner-driven approaches.

Two disciplines that generally apply a consumer-based planning strategy are health communication and social marketing. Social marketing, in particular, is defined and characterized by its consumer orientation. Though they are generally considered distinct disciplines, they both craft communication strategies, develop interventions, and perform evaluations to improve programs, only after they identify who their consumers are, what they need, how they will respond and change most effectively, and if programs can truly meet the consumers' needs.

Health Communication

Health communication is broadly defined as any type of human communication concerned with health (Rogers, 1996). It has also been interpreted as the art and technique of informing, influencing, and motivating individual, institutional, and public audiences about important health issues (USDHHS, 1998). Health communication is also commonly defined by its applications, including media advocacy, risk communication, entertainment education, print material, and interactive communication (Maibach & Holtgrave, 1995). Used appropriately, health communication can influence attitudes, perceptions, awareness, knowledge, and social norms, which all tend to act as precursors to behavior change. To accomplish these outcomes, health communication uses interpersonal, small group, organizational, community, and mass media channels.

An early work that did much to direct the health communication movement was developed by the Office of Communications at the National Cancer Institute and titled *Making Health Communication Programs Work: A Planner's Guide* (USDHHS,

1989). It was suggested in this guide that disciplines such as health education, social marketing, and mass communication collectively defined health communication. More recently, it has been suggested that four prominent disciplines define health communication: social marketing, public relations, advocacy, and negotiation (Ratzan, 1999a). It is generally agreed that health communication is multidisciplinary in nature.

Although communicating information about health and disease has occurred for thousands of years, the health communication discipline itself is quite young. Because of the multi- and interdisciplinary nature of health communication, relatively few of those who perform health communication tasks have been formally trained in an academic program. But several ongoing academic and professional efforts are serving to develop health communication as a discipline unto itself (Fowler et al., 1999). In fact, health communication has emerged sufficiently to lay claim to improvements in health and reductions in disease. For example, it has been reported that health communication played a primary or contributing role in the completion of 219 of 300 objectives within *Healthy People 2000* (USDHHS, 1998).

Today, we find ourselves in a new age of communication that holds the potential to drive a health revolution (Ratzan, 1999b). At the same time, we know that transmission of information or mere data do not equal effective communication (Ratzan, 1999b). To the contrary, driving a health revolution will require that those who perform health communication use strategic approaches based on established communication and behavioral theories, and incorporate consumer feedback to create targeted interventions and messages.

Social Marketing

Social marketing has been defined as a program-planning process designed to influence the voluntary behavior of a specific audience segment to achieve a social rather than a financial objective. Borrowing from commercial marketing principles, the process offers benefits the audience wants, reduces barriers the audience faces, and uses persuasion to influence intentions to act favorably (Albrecht, 1997).

A frequent misinterpretation of social marketing is that it is limited to narrow interventions, such as communication or advertising strategies. Used correctly, social marketing is best viewed as a planning framework that positions consumers at the core of all activity. Although it is not necessarily a complicated process, it can represent a time-consuming and costly process.

Social marketing strategies have been used in varying degrees for nearly 30 years in international and domestic settings, with the primary intent to improve health conditions and quality of life in general. Early international social marketing interventions focused primarily on immunizations, family planning, agricultural reforms, and nutrition (Walsh et al., 1993). Social marketing activity in the United States has focused on diverse issues, including the prevention of AIDS (Dejong, 1989; Fisher et al., 1996; Harvey, 1994), prevention of cardiovascular disease (Glascoff, 1986; Samuels, 1993), low-fat eating (Ngo, 1993), the Five-a-Day

Campaign (Loughrey et al., 1997), prevention and treatment of drug use (Black et al., 1993; Black & Smith, 1994), and breast cancer screening (Bryant et al., 1996).

Based on the results of a Delphi survey conducted among leading social marketing authorities (Maibach, Shenker, & Singer, 1997), 10 key elements displayed in Figure 2.5 best characterize social marketing. What becomes readily apparent is that social marketing attempts to strategically understand the consumer and ensure that interventions are not only based on consumer input but also tested with consumers before being implemented. This is significantly different from traditional health promotion practice.

Two models that capture the critical characteristics of health communication and social marketing are CDCynergy and SMART, respectively. They both focus on targeted audiences, rely heavily on consumer data for decision making, and attempt to continually return to the consumer for feedback and program improvement.

CDCynergy

Perhaps the most comprehensive and theoretically based health communication planning model is **CDCynergy,** or **Cynergy** for short, developed by the Office of Communication at the Centers for Disease Control and Prevention (CDC). Although it is a CD-ROM tool, its contents resemble most planning models and contain the basic components outlined in Figure 1.3, and included in both the PRECEDE-PROCEED and MATCH models. However, it does pay closer attention to audience analysis and feedback, segmentation principles, and targeted communication strategies.

CDCynergy was developed primarily for public health professionals at CDC who have responsibilities for health communication. However, because of widespread interest in the model, CDC made it available to other health professionals who found the model useful for health promotion in community, worksite, school,

---

FIGURE 2.5   *Key Elements That Best Characterize the Practice of Social Marketing*

- Audience-centered program development
- Promotion of voluntary behavior change
- Audience segmentation and profiling
- Formative research to develop and test programs
- A range of product development based on audience research
- Product distribution based on audience research
- Program promotion through channels identified in audience research
- Process evaluation
- Outcome evaluation
- Audience and community involvement in the planning process

Source: Maibach, Shenker, and Singer (1997).

and health care (including managed care) settings. Although it is considered public domain (meaning restrictions are not placed on copying or general use), CDC currently requires training before releasing a copy of the CD-ROM. However, a CDCynergy workbook and the CD-ROM, from which this review is based, can provide the planners with most, if not all, necessary information. At the time this textbook was being prepared, plans were underway to update the current version (1.1).

Cynergy uses six phases to help planners acquire a thorough understanding of a health problem and who it affects; explore a wide range of possible strategies for influencing the problem; systematically select the strategies that show the most promise; understand the role communication can play in planning, implementing, and evaluating selected strategies; and develop a comprehensive communication plan (CDC, 1999a, p. 3). Figure 2.6 displays the six sequential yet interrelated phases, which are designed to build on the previous phases and prepare program planners for subsequent phases.

The first phase of CDCynergy is called Problem Definition and Description. Like other planning models, CDCynergy initially relies on good epidemiologic data and professional expertise to identify a primary health problem or contributing factor that merits attention and resources. Although programs and interventions are not generally implemented in a consumer-based model before obtaining adequate consumer input, an initial focus based on epidemiology or other good information is important to set the planning process in the right direction. Phase 1 requires the planner to state the problem and determine if the organization has the authority, capacity, and justification to address the problem (CDC, 1999a).

A short written problem statement assesses the difference between what is occurring and what should occur in relation to the identified health problem. Using epidemiologic data, the problem is described in terms of who is affected and to what extent, where the problem exists geographically, when it occurs, and any related trends that may be evident.

In addition to describing the scope and magnitude of the problem, Phase 1 examines whether the organization is in a good position to address the problem. To help make this determination, Cynergy walks planners through several questions. One series of questions pertains to the health problem's relevance to the organization. In other words, does the organization have authority or a mandate to address the problem? Is it a priority for the organization or part of its mission, and is there any kind of public demand for the organization to address the problem? In essence, planners must provide a rationale for why the problem should be addressed in general, and why the organization specifically should address the problem.

Finally, the organization assesses whether it has the capacity to address the problem. It does this by analyzing things such as human resources, including knowledge and expertise, technology resources, and the political climate in general. If the organization cannot adequately respond to these questions, it is important to stop the Cynergy planning process and either identify a more appropriate problem or use a more appropriate planning approach.

FIGURE 2.6   *CDCynergy Phases and Steps*

Phase 1:   *Problem Definition and Description*
- Define the problem and make sure it is relevant to your program.
- Consider resources and the variables that are working both for and against your project (e.g., you may have a lot of organizational support, but little time and money).

Phase 2:   *Problem Analysis*
- Determine the factors that contribute to the health problem.
- Select target population groups.
- Set goals.
- Determine the role of communication in the intervention strategies selected. (If communication has a role, either as the main intervention activity or as a support activity, then continue to Phase 3).

Phase 3:   *Communication Program Planning*
- Choose primary and secondary target audiences.
- Set communication objectives.
- Investigate promising settings, channels, activities, materials, and message variables in preparation for testing in Phase 4.

Phase 4:   *Program and Evaluation Development*
- Develop and test messages and choose how to communicate them.
- Plan and document your communication effort as well as your evaluation.

Phase 5:   *Program Implementation and Management*
- Implement your effort, responding to such issues as midcourse adjustments and media interest in your topic.

Phase 6:   *Feedback*
- Communicate to others the lessons learned.
- Plan for what to do next.

Source: Centers for Disease Control and Prevention (1999a).

At the conclusion of Phase 1, program planners end up with a brief description of the problem, a rationale for why the organization is addressing the problem, and a list of factors that justify the organization's involvement with the problem (CDC, 1999a). This problem definition and description can then provide a rationale to justify a program to supervisors, funding agencies, decision makers, the public, the press, constituents, or program partners. It gives program planners confidence in decision making and provides a clear direction and foundation for subsequent phases.

Whereas Phase 1 identifies the problem and provides a rationale for why an organization is doing something about the problem, Phase 2, Problem Analysis, guides program planners in describing the problem in more detail. The first task in this phase is identification of factors that directly or indirectly contribute to the problem, including biology, behavior, the environment, policies (or lack of policies), other barriers, and resources. A thorough understanding of contributing factors allows the planners to more effectively identify appropriate interventions.

An example of contributing factors is provided in the CD-ROM itself and relates to a problem statement that reads: "People are not getting tested and treated for H. pylori" (CDC, 1999b, Phase 2). Contributing factors could include a lack of awareness on the part of ulcer sufferers related to the link between H. pylori and ulcers. Perhaps there is contentment on the part of those with ulcers to continue to treat symptoms. Or perhaps there is a lack of willingness among health insurers to pay for testing or treatment. In addition, ulcer sufferers may feel they cannot complete antibiotic treatment because of inconvenience or negative side effects (CDC, 1999b).

Once contributing factors are adequately identified, potential target population groups are identified. Continuing with the H. pylori example, a number of target groups may be appropriate, including ulcer sufferers, primary care physicians, health insurance companies, and managed care organizations. The critical factor is that these groups must share one or more characteristics that are linked to the problem, and they must be large enough and different enough from other groups to justify separate analyses (CDC, 1999b).

After target population groups have been selected, goals (general statements of intent) (see Chapter 6 for more information about goals) are developed and broad strategies or interventions are considered. Cynergy uses four general categories of intervention activities: communication (which includes many traditional health education interventions), engineering, policy, and health services. If communication is selected as a primary strategy, Cynergy proceeds to establish communication objectives and link these objectives with specific communication strategies. If another type of method is selected as a primary intervention activity, communication takes a secondary role in supporting the primary activity.

Finally, Phase 2 helps the program planners examine partners and potential partners to engage in the identified goals and preliminary strategies. At the conclusion of Phase 2, the planners have a summary of contributing factors related to the health problem, a list of relevant population groups, a rationale for the selected strategy, and a list of partners and potential partners (CDC, 1999a).

Phase 3, Communication Program Planning, represents the heart and soul of health communication planning. In this phase, segmentation occurs to identify primary and secondary target audiences; communication objectives are written; settings, channels, activities, and materials are selected; and message variables are identified.

After target population groups are identified in Phase 2, the program planners more fully describe these groups in Phase 3. The groups are characterized in terms of demographic variables (gender, age, ethnicity, income, education, etc.), geodemographics variables (where people live, population density, access to health care and insurance, etc.), psychographic variables (consumer beliefs, values, preferences, personality traits), and health beliefs and behaviors. With this information in hand, the planners identify the most appropriate population group, which becomes the primary target audience.

Once a primary target audience has been selected, consumer research is performed to collect more specific data about individuals in the audience. It is important to identify the primary target audience before collecting this type of data. Otherwise, a great deal of time, energy, and resources stand to be underutilized or wasted. Techniques such as focus groups and a variety of survey methods can be used to identify the wants and needs of consumers, as well as barriers, factors that compete for their time and energy, and preferences for program methods, messages, and program distribution points.

Phase 3 also requires identifying secondary audiences, which are groups of people who can reach and influence members of the primary target audience. For example, if the primary target audience is 12- to 15-year-old youth who smoke cigarettes, a secondary target audience might be their parents or their peers. Phase 3 also requires the development of communication objectives, which describe the effects communication strategies will have on the target audience.

Other important communication variables addressed in Phase 3 include exploring possible settings, channels, and activities. Identifying an appropriate setting requires program planners to determine when and where the audience is most attentive and open to communication efforts. Examples include a worksite, where employees might see a poster; schools, where public announcements may be broadcast over the public announcement system; homes, where television may be viewed; or cars, where radios are heard. A *channel* is the route of message delivery (interpersonal, small group, organizational, community, mass media, etc.). An *activity* is a method used within a channel to deliver a message (e.g., the activity of holding training classes to help seniors start their own walking clubs). Once activities are identified, the planner must also identify needed materials to support the communication activities (CDC, 1999b, Glossary).

Finally, Phase 3 considers message variables gleaned from consumer research that will appeal to the primary target audience. These variables include style, tone, the message source, and type of appeal. *Style* pertains to visual presentation and the format that is used to convey the message (use of cartoon figures versus graphs, or using flowery embellished text versus short or direct text). *Tone* refers to the manner in which a message is expressed (positive, alarming, sensible, sophisticated, funny, etc.). The *message source* is the delivery person (i.e., physician, peer, government, community insider, celebrity, etc.) (CDC, 1999b, Glossary).

The end result of Phase 3 will be a briefing document that includes identification of the primary target audience and a rationale for its selection; a profile of the target audience; communication objectives, promising settings, channels, and activities for communication with the target audience; a list of materials program planners may need; and a summary of preferred message variables (CDC, 1999b).

Phase 4, Program and Evaluation Development, addresses developing communication concepts and evaluation together. This involves using the consumer research data from Phase 3 to develop communication concepts, messages, and materials, and to decide how to communicate messages. Pretesting is performed after each of these steps. Once concepts, messages, and materials are developed and pretested, an implementation plan is developed. This includes creating tasks and time lines, assignments, and target dates; identifying resources that are required; and developing progress checks (CDC, 1999a).

The evaluation portion of Phase 4 addresses both formative and summative evaluation. (See Chapter 13 for more information on formative and summative evaluation.) This means that those who perform evaluation are examining how well the program is being implemented and how well the consumers are responding to the communication strategies. They also determine whether changes in contributing factors related to the health problem are being made as a result of accomplishing the communication objectives. Phase 4 includes measurements of the reach and exposure of communications, cost analysis, and testing theories that are linked with the communication strategies. It also generates a summary of the programs messages and materials, an implementation plan, and an evaluation plan (CDC, 1999a).

Phase 5, Program Implementation and Management, pertains to program management and focuses primarily on logistical and communication issues. Logistical issues are composed of things like keeping the program on task and on budget, making appropriate reports, and communicating progress to the appropriate people. This involves communicating with internal staff to make sure everyone understands what the program is trying to accomplish and where it is in its progress.

Communication issues pertain to the maintenance of relationships with partners and working with the media. This requires communication with external staff and partners to make sure everyone is informed and valued in their roles, and that activities don't compete against each other to undermine the overall effort (CDC, 1999a). It also means that the program planners take advantage of breaking news or release of new research on the selected health problem, and can respond to all media inquiries. At the end of Phase 5, the planners will have developed a mechanism for internal and external communication related to program implementation and management.

The sixth and final phase of Cynergy, Feedback, addresses issues such as lessons learned during the course of program implementation and delivery, how these learned lessons can be shared with others, and how this new discovery can be redirected back into the program. This includes the creation of a dissemination plan for key findings.

Careful observance and completion of all steps in the phases of the Cynergy model will result in a strategic communication plan that is science and audience based. This will greatly increase the likelihood of achieving program goals and objectives and reducing the related health problem.

SMART

Although social marketing has been used to improve health for over 30 years, relatively few social marketing planning frameworks exist. Glanz, Lewis, and Rimer

(1997) have proposed types of planning processes related to social marketing. Bryant (1998) and Andreason (1995) have also outlined a sequential process to facilitate social marketing activity. An attempt has also been made to synthesize existing social marketing frameworks into a standardized sequence of phases or steps (Walsh et al., 1993). **SMART (Social Marketing Assessment and Response Tool)** (Neiger, 1998), influenced primarily by Walsh and colleagues (1993), is also a composite of these planning frameworks but differs in sequence of steps, certain content areas, and consistency with models most often used in health promotion settings. A careful review of the model also provides an excellent overview of social marketing in general.

As displayed in Figure 2.7, SMART is composed of seven phases. Like other social marketing planning frameworks, the central focus of SMART is consumers. The heart of this model, composed of Phases 2 through 4, pertains to acquiring a rich understanding of the consumers who will be the recipients of a program and its interventions. These three phases seek to understand consumers before methods and interventions are developed. Unlike sales or forced approaches that are so often used in health promotion, a social marketing approach represents an honest attempt to respond directly to consumer feedback.

Preliminary planning is critical for any type of health promotion program. It is also the first phase of SMART. Preliminary planning allows program planners to objectively assess all health problems and determine which one is most appropriate to address. This is most often accomplished through analysis of epidemiologic data, including various mortality and morbidity rates and associated risk factor data. It also includes objective priority setting with predetermined criteria. Sometimes, program planners do not undergo a process to select a priority health problem because the decision has already been made or the organization is dedicated to a specific health problem (e.g., the American Heart Association). Once a single health problem is determined, it is defined in terms of behaviors. Risk factors, or contributing factors, then become the focus of the social marketing process. This is similar to most health promotion programs.

Although goals are outlined in Phase 1, objectives are not. This makes sense from a social marketing perspective, since consumer research has not yet been performed. The goals are general statements of intent or direction, but they do not specify program components and direct the planner into specific courses of action.

Another task in Phase 1 is to develop preliminary plans for evaluation. Theoretically, it will make sense to most health educators to consider evaluation early in the planning process. In reality, evaluation is too often an afterthought, if it is performed at all. Preliminary decisions regarding evaluation outcomes must be made up front in order to account for expertise, time, and budget requirements. Therefore, it is also important to determine how preprogram (pretest or baseline) and postprogram (posttest) data will be collected and to identify valid survey or data collection instruments. Planners can also control for various kinds of bias or error in data collection if these basic evaluation concepts are considered before the program is implemented.

Finally, program costs need to be projected before the social marketing project begins. Social marketing can be an expensive proposition in terms of staff

FIGURE 2.7 *The SMART Model*

Phase 1: *Preliminary Planning*
- Identify the focus of interest.
- Name the problem in terms of behaviors.
- Develop goals.
- Outline preliminary plans for evaluation.
- Project program costs

Phase 2: *Consumer Analysis*
- Identify and segment the target population.
- Identify formative research methods.
- Identify consumer wants, needs, and preferences.
- Develop preliminary ideas for preferred interventions and communication strategies.

Phase 3: *Market Analysis*
- Examine the fit between the focus of interest and the target population.
- Establish and define the market mix (4 Ps).
- Assess the market to identify competitors (behaviors, messages, programs, etc.) and allies (support systems, resources, etc.).

Phase 4: *Channel Analysis*
- Identify which communication channels are best suited for the target population.
- Assess options for program distribution.
- Identify program partners.
- Determine how many channels should be used.

Phase 5: *Develop Materials and Pretest*
- Develop program interventions and materials using information derived from consumer, market, and channel analysis.
- Interpret the marketing mix into a program strategy that clearly communicates exchange and societal good.
- Pretest and refine the program.

Phase 6: *Implementation*
- Communicate with partners and clarify involvement.
- Activate communication and distribution.
- Document procedures and compare progress to time lines.
- Refine the program continually.

Phase 7: *Evaluation*
- Assess the degree to which the target population is receiving the program.
- Assess the immediate impact on the target population and refine the program as necessary.
- Ensure that program delivery is consistent with protocol.
- Analyze changes in the target population.

Source: Adapted from Walsh et al. (1993) by Neiger (1998).

costs and direct expenses. When performed correctly, a social marketing project can easily take a year before implementation even begins. Program planners and organizations must decide if they are ready to make these kinds of time and financial commitments. Planning for both cost-benefit and cost-effectiveness analyses, outlined in Chapter 14, are appropriate in this phase.

At the end of Phase 1, the social marketing planners have (1) identified the focus of interest in terms of modifiable behaviors, (2) developed goals that provide general direction, (3) outlined preliminary plans for evaluation, and (4) estimated total project costs. Based on this information, the planners and organizations can make an educated decision about the potential costs and benefits of the project.

Phase 2 of SMART is consumer analysis. In social marketing language, the process of performing consumer analysis is formative research. **Formative research,** as defined in social marketing, is a process that identifies differences among subgroups within a population, targets a subgroup, identifies the wants and needs of the subgroup, and identifies factors that influence its behavior, including benefits, barriers, and readiness to change (Bryant, 1998).

As discussed in CDCynergy, it is important to narrow a large, and perhaps unwieldy, population into smaller segments that make a project more manageable. Segmentation also allows a planner to focus on a subpopulation that is either at highest risk or, for other important reasons, is the most appropriate target for social marketing interventions. At times, and perhaps too often, health promotion programs are distributed and implemented to anyone and everyone in the population. Dismal results are then discouraging and perplexing. In contrast, programs that segment populations based on factors such as readiness to change, interest, learning style, support, self-efficacy, and locus of control hold more promise for successful outcomes (Albrecht & Bryant, 1996).

Segmentation can be performed with demographic, psychographic, attitudinal, or behavioral methods. Attitudinal variables involve judgments about products and services, benefits sought, and readiness to change. Behavioral variables include rationale for purchase decisions, product use, user status, and loyalty level (Albrecht & Bryant, 1996). (See Chapter 11 for more information on segmentation.)

Once a target audience has been segmented, and only after segmentation has occurred, does the bulk of formative research occur—that is, actually talking to consumers in the target audience about their wants, needs, and preferences. A commonly used method is focus groups. In-depth interviews, key informant interviews, public hearings, opinion polls, and a variety of other survey techniques can also be used to collect information about the target audience. The purpose of these techniques is to find out what consumers think about the health problem that has been identified and the related behaviors or contributing factors. (See Chapter 5 for different techniques of data collection.)

It is important to remember that no single type of data collection technique is necessarily best in performing formative research. To the contrary, it is helpful to use multiple methods to gain a better perspective of the target audience. It is a mistake for those who engage in social marketing to perform one or two focus groups in the name of consumer analysis and allege they understand their consumers. In fact,

Beckwith (1997) criticized focus groups, claiming dominant people control discussions and that they reveal more about group dynamics than market dynamics.

At the conclusion of Phase 2, a target population is identified. Adequate formative research has been performed yielding data about major themes, directions, and consumer preferences related to interventions and communication messages. Although Phases 2 through 4 are often performed simultaneously, information collected in Phase 2 can provide context for the other two phases. For example, knowing about consumer preferences related to some type of behavior change allows planners to more effectively understand consumer preferences related to the market mix and communication strategies.

Phase 3, Market Analysis, examines the fit between the focus of interest (desired behavior change) and important market variables within the target audience. *Marketing mix* is a term that is often used in both commercial and social marketing. It is composed of four components, also known as the 4Ps: product, price, place, promotion. (See Chapter 11 for a discussion of the 4Ps.)

All of the factors in the market mix are analyzed in context of the target audience and provide additional issues that should be addressed in the formative research process. Market analysis also analyzes the marketplace to identify competitors and allies. For example, a competitor in social marketing may be anything that vies for the necessary resources to engage in the behavior as prescribed. If the product is an exercise program that combines strength training and cardiovascular endurance, a competitor may be a toning program that focuses on different outcomes. A busy schedule may be a competitor. An ally may be a supportive workplace that encourages and even promotes exercise behavior.

At the conclusion of this phase, consumer analysis is enriched by a better understanding of important market variables that influence consumers. Combined with consumer analysis and channel analysis, market analysis provides a powerful combination of useful information about consumers, the environment they live in, and strengths and weakness associated with potential social marketing interventions.

The fourth phase of SMART is Channel Analysis. Since preliminary message design is addressed through formative research in Phase 2, what remains is consumer feedback on channel selection. Although communication may not be the focal point of a social marketing campaign, it will play a secondary role in communicating important messages about the product. Formative research includes specific questions about the type of communication channels consumers believe are most appropriate for the behavior change in question. As described in CDCynergy, communication channels include interpersonal, small group, organizational, community, and mass media channels. Channels also relate to place in the market mix or how the product is accessed. In other words, the channel must be appropriate for the way the product is distributed. For example, if the product is increased vegetable consumption and the place is the worksite cafeteria, an appropriate channel might be an organizational newsletter.

In most cases, the use of multiple channels increases the likelihood that the messages will be heard and acted upon. However, if the message is not consumer oriented and is not adequately supported by an effective market mix, the channel itself is relatively unimportant. That is why all these factors are planned in unison.

Finally, Phase 4 considers which potential partners, if any, might collaborate in sharing the burden of communication. For example, if mass media is an appropriate channel, and consumer-oriented public service announcements are used in the communication strategy, perhaps television and radio stations would be willing to donate air time. One problem frequently experienced in social marketing is that multiple organizations with similar missions communicate competing, albeit only slightly different messages. In extreme cases, the messages can be nearly polar opposites. For this reason alone, it is important to develop communication partners. At the conclusion of Phase 4, communication channels are identified that are consistent with preliminary messages, and product distribution points and potential communication and intervention partners are identified.

Phase 5 of SMART consists of developing and pretesting the intervention materials. Once formative research is performed, it is critical that the data are transferred or infused adequately into the design of programs, interventions, and communication strategies. To do this, data must be analyzed and categorized adequately to assure that planners understand what they have seen, heard, and observed. As program planners meet to design programs and materials, they should keep formative research data in front of them and refer to it often. Discussion and decisions should reflect all data and represent a consensus among all planners. In other words, materials and methods should represent what was learned in formative research.

Once a program prototype is developed, it is imperative to return to the target audience and test the concepts before implementing a widespread campaign. In fact, social marketing represents a process of continually returning to the consumers until the program and all its support mechanisms are consistent with their views and preferences. Several mechanisms are available to perform pretesting. One example is a pilot test where the program can be implemented with the target audience on a smaller, less expensive scale. Theater testing or focus groups can also be used to test communication messages, key components of interventions, and program formats and sequences. A theater test gathers a representative sample of the target audience to react, usually to audio- or audiovisual materials (USDHHS, 1989).

Phase 6 of SMART is implementation. Implementation in social marketing is closely related to the implementation factors addressed in CDCynergy. This phase is concerned with clarifying everyone's role, including external partners. This means that procedures are communicated and documented, and that time lines are developed and followed. In this phase, the communication and distribution plans are activated and the actual program and its interventions are offered. In addition, the program is refined continually, based on consumer feedback.

The seventh and final phase of SMART is evaluation. The preliminary evaluation strategies that were identified in Phase 1 now take effect. Evaluation always has at least two major objectives: improve the quality of the program and determine the effectiveness of the program. With respect to quality, program planners assess the degree to which the target audience, within the larger population, is actually receiving the program or interventions. Planners also assess the immediate impact the program is having and whether the interventions and related support strategies are acceptable and motivational to the target audience. Planners also ensure that program delivery is consistent with program protocol or at least consistent with developed time lines.

Ultimately, social marketing, and all the related work, is of little value unless behavior change occurs and health is improved. Evaluation also concerns itself with measuring these outcomes. Effective planners and evaluators also make sure that evaluation results are folded back into the program so that it can be improved before it is too late.

Other Planning Models

As noted at the beginning of this chapter, there are other planning models available to planners in addition to the PRECEDE-PROCEED, MATCH, CDCynergy and SMART models. Because these models are not currently used as much as those already presented, they are presented here in abbreviated form. If you are interested in learning more about these models, check the original sources or consult an earlier edition of this book (McKenzie & Smeltzer, 1997).

The Planning, Program Development, and Evaluation Model (PPDEM)

The Planning, Program Development, and Evaluation Model (PPDEM) (Timmreck, 1995) is a planning model that is comprised of 10 steps. The first step is the creation of a mission statement. The mission statement (general idea or main purpose) "is usually based on a general observation, an obvious seen need or interest, or a need assessment result" (Timmreck, 1995, p. 30). The second step is aimed at community and organizational assessment. More specifically, it is comprised of a complete assessment and evaluation of organization, inventory of resources, and review of regulations and policies. *Complete assessment* refers to completing both an internal (organizational) and external (community outside the organization) assessment. An inventory of resources examines the available resources to carry out a program, whereas the review of regulations and policies examines the government or organization statements in place that could restrict, block, or place requirements on program development (Timmreck, 1995).

Step 3 of the PPDEM includes the writing of goals and objectives for the needs assessment or program feasibility studies. Such a step forces the planners "to clearly think through what needs to be done and how to put needed activities into action" (Timmreck, 1995, p. 63). Step 4 is carrying out the needs assessment.

The fifth step is comprised of determining the gaps in existing services and programs, and setting priorities for a program based on an analysis of the needs assessment data. Step 6 consists of writing the goals and objectives for the proposed program after the project has been approved by the administration (Timmreck,

1995). With the goals and objectives in place, step-by-step activities and procedures (Step 7) need to be considered. This step would also include a decision on whether the proposed program should be pilot tested. Step 8 revolves around the creation of the time lines for implementation. The time lines would be for both "the step-by-step activities and the other matters that need to be accomplished" (Timmreck, 1995, p. 142) during program planning, implementation, and evaluation.

Step 9 of the PPDEM is the implementation step. It is the point at which time the program is put into effect. This step includes all the logistics that are needed during implementation. The final, or tenth step, of this model is evaluation and feedback. Like the other models already presented in this chapter, it includes a determination if the program objectives are being met and approaches evaluation from the three levels of process, impact, and outcome.

Model for Health Education Planning (MHEP)

The Model for Health Education Planning (MHEP) (Ross & Mico, 1980), first developed by Mico in 1966 and periodically updated, analyzes planning through six phases and the dimensions of content (subject matter), method (steps and techniques), and process (interactions). Phase 1 is the initiation of the planning activity. To carry out this phase, planners must

1. Understand the target population's problem and something about its system.
2. Enter into an initial contract.
3. Make the client aware that a problem exists.

Phase 2 of the MHEP involves completing a needs assessment. Ross and Mico (1980) suggest that to complete a needs assessment, planners should first identify how the problem was measured in the past, determine what data need to be collected now and how best to gather them, collect and analyze the data, and finally describe the nature and extent of the problem.

Phase 3 of the model deals with goal setting. The goals should be based on the problems identified in the needs assessment. They should be appropriate and realistic, and should include input from those who will be affected. Also, in this goal-setting phase, planners should develop strategies for implementing the goals. Phase 4, called planning/programming, "converts the agreed-upon strategies into a rational implementation plan or program, designs systems and tools for managing the activity, and negotiates commitments among those involved" (Ross & Mico, 1980, p. 224).

The final two phases of the MHEP are implementation (Phase 5) and evaluation (Phase 6). In Phase 5, planners offer the program, provide any needed assistance to facilitators and participants, and keep track of the progress. Phase 6, as described by Ross and Mico (1980), includes the following steps:

1. Clarifying the evaluation measures
2. Collecting and analyzing evaluation data
3. Providing appropriate feedback
4. Redefining the problem and standards

Comprehensive Health Education Model (CHEM)

The Comprehensive Health Education Model (CHEM) (Sullivan, 1973) comprises six major steps and several suggested procedures within each of the steps. The first step is to involve people. Step 1 includes identifying the target population and those needed to carry out the program, determining the roles of those involved, and establishing the necessary relationships among the people.

Step 2 involves setting the ultimate goals for the program. In Step 3, defining the problems, planners determine the gaps between what is and what could be. Once they have identified the problems, planners need to determine what problems to tackle. Next, they design the program plans (Step 4). This includes identifying the most appropriate approach; setting specific operational objectives; defining a timetable, activities, and resources; conducting a pretest; and developing evaluation procedures. The fifth step consists of obtaining the necessary resources to implement the program and then implementing it. In the sixth and final step, planners evaluate the program, based on the program objectives. Results of the evaluation then provide data for later decision making regarding the program.

Model for Health Education Planning and Resource Development (MHEPRD)

A less well-known model than those already presented is the Model for Health Education Planning and Resource Development (MHEPRD) introduced by Bates and Winder (1984). The creators of this model state that it can be distinguished from others because it separates process from end results, and because of the use of evaluation. Each of the five major components in the MHEPRD—health education plans, demonstration programs, operational programs, research programs, and information and statistics—represents an end result of the planning process. The creators do not see evaluation as a separate phase of the model. Instead, it plays an integral part in each phase by testing and validating program assumptions throughout the entire process (Bates & Winder, 1984).

In Phase 1 of the model, health education plans are an end result of a needs assessment (or, as Bates and Winder call it, a "policy-analysis process") and ongoing evaluation of information and statistics. The plans developed in Phase 1 are treated as hypotheses to be tested in Phase 2. To validate their effectiveness, planners create demonstration programs. Phase 3 examines the results of the demonstration programs to determine which should continue and thus become operational programs. This phase also includes the development of an implementation plan that reflects the experiences learned during the demonstration. This process should yield operational programs that are based on a sound rationale of research, planning, and demonstrations.

Phase 4 implements the operational programs. During this phase, steps that are commonly used in a research project are put to use. The problems that surface during implementation provide the basis for research questions for the program planners. The planners, in turn, formulate possible answers to the questions through appropriate experimentation. The data generated through the experimentation are used for

TABLE 2.3   *Summary of Health Education/Promotion Planning Models (by author and year)*

PRECEDE-PROCEED (Green & Kreuter, 1999)	CDCynergy (CDC 1999a)	SMART (Neiger, 1998)	MATCH (Simons-Morton et al., 1988)
Phase 1 Social assessment	Phase 1 Problem definition and description	Phase 1 Preliminary planning	Phase 1 Goals selection
Phase 2 Epidemiological assessment	Phase 2 Problem analysis	Phase 2 Consumer analysis	Phase 2 Intervention planning
Phase 3 Behavioral and environmental assessment	Phase 3 Communication program planning	Phase 3 Market analysis	Phase 3 Program development
Phase 4 Educational and ecological assessment	Phase 4 Program and evaluation development	Phase 4 Channel analysis	Phase 4 Implementation preparations
Phase 5 Administrative and policy assessment	Phase 5 Program implementation and management	Phase 5 Develop materials and pretest	Phase 5 Evaluation
Phase 6 Implementation	Phase 6 Feedback	Phase 6 Implementation	
Phase 7 Process evaluation		Phase 7 Evaluation	
Phase 8 Impact evaluation			
Phase 9 Outcome evaluation			

future policy analysis and planning. Thus, the planning process becomes cyclic in nature since it always builds on previous planning. As the process continues, the result should be better organized and more effective health education services (Bates & Winder, 1984).

Generic Health/Fitness Delivery System (GHFDS)

The final model to be presented in this chapter is the Generic Health/Fitness Delivery System, or GHFDS (Patton et al., 1986). As its name suggests, this model

TABLE 2.3   Continued

PPDEM (Timmreck, 1995)	MHEP (Ross & Mico, 1980)	CHEM (Sullivan, 1973)	MHEPRD (Bates & Winder, 1984)	GHFDS (Patton et al., 1986)
Step 1 Mission statement	Phase 1 Initiate	Step 1 Involve people	Health education plans	Needs assessment
Step 2 Complete assessment and evaluation	Phase 2 Needs assessment	Step 2 Set goals	Demonstration programs	Goal setting
Step 3 Writing goals and objectives for needs assessment	Phase 3 Goal setting	Step 3 Define problems	Operational programs	Planning
Step 4 Needs assessment	Phase 4 Planning and programming	Step 4 Design plans	Research programs	Program implementation
Step 5 Determine and set priorities	Phase 5 Implementation	Step 5 Conduct activities	Information and statistics	Evaluation
Step 6 Writing goals and objectives for project	Phase 6 Evaluation	Step 6 Evaluate results	Evaluation process	Educational component
Step 7 Step-by-step activities and procedures			Various other processes	Service component
Step 8 Determine time line charts				
Step 9 Implementation of the project				
Step 10 Evaluation and Feedback				

was not developed specifically for health education but can easily be applied to it. This goal-oriented planning model suggests five steps: needs assessment, goal setting, choice of strategies to meet goals, delivery of program, and evaluation. Each of the steps has two components, education and service. The education component provides a cognitive experience in each step, while the service component provides a hands-on experience. This approach to program planning is dynamic and interactive. It provides constant insight and feedback so as best to meet the needs of those in the target population. Input from a previous step in the GHFDS modifies the approach used in delivering the later steps in the model. Feedback from the later steps becomes most useful in modifying program delivery (Patton et al., 1986).

Summary

A model can provide the framework for planning and evaluating a health promotion program. Several different planning models have been developed and revised over the years. The planning models for health education/promotion presented in this chapter are the following:

1. PRECEDE-PROCEED (Predisposing, Reinforcing, and Enabling Constructs in Educational/Environmental Diagnosis and Evaluation; Policy, Regulatory, and Organizational Constructs in Educational and Environmental Development)
2. MATCH (Multilevel Approach To Community Health)
3. CDCynergy
4. SMART (Social Marekting Assessment and Response Tool)
5. PPEDM (The Planning, Program Development, and Evaluation Model)
6. MHEP (Model for Health Education Planning)
7. CHEM (Comprehensive Health Education Model)
8. MHEPRD (Model for Health Education Planning and Resource Development)
9. GHFDS (Generic Health/Fitness Delivery System)

To date, probably the best-known model and the one most often used in health promotion is the PRECEDE-PROCEED model. MATCH has also been a time-honored model. The newer models of CDCynergy and SMART are starting to take hold and are being used more and more. And finally, there are several other that have made and continue to make valuable contributions (Table 2.3).

Questions

1. Why is it important to use a model when planning?

2. Name the nine models presented in this chapter, and list one distinguishing characteristic of each.

3. Of the models presented, which one has been most commonly used? Name the different phases of this model.

4. How are the CDCynery and SMART models different from the others presented in this chapter?

5. What five or six components seem to be common to all the models? (Note that the names of the components may not be the same, but the concepts are.)

Activities

1. After reviewing the models presented in this chapter, create your own model by identifying what you think are the common

key components of the models. Provide a rationale for including each component. Then draw a diagram of your model and put it on a transparency so that you can share it with the class. Be prepared to explain your model.

2. In a one-page paper, defend what you believe is the best planning model presented in this chapter.

3. Using a hypothetical health problem for a specific target population, in a written paper explain the steps/phases for one of the models presented in this chapter.

4. List and describe any potential advantages and disadvantages of using a consumer-based planning model in health promotion. How do these advantages and disadvantages compare with more traditional planning models used in health promotion? Be prepared to discuss your ideas in class.

5. Identify a public service announcement on television or radio, or obtain a copy of one from a nearby health agency. Analyze factors such as style, tone, message source, and type of appeal. Based on your analysis, was the public service announcement developed appropriately for the intended audience? Summarize your comments in a one-page paper.

6. USing either the CDCynergy or SMART model, identify a relevant health problem, target a specific audience, perform or gather appropriate consumer research, and develop ideas for appropriate intervention and communication strategies. Summarize your findings in a three-page paper.

Activities on the Web

1. Visit the website for the Institute of Health Promotion Research at the University of British Columbia <http://www.ihpr.ubc.ca> and locate the bibliography for published articles that use the PRECEDE-PROCEED model. Identify at least two articles that apply the model to the topic that you are considering for development in your program planning class. Locate and read the two articles and write a summary of each.

2. Visit the website for the library at your school. Using the available search program (i.e., First Search, Web Cat), locate any sources that relate to any of the planning models identified in this chapter. Print out the sources that you find and take them to class to share.

3. Visit the website for the Office of Communication in the Office of the Director at the Centers for Disease Control and Prevention <http://www.cdc.gov/od/abtoc.htm>, Go to HealthComm KEY. Answer the following questions: (a) What is the HealthComm KEY database? (b) How are the articles summarized for the database? (c) How can you use the HealthComm database?

4. Visit the website for the Novartis Foundation for Sustainable Development <http://foundation.novartis.com/social_marketing.htm>. Read a short course in social marketing and summarize three to five points that best characterize social marketing from your perspective.

5. Visit the website for the National Cancer Institute's document, Making Health Communications Work <http://rex.nci.nih.gov/NCI_Pub_Interface/HCPW/HOME.HTM>. Read the Health Communications Process: Overview. Write a one-page summary of health communications.

3

Starting the Planning Process

After reading this chapter and answering the questions at the end, you should be able to:

- Explain the importance of gaining the support of decision makers.
- Develop a rationale for planning and implementing a health promotion program.
- Identify the individuals who could make up a planning committee.
- Explain what program parameters are and the impact they have on program planning.

Key Terms

advisory board
institutionalized
organizational culture
parameter

pilot program
planning committee
program ownership
stakeholders

steering committee
vendor

Planning a health promotion program is a multiphase process. "To *plan* is to engage in a process or a procedure to develop a method of achieving an end" (Breckon, Harvey, & Lancaster, 1998, p. 145). However, because of the many different variables and circumstances of any one setting, the multiphase process of planning does not always begin the same way. There are times when the need for a program is obvious and everyone knows that a new program should be put in place. There are other times when a program has been successful in the past and just needs to be changed or reworked slightly before being implemented again. And there are situations where planners have been given the autonomy and authority to create the needed programs. But when the need is not so obvious, or when there has not been success in the past, or when the autonomy is not present, the planning process begins with the planners needing to gain the support of key people in order to ensure that the planning process proceeds as smoothly as possible. This chapter presents the initial steps of obtaining the support of decision makers, identifying those who may be interested in helping to plan the program, and establishing the parameters in which the planners must work.

Gaining Support of Decision Makers

No matter what the setting of a health promotion program—whether a business, an industry, the community, a clinic, a hospital, or a school—it is most important that the program have support from the highest level (the administration, chief executive officer, church elders, board of health, or board of directors) (Chapman, 1997; Wolfe, Slack, & Rose-Hearn, 1993) of the "community" for which the program is being planned. These top-level people in decision-making positions are able to provide the necessary resource support for the program.

> "Resources" usually means money, which can be turned into staff, facilities, materials, supplies, utilities, and all the myriad number of things that enable organized activity to take place over time. "Support" usually means a range of things: congruent organizational policies, program and concept visibility, expressions of priority value, personal involvement of key managers, a place at the table of organizational power, organizational credibility, and a role in integrated functioning. (Chapman, 1997, p. 1)

There will be times when the idea for, or the motivating force behind, a program comes from the top-level people. When this happens, it is a real boon for the program planners because they do not have to "sell" the idea to these people to gain their support. However, this scenario does not occur frequently.

Often, the idea or the big push for a health promotion program comes from someone other than one who is part of the top level of the "community." The idea could start with an employee, an interested parent, a health educator within the organization, a member of the parish or congregation, or a concerned citizen. The idea might even be generated by an individual outside the "community," such as a **vendor** trying to sell a program to a business. When the scenario begins at a level below the decision makers, those who want to create a program must "sell" it to the decision makers. In other words, in order for resources and support to flow into health promotion programming, decision makers need to clearly perceive a set of values or benefits associated with the proposed program (Chapman, 1997). Without the support of decision makers, it becomes more difficult, if not impossible, to plan and implement a program. Behrens (1983) has stated that health promotion programs in business and industry have a greater chance for success if all levels of management, including the top, are committed and supportive. This is true of health promotion programs in all settings, not just programs in business and industry.

If they need to gain the support of decision makers, program planners should develop a rationale for the program's existence. Why is it necessary to "sell" something that everyone knows is worthwhile? After all, does anyone doubt the value of trying to help people gain and maintain good health? The answer to these and similar questions is that few people are motivated by health concerns alone. Decisions by top-level management to develop new programs are based on a variety of factors, including finances, policies, public image, and politics, to name a few. Thus, to "sell" the program to those at the top, planners need to develop a rationale that shows how the new program will help those at the top to meet the organization's goals and, in turn, to carry out its mission. In other words, program planners need to position their program rationale politically, in line with the organization. To do this, planners need to amass as many "political data" (data that help to align the program with the organization's mission) as possible; this will enable them to put together a sound rationale to "sell" program development. There are several different sources of information (see Figure 3.1) that can be used in developing a rationale. One source would be the results of a needs assessment showing that such a program is needed and wanted. An example of such a situation is the result of a Gallup poll conducted for the American Cancer Society that indicated that there was overwhelming support for comprehensive school health education from adolescent students (ages 12–17), parents, and school administrators (Seffrin, 1994). However, more than likely, a formal needs assessment will not yet have been completed at this point in the planning process. Often, a complete assessment does not take place until permission has been given for planning to begin. However, if an assessment has been completed for this or another related or similar program, data from it can be used to help develop the rationale.

Epidemiological data about a specific health problem are a second information source for building a rationale. These data gain additional significance when it can be shown that the described health problem(s) are the result of modifiable health behaviors and that spending money to promote healthy lifestyles and prevent health problems makes good economic sense. Seffrin (1994, p. 399) presents a good example when he talks about the impact of cigarette smoking on the 48 million smokers in the United States and the United States population in general. He writes, "Not only does tobacco addiction exact an unacceptable burden in health care costs—about $65 billion annually—and a true carnage in human lives—20% of all deaths in 1993—it also strips one-fourth of our population of significant free-

---

FIGURE 3.1 *Summary of Information Sources for Building a Rationale*

1. Needs assessment data
2. Epidemiological data about a specific health problem
3. Values and benefits that are important to decision makers
4. Compatibility between the proposed program and the health plan of a state or the nation
5. Protecting human resources

---

dom of choice through addiction, and sets an unnecessary and undesirable limit on each smoker's human potential." Examples of another 18 commonly seen health problems (e.g., breast cancer, cervical and colorectal cancer, coronary heart disease, HIV/AIDS transmission, low birth weight, and tuberculosis) in the United States and their related economic impact are presented in a publication titled *An Ounce of Prevention…What Are the Returns?* (CDC, 1999). Further, Goetzel and colleagues (1998) and Riedel (1999) present very useful data on the relationship between modifiable health risks and health care expenditures. Goetzel (1998) present data on such health risks as depression, high stress, high blood glucose levels, and abnormal blood pressure, to name a few, and Riedel (1999) provides an informative overview of the cost-effectiveness of health promotion.

A third source of evidence on which a program rationale can be built is on the values and benefits of such a program to the decision makers. Obviously, these values and benefits vary, depending on the settings and what is important to decision makers. Chapman (1997) outlines the values and benefits associated with health promotion programming in which supporting data and/or documentation exist or can be collected. Further, the values and benefits he presents focus on four different types of programming: for worksites, communities, individuals, and managed care organizations. Chapman's work is presented in Table 3.1

When planners use the value and benefits information associated with the "reduction in health care costs" as part of their rationale, they should do so with caution (Edington & Yen, 1992; Goetzel et al., 1998; Sciacca et al., 1993; Warner 1987; Warner et al., 1988).

> To establish a cost-based, as well as a health-based, reason for performing more prevention and health promotion, several types of empirical evidence must be gathered and broadly communicated to clinicians, health plan managers, employers, and consumers. First, researchers must demonstrate that poor health habits and modifiable risk factors impose a financial burden, ie [sic], that individuals possessing these risk factors cost more than those without these risks, even in the short run. Second, researchers need to demonstrate that improvements in risk factors result in a reduction in cost. Third, researchers need to demonstrate that health habits can be changed and that the resultant lower risk can be maintained over time. Finally, researchers need to demonstrate that the benefits of changing habits and lowering health risk out-weigh the costs. This involves conducting cost-effective and cost-benefit studies that demonstrate the relative value of prevention activities when compared with the costs of illness treatment or doing nothing. Consequently, the challenges associated with documenting a financial payback for prevention and health promotion are significant. (Goetzel et al., 1998, pp. 843–844)

The first step in this process of establishing the relationship between the presence of modifiable risk factors and increased medical expenditures has been presented (Goetzel et al., 1998). However more research in this area is needed before planners can use "the reduction in health care costs" argument with absolute assurance in their rationale for health promotion programming.

A fourth source of data in other successful programs that have been conducted in similar settings. For example, planners may know of other successful programs in

TABLE 3.1   *Values or Benefits Associated with Health Promotion Programming*

Focus	Value or Benefit Statement	Supporting Data and/or Documentation
Worksite	Increased worker morale	Studies using survey instruments that measure employee morale, industry or trade association data, human resource annual surveys with carefully selected questions
	Potentially greater employer loyalty	Survey results and patterns over time, use of loyalty proxy questions, and survey or focus group findings
	Improved employee resiliency and decision making quality	Studies from the psychological and exercise physiology literature
	Positive public and community relations	Recognition awards for local or peer employers, coalition or community consortium activities, industry and trade showcase or write-ups
	Increased worker productivity	Business and industrial management studies, selected studies from the worksite health promotion literature, local or trade data using collective productivity indicators
	Informed, health care cost-conscious workforce	Studies and anecdotal articles about consumer activism, scores from consumer health knowledge surveys, survey results on self-efficacy and consumerism
	Recruitment tool	Social psychology literature and business survey literature, selected labor market survey data
	Retention tool	Social psychology literature and business survey literature, selected labor market survey data
	Opportunity for cost savings via: Reduced sick leave absenteeism	A large number of worksite health promotion studies that address sick leave absenteeism effects, survey data from National Institutes of Occupational Health & Safety (NIOSH) and from trade and industry associations
	Opportunity for cost savings via: Reduced short- and long-term disability claims	A few articles on worksite health promotion programs and their impact on disability days, benefits and business surveys, risk management literature
	Opportunity for cost savings via: Decreased health care utilization	A moderate number of articles on the evaluation of worksite health promotion programs and their impact on health care

TABLE 3.1 **Continued**

Focus	Value or Benefit Statement	Supporting Data and/or Documentation
		costs, the medical care research literature and the managed care research literature, which also contain a variety of references; another major set of references are the actuarial studies that have been done on the relationship of health risks to health costs
	Opportunity for cost savings via: Reduced premature retirement	Studies of early medical or disability retirement from the benefits, disability management, and actuarial literature
	Opportunity for cost savings via: Decreased overall health benefit costs	Worksite health promotion evaluation literature, business and benefits management literature, trade or competitor information
	Opportunity for cost savings via: Fewer on-the-job accidents	Worksite health promotion evaluation literature, risk management literature, safety literature, NIOSH publications, publications of the Bureau of Labor Statistics
	Opportunity for cost savings via: Lower casualty insurance costs	Casualty underwriter's publications and risk management literature
	Opportunity for cost savings via: Smaller total workforce	Business literature plus projections at various sick leave and disability reduction levels, review of personal replacement cases that have occurred in the last 2 to 5 years
	Opportunity for cost savings via: Reduced medical leave time	Occupational health literature and payroll system coding data
	Opportunity for cost savings via: Reduced occupational medical costs	Occupational health literature and occupational health unit data
Community	Provides a model for other local organizations	Community health promotion literature and community organization literature plus Robert Wood Johnson Community Snapshots Project
	Contributes to establishing good health as a norm	Community health promotion literature and cultural change literature plus Centers for Disease Control and Prevention publications
	Complements and reinforces national and local public health initiatives	Office of Disease Prevention and Health Promotion publications and Objectives for the Nation: 2000 plus local public health reports and plans

(continued)

TABLE 3.1 Continued

Focus	Value or Benefit Statement	Supporting Data and/or Documentation
	Improves quality of life of citizenry	Community Health Care Forum materials and National League of Cities publications
	Helps control (and possibly reduce) the economic and social burden on all taxpayers from premature mortality and morbidity	Compression of morbidity literature and community health promotion literature plus Health Care Financing and Agency for Health Services Research publications and studies
	Helps improve the general economic well-being of communities through the improvement in general health status and productivity	Community health promotion literature and national econometric studies and analyses
Individual	Increased morale via employer's, provider's, or community's interest in their health and well-being	Social psychological and psychological literature
	Increased knowledge about the relationship between lifestyle and health	Attitude and correlated research within the health promotion and health education literature
	Increased opportunity to take control of their health and medical treatment	Consumer satisfaction surveys and national market research studies plus self-efficacy literature
	Improved health and quality of life through reduction of risk factors	Literature surrounding the use of SF12 and SF36 and self-reported perception of health status
	Increased opportunity for support from co-workers and environment	Social psychological literature, health education research literature, and cultural change literature
	Reduced work absences	Attitude and correlated research within the health promotion and health education literature
	Reduced out-of-pocket and premium costs for medical care	Attitude and correlated research within the health promotion and health education literature plus Bureau of Commerce and Census publications
	Reduced pain and suffering from illness and accidents	Attitude and correlated research within the health promotion and health education literature
Managed Care Organizations	Greater member satisfaction	Perceived value of health benefit literature, Health Plan Employer Data Information Set (HEDIS) literature

TABLE 3.1   **Continued**

Focus	Value or Benefit Statement	Supporting Data and/or Documentation
	Increased market share through differentiation	Managed care marketing literature and strategic planning literature for the managed care industry
	More appropriate utilization by consumers and patients	Medical self-care literature, case management literature, medical care literature, and demand management literature
	Reduced utilization and cost through improvements in morbidity	Compression of morbidity literature, epidemiology literature, managed care and demand management literature
	Improved price competitiveness	Managed care literature, financial analysis of managed care industry literature, and benefit survey literature
	Improved HEDIS performance	National Committee on Quality Assurance publications and particularly HEDIS Version 3.0

Source: Chapman (1997), pp. 4–5. Reprinted by permission.

surrounding communities, companies, churches, or schools; the people associated with those programs may be able to provide data they generated or may be willing to share their thoughts on how they "sold" their program to those at the top. Of course, planners can always refer to successes reported in the professional literature.

A fifth source of information for a rationale is a comparison between the proposed program and the health plan for the nation or a state. Comparing the health needs of the target population with those of other citizens of the state or of all Americans, as outlined in the goals and objectives of the nation (OPHS, 1998), should enable program planners to show the compatibility between the goals of the program and those of the nation's health plan. A discussion of these national health goals and objectives is presented in Chapter 6.

When preparing a rationale to gain the support of decision makers, program planners should emphasize the importance of people as a resource to any "community." Andrew J. J. Brennan, director of Metropolitan Life Insurance Company's Center for Health Help, sums up this point nicely by stating, "People are our company's single biggest asset. It makes good business sense to invest wisely in our employees' good health" (quoted in Novelli & Ziska, 1982). Stated another way, "Fit and healthy people are more productive, are better able to meet extraordinary demands and deal with stress, are absent less, reflect better on the company or community as exemplars, and so forth" (Chapman, 1997, p. 6).

Creating a Rationale

Planners must realize that gaining the support of decision makers is initially the most important step in the planning process and should not be taken lightly. Many program ideas have died at this stage because the planners were not well prepared. Before making an appeal to decision makers, planners need to be thoroughly prepared. "The 'selling job' should be backed by a soundly researched idea" (McKenzie, 1988, p. 149). Therefore, planners need to put much care into developing their rationale. No formula or recipe has been put forward for writing a rationale, but through experience, the authors have found a logical format for putting ideas together (see Figure 3.2). Begin the rationale by titling it and indicating who contributed to its authorship. The first paragraph or two of the rationale

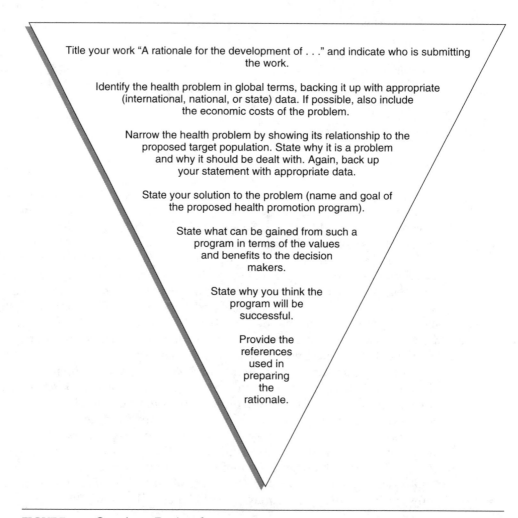

FIGURE 3.2 *Creating a Rationale*

should identify the health problem in global terms. This is where you can use epidemiological and other needs assessment data. If you can, also include the economic costs of such a problem; it will strengthen your rationale. Most local health problems are also present on the international, national, and/or state levels. Presenting the problem at these higher levels shows decision makers that dealing with the health problem is consistent with the concerns of others.

Showing the relationship of the local health problem to the "bigger problem" at the international, national, and/or state levels is the next logical step in presenting the rationale. Thus, the next portion of the rationale should identify the local health problem and state *why* it is a problem and *why* it should be dealt with.

At this point in the rationale, you should state your solution to the problem. In other words, state the name and purpose of the proposed health promotion program. The statement of the purpose of the program should be followed by a statement of what can be gained from the program. The benefits of the program should be given in terms that are meaningful to the decision makers. (See Figure 3.3 for methods to determine the values and benefits that should be emphasized in your rationale.) This can be done by:

1. Comparing the proposed program with other successful programs
2. Stating the values and benefits (see Table 3.1) that are important to the decision makers
3. Stating that the program will protect human resources

Next, state why you believe this program will be successful. It can be helpful to point out the similarity of this target population to others with which similar programs have been successful. Using the argument that the "timing is right" for the program can also be useful.

FIGURE 3.3 *Methods for Determining the Values and Benefits That Should Be Emphasized*

1. Examine recent or past meeting minutes, decisions, or comments that are relevant to the value placed on health and prevention.
2. Find out from the individuals in a position to know, why past decisions related to budget or employee benefits were made by the managers involved.
3. Review past formal reports or evaluations of health programs and benefits that have been commissioned or carried out on behalf of the decision makers.
4. Conduct an informal survey of the most influential decision makers to get some sense of their own as well as their perception of the value priorities of the other decision makers involved.
5. Conduct a formal survey of all or a portion of the key decision makers involved to determine what is the most important to them
6. Analyze the implementation questions that have been raised in the past on similar programs or topics.

Source: Chapman (1997), p. 2. Reprinted by permission.

Finally, make sure to include a list of the references used to prepare the rationale. This shows decision makers that you have researched your idea. (See the examples of rationales presented in the Activities section at the end of the chapter.)

Identifying a Planning Committee

The number of people involved in the planning process is determined by resources and circumstances of a particular situation. There are times when just a single person will do the planning, while other times there may be several involved. "One very helpful method to develop a clearer and more comprehensive planning approach is to establish a committee" (Gilmore & Campbell, 1996, p. 16). Identifying individuals who would be willing to serve as members of the **planning committee** (sometimes referred to as a **steering committee** or **advisory board**) becomes one of the planner's first tasks. The number of individuals on a planning committee can differ depending on the setting for the program and the size of the target population. For example, the size of a planning committee for a safety belt program in a community of 50,000 people would probably be larger than that of a committee planning a similar program for a business with 50 employees. There is no ideal size for a planning committee, but the following guidelines, which have been presented earlier (McKenzie, 1988) and are given here in a modified form, should be helpful in setting up a committee.

1. Select individuals who represent a variety of groups in the target population. If possible, the committee should have representation from all segments of the target population (e.g., administrators/students/teachers, age groups, health behavior participants/nonparticipants, labor/management, race/ethnic groups, different sexes, socioeconomic groups, union/nonunion members, etc.). The greater the number of individuals who are represented by committee members, the greater the chance of the target population's developing a feeling of **program ownership.** With program ownership will come better planned programs, greater support for the programs, and people who will be willing to help "sell" the program to others because they feel it is theirs (Strycker et al., 1997).
2. Select willing individuals who are interested in seeing the program succeed. Select a combination of "doers" and "influencers." Doers are people who will be willing to roll up their sleeves and do the physical work needed to see that the program is implemented. Influencers are those who with a single phone call or signature on a form will enlist other people to participate or will help provide the resources to facilitate the program. Both doers and influencers are important to the planning process.
3. Ensure that the committee includes an individual who has a key role within the organization sponsoring the program—someone whose support would be most important to ensure a successful program and institutionalization.

4. Include representatives of other **stakeholders** (people who have a stake in the program being planned) not represented in the target population.
5. Reevaluate committee membership regularly to ensure that the composition lends itself to fulfilling program goals and objectives.
6. Add new individuals periodically to generate new ideas and enthusiasm. It may be helpful to set a term of office for committee members. If terms of office are used, it is advisable to stagger the length of terms so that there is always a combination of new and experienced members on the committee.
7. Be aware of the politics that are always present in an organization or target population. There are always some people who bring their own agendas to committee work.
8. Make sure the committee is large enough to accomplish the work, but small enough to be able to make decisions and reach consensus. If necessary, subcommittees can be formed to handle specific tasks.

The actual means by which the committee members are chosen varies according to the setting. Commonly used techniques include:

1. Asking for volunteers by word of mouth, a newsletter, a needs assessment, or some other widely distributed publication
2. Holding an election, either throughout the community or by subdivisions of the community
3. Inviting people to serve
4. Having members appointed by a governing group or individual

Once the planning committee has been formed, someone must be designated to lead it. This is an important step (Strycker et al., 1997). The leader (chairperson) "should be interested and knowledgeable about health education programs, and be organized, enthusiastic, and creative" (McKenzie, 1988, p. 149). One might think that most program planners, especially health educators, would be perfect for the committee chairperson's job. However, sometimes it is preferable to have someone other than the program planners serve in the leadership capacity. For one thing, it helps to spread out the workload of the committee. Planners who are not good at delegating responsibility may end up with a lot of extra work when they serve as the leaders. Second, having someone else serve as the leader allows the planners to remain objective about the program. And third, the planning committee can serve in an advisory capacity to the planners, if this is considered desirable. Figure 3.4 illustrates the composition of a well-chosen planning committee.

Parameters for Planning

Once the support of the decision makers has been gained and a planning committee formed, planners must identify the **parameters** within which they can work. There are several questions to which planners should have answers before they

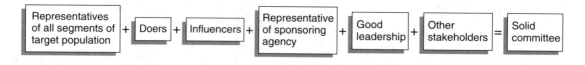

FIGURE 3.4 *Make-Up of a Solid Planning/Steering Committee*

become too deeply involved in the planning process. In an earlier work (McKenzie, 1988), six such questions were presented, using the example of school-site health education/promotion programs. The six questions are modified for presentation here. It should be noted, however, that not all of the questions would be appropriate for every program because of the different circumstances of each setting.

1. What is the decision makers' philosophical perspective on health promotion programs? What are the values and benefits of the programs to the decision makers? (Chapman, 1997). Do they see the programs as something important or as "extras"?
2. What type of commitment to the program are the decision makers willing to make? Are they interested in the program becoming **institutionalized**? That is, are they interested in seeing that the "program becomes imbedded within the host organization, so that the program becomes sustained and durable" (Goodman et al., 1993, p. 163)? Or are they more interested in providing a one-time or **pilot program**? (*Note:* Goodman et al. [1993] have developed a scale for measuring institutionalization.)
3. What type of financial support are the decision makers willing to provide? Does it include personnel for leadership and clerical duties? Released/ assigned time for managing the program and participation? Space? Equipment? Materials?
4. Are the decision makers willing to consider changing the **organizational culture**? For example, are they interested in "well" days instead of sick days? Would they like to create employee smoking and safety belt policies? Change vending machine selections to more nutritious foods? Set aside an employee room for meditation? Develop a health promotion corner in the organization library?
5. Will all individuals in the target population have an opportunity to take advantage of the program, or will it only be available to certain subgroups?
6. What is the authority of the planning committee? Will it be an advisory group or a programmatic decision-making group? What will be the chain of command for program approval?

After the parameters have been defined, the planning committee should understand how the decision makers view the program, and should know what type and amount of resources and support to expect. Setting the parameters early will save the planning committee a great deal of effort and energy throughout the planning process.

Summary

Gaining the support of the decision makers is an important initial step in program planning. Planners should take great care in developing a rationale for "selling" the program idea to these important people. A planning committee can be most useful in helping with some of the planning activities and in helping to "sell" the program to the target population. Therefore, the committee should be composed of interested individuals, "doers" and "influencers," who are representative of the target population. If the planning committee is to be effective, it will need to be aware of the parameters set for the program by the decision makers.

Questions

1. Why is the support of the decision makers important in planning a program?

2. What kinds of reasons should be included in a rationale for planning and implementing a health promotion program?

3. How important is "selling" the idea of a program to decision makers?

4. What items should be addressed when creating a program rationale?

5. Who should be selected as the members of a planning committee?

6. What are *parameters?* Give a few examples.

7. Why is it important to know the parameters at the beginning of the planning process?

Activities

1. Write a two-page rationale for "selling" a program you are planning to decision makers, using the guidelines presented in this chapter.

2. Write a two-page rationale for beginning an exercise program for a company with 200 employees. A needs assessment of this target population indicates that the number-one cause of lost work time of this cohort is back problems and the number-one cause of premature death is heart disease.

3. For a program you are planning, write a two-page description of the individuals (by position/job title, not name) who will be

asked to serve on the planning committee, and provide a rationale for asking each to serve.

4. Provide a list (by position/job title, not name) and a rationale for each of the 10 individuals you would ask to serve on a communitywide safety belt program. Use the town or city in which your college/university is located as the community.

5. Following are two program rationales written by former students at Ball State University. Read each of the rationales and then select one to critique using the guidelines presented in this chapter. Critique by

describing the following: (a) the strengths of the rationale, (b) the weaknesses, and (c) how you would change the rationale to make it stronger. Be critical! Closely examine the content, reasoning, and references.

Example 1
A Rationale for Offering a Violence Education Program in the Schools[*]

During the past ten years, many programs have been implemented in an attempt to curb the use of tobacco products by our country's high school students. As a result, the nation has witnessed a reduction in such activity. Also, programs to increase awareness about drinking and driving have been introduced in abundance. A dramatic decrease has followed there as well. But the amount of crime and violence in our nation's schools and the number of deviant acts committed by our nation's adolescents have continued to rise throughout the 1980s with relatively little intervention by comparison, though the issue is of equal if not greater importance. It is reported that 91% of all high school seniors worry about crime and violence, an increase of over 10% since 1980 (*Sourcebook of Criminal Justice Statistics,* 1992). The number of inmates under the age of eighteen in U. S. state prisons increased from 2,057 in 1986 to 4,552 in 1991 (U.S. Bureau of Justice Statistics, 1992). Although the problem has been addressed in *Healthy People 2000,* very few programs are currently being implemented at the school level to aid in rectifying the problem.

Many reasons have been proposed for the increase in juvenile crime. Some of the more commonly cited reasons are family breakdown and lack of parental supervision, increased prevalence of gang activity, violence portrayed in movies and on television, increased availability of drugs, and the "softness" of the court system regarding juvenile punishment. Other reasons cited include the fast pace of life in the United States, and increased levels of stress on the family as a result of economics and divorce (Smith & Gunason, 1994). While not in a position to solve all of these social problems, the public schools are in a position to offer anti-violent and positive conflict-resolution alternatives in a comprehensive health education program.

Who stands to gain from such a program? First and foremost, students can gain a future from such a program. Students who commit major criminal violations reduce their chances of landing a job with adequate upward mobility to support a household, while dramatically decreasing their overall job opportunities. Without this ability to choose a profession, their futures are often thrust upon them by circumstance. As crime and violence in the schools are reduced, a better education is also made possible. Where gangs are prevalent, 35% of students report that they feared an attack at school (Smith & Gunason, 1994). Optimal learning does not take place under such circumstances. Teachers also find it difficult to perform adequately under the constant demands of disciplinary action. When violence runs rampant in the school systems, the students and teachers are unable to concentrate solely on education.

Taxpayers also stand to gain immensely from an anti-violent conflict-resolution program in the schools. It is estimated that hospital costs and long-term rehabilitation costs for treating gunshot wounds amounted to $14.4 billion in 1985 (Smith & Gunason, 1994). Taxpayers paid for 80% of these costs. Gunshot wounds are now the second leading cause of death among individuals between the ages of ten and thirty-four (Smith & Gunason, 1994). With 48% of males reporting carrying a weapon to school in Indiana, and weapon law violations among blacks increasing by an estimated 103% since 1980, the cost to taxpayers will continue to increase unless intervention programs are planned and implemented in the near future (Ellis & Torabi, 1992; Smith & Gunason, 1994).

[*]This rationale was written by Brian Allred and Jenni Robison while they were graduate students at Ball State University, Muncie, Indiana. Reprinted by permission.

Another burden to the taxpayers is the state detention centers—in Indiana, $31 million was spent in one year in caring for youngsters in these centers. The cost to the Indiana taxpayer for adolescents needing these facilities is nearly $30,000 per day (Smith & Gunason, 1994).

Finally, the community at large benefits from a school-based program. Economically, the community becomes recognized as safer, encouraging more individuals to purchase housing in the community and thus creating a larger base for companies wishing to do business in the community. The result is greater economic freedom and opportunity. Socially, the community benefits by the reduced amount of fear of and contempt for the younger generations. Such a program reinforces the idea that our children are indeed our future, and that it is well worth it to invest in that future, not only for their sake, but for the sake of the country as a whole.

References

Ellis, N. T., & Torabi, M. (1992). *The Indiana student health survey: Surveillance of 9th and 12th grade youth health behaviors.* Indianapolis, IN: Indiana Department of Education.

Smith, D. L., & Gunason, S. (Ed.). (1994). *Kids, crime, and court: The juvenile justice system in Indiana.* Indianapolis, IN: Indiana Youth Institute. *Sourcebook of Criminal Justice Statistics.* (1992). Washington, D.C.: Government Printing Office.

U.S. Bureau of Justice Statistics. (1992). Washington, D.C.: Government Printing Office.

Example 2
A Rationale for "Mind, Body, and Soul": A Health Education Program at First Presbyterian Church, Muncie, IN[*]

The health status of Americans has improved greatly in the last 50 years as evidenced by the decrease in the number of cases of communicable disease, increased life expectancy, and the declining death rates (NCHS, 1997). However, the health status of Americans could be further improved if Americans were willing to make additional changes. We now know that better control of behavioral risk factors alone—such as lack of exercise, poor diet, use of tobacco and other drugs, and alcohol abuse—could prevent between 40 and 70% of all mature deaths, one-third of all acute disabilities, and two-thirds of chronic disabilities (USDHHS, 1990).

Closer to home, recent data also indicate that the health status of Hoosiers has improved but they too could do more to improve their health. In 1996, 32% of the adults (>17 years of age) in Indiana were overweight, 29% were current smokers, and 66% were classified as having a sedentary lifestyle (ISDH, 1998). The data from Indiana are also consistent with the data that were collected from the members of the adult education class, the Mariners, at First Presbyterian Church in Muncie, IN. The data collected using a health risk appraisal (HRA) (Healthier People Software, no date) and a health and spirituality questionnaire (developed by health science students from Ball State University) indicated that the Mariners were interested in educational programs on faith and its relationship to health, humor and healing, and stress management (including prayer as a means of stress reduction). In addition, there appears to be a need for or an interest in programs associated with aging (including Alzheimer's disease), the family, nutrition, weight control, and exercise.

It seems logical to try to address some of the health needs and interests of those in the Mariners class through the Christian Education program of the church. For a long time, religious organizations have functioned as "healing" institutions as evidenced by the mental health issues addressed through pastoral counseling (Ransdell & Rehling, 1996). The idea of addressing the health needs and interests of a

---

[*]This rationale was written by the undergraduate students enrolled in the program planning classes at Ball State University, Muncie, Indiana.

target population in combination with spiritual practices has been encouraged. "In recent years, both the validity of spiritual and religious practices as well as the potential to the overall health and well-being have not only been acknowledged by modern medicine, but encouraged as mechanisms for health enhancement" (Droege, 1996, p. 7). And further, it makes good sense to offer health related programs at church since the Bible "provides a very powerful foundation for the development of health programs within the spiritual framework of the church" (Jackson, 1991, pp. 8–9). In a more practical sense, religious organizations have a number of important potential advantages for involvement in health education/promotion programs because religious organizations: 1) tend to involve large numbers of entire families, 2) are often the center of the neighborhood and a natural gathering place, 3) have a long history of outreach and helping others, 4) often have a talented and multi-disciplinary membership, 5) have been found to be receptive to the efforts of primary prevention, and 6) have the facilities to accommodate such programs (Lasater, Carleton, & Wells, 1991). In addition, religious organizations are good settings for health education/ promotion programs because when people attend they do so with the expectation of learning; religious organizations are accepted as educational institutions (Lasater, Carleton, & Wells, 1991). Consequently, the church is a natural community arena for health education/promotion programs that focus on behaviors which are then reinforced by the social support and social networks that exist in churches (Levin, Larson, & Puchalski, 1997; Thomas, Quinn, Billingsley, & Caldwell, 1994).

There are several benefits that can be anticipated from the Mind, Body, and Soul program offered at First Presbyterian Church. First and foremost, it should be expected that the Mariners class members will increase their knowledge about the topics presented. Such knowledge will be

beneficial to both the Mariners class members and the people—family and friends—with whom they come in contact. Second, such a program will introduce participants to topics that have not been addressed before in the class. Third, the program will provide participants with an opportunity to apply spiritual and religious concepts to everyday living. And fourth, such a program may attract other members of the congregation to the Mariners class that have not attended in the past.

The Mind, Body, and Soul program for the First Presbyterian Church Mariners class has great potential for being successful for several reasons. First as noted earlier, the Bible provides a solid base on which to build a health education/promotion program (Jackson, 1991). A number of the scriptures support the healing power of faith (Lloyd, 1994). Class members are interested in learning more about the Bible. Second, the majority of similar other church-based health promotion programs have been highly successful (Cook, 1993). And finally, the program will be well planned and will meet the needs and interests of the class members. Ransdell and Rehling (1996) have indicated that such programs have a better chance of being successful.

References

Cook, D. A. (1993). Research in African American churches: A mental health imperative. *Journal of Mental Health Counseling, 17:* 320–333.

Droege, T. (1996). Spirituality and healing. *Faith and Health,* Summer: 7.

Healthier People Software. (no date). *Healthier People: Health Risk Appraisal Program.* Memphis, TN: Author.

Indiana State Department of Health (ISDH). (1998). *Indiana Health Behavior Risk Factors.* Indianapolis, IN: Author.

Jackson, C. (1991). Healthy spirits, souls, and bodies. *Spirit of Truth,* June: 8–9.

Lasater, T. M., Carleton, R. A., & Wells, B. L. (1991). Religious organizations and large-scale health related lifestyle change programs. *Journal of Health Education, 22:* 233–239.

Levin, J. S., Larson, D. B., & Puchalski, C. M. (1997). Religion and spirituality in medicine: Research and Education. *The Journal of the American Medical Association, 278:* 792–793.

Lloyd, J. J. (1994). Collaborative health education training for African American health ministers and providers of community services. *Educational Gerontology, 20:* 265–276.

National Center for Health Statistics (NCHS). (1997). *Health, United States, 1996–97 and Injury Chartbook* (DHHS pub. no. PHS 97–1232). Hyattsville, MD: Author.

Ransdell, L. B., & Rehling, S. L. (1996). Church-based health promotion: A review of the current literature. *American Journal of Health Behavior, 20*(4): 195–207.

Thomas, S. B., Quinn, S. C., Billingsley, A., & Caldwell, C. (1994). The characteristics of northern black churches with community outreach programs. *American Journal of Public Health, 84:* 575–579.

U.S. Department of Health and Human Services (USDHHS). (1990). *Prevention '89/ '90.* Washington, D.C.: U.S. Government Printing Office.

Activities on the Web

1. Assume that you are responsible for putting together a rationale for a health promotion program about stroke awareness. Visit the website of the American Heart Association <http://www.americanheart.org> and identify five facts about stroke that could be used in the first few paragraphs of your rationale. What are the five facts you have chosen to include in your rationale? Create a bibliographic reference for the site.

2. Many different individuals and agencies maintain excellent health education websites. Here are four:
   a. U.S. Department of Health and Human Services' "healthfinder" <http://www.healthfinder.gov/>
   b. Johns Hopkins Health Information <http://www.intelihealth.com>
   c. Former Surgeon General Koop <http://www.drkoop.com/>
   d. Mayo Clinic's Health Oasis <http://www.mayohealth.org/>

   Using any or all of these sites, locate information that could be used to help develop the rationale for the program you are planning. Using this information, write one paragraph that could be included in your rationale. Be sure to provide the bibliographic source for the information you find.

3. Four good websites for helping to assemble statistical data for a program rationale are:
   a. Statistical Abstracts of the United States <http://www.census.gov/stat_abstract>
   b. U.S. Bureau of the Census <http://www.census.gov/>
   c. World Health Organization Statistical Information System (WHOSIS) <http://www.who.org/whosis/>
   d. Association of State and Territorial Health Officials <http://www.astho.org/state.html>

   Using data from any or all of these websites, develop a first paragraph for the rationale you are creating.

4. If you are planning a program for the worksite setting, visit the website for the Wellness Councils of American and Canada <http://www.welcoa.org>. Using this site, locate information that could be used to help develop the rationale for the program you are planning. Using this information, write one paragraph that could be included

in your rationale. Be sure to provide the bibliographic source for the information you find. Also, print out a copy of the Wellness Councils' home page and attach it to your paragraph.

5. If you are planning a program for a multicultural target population, visit the website for the U.S. Department of Health and Human Services, Office of Minority Health Resource Center's "Initiative to Eliminate Racial and Ethnic Disparities in Health" <http://www.raceandhealth.omhrc>. Using this site, locate information that could be used to help develop the rationale for the program you are planning. Using this information, write one paragraph that could be included in your rationale. Be sure to provide the bibliographic source for the information you find. Also, print out a copy of the Initiatives' home page and attach it to your paragraph.

4

Assessing Needs

After reading this chapter and answering the questions at the end, you should be able to:

- Define needs assessment.
- Explain why a needs assessment must be completed.
- Differentiate between primary and secondary data sources.
- Locate secondary data sources that are in print and on the World Wide Web.
- Explain how a needs assessment can be completed.
- Conduct a needs assessment on a given group of people.

Key Terms

APEX/PH
assessment
browser
community analysis/
   community diagnosis
Delphi technique
eyeballing data
health assessment
home page
key informants

needs assessment
networking
opinion leaders
primary data
proxy measure
reliable
search engine
secondary data
segmenting
self-directed assessments

service demands
service needs
significant others
subject archive
target population
Uniform Resource Locator
   (URL)
valid
website
World Wide Web (WWW)

Once the planning committee is in place, the next step in the planning process is to identify the need(s) or problem(s) of those to be served—the **target population.** Assessing the needs of the target population may be the most critical step in the planning process because it "provides objective data to define important health problems, set priorities for program implementation, and establish a baseline for evaluating program impact" (Grunbaum et al., 1995, p. 54). Without determining the needs, resources can be wasted on unwarranted programing. Many fine programs have failed because there was no need for them. An example of such a scenario might be a program planned by a voluntary health agency that has a national goal to offer more smoking cessation programs in the workplace. If we look at the national figures, there may appear to be a need for such a program. Approximately 25% of the adult population in the United States today smokes; that figure is even higher among skilled and unskilled labor. So it appears that there is a need on the national level. But it is necessary to consider the local level, where the program must be implemented. What about Blue Earth County, Minnesota? Delaware County, Indiana? Wood County, Ohio? Do 25% of the adults in these counties smoke? What percentage of county residents who work in industry smoke? Do those smokers want to quit? Do employers mind if their employees smoke? Is there really a need for smoking cessation programs in the worksites of these counties? No one can say for sure until a needs assessment has been completed, and even then the need for such a program may not be clear.

What Is a Needs Assessment?

Up to this point, we have used the term **needs assessment** several different times, without defining it. Now, let's take a closer look at the term and what it means. First, it should be noted that other terms have been used in a similar context. Dignan and Carr (1992) used the terms **community analysis/community diagnosis,** whereas Green and Kreuter (1999) used the term **assessment** with the first five phases of the PRECEDE-PROCEED model. All these terms are used to describe the process by which those who are planning programs can determine what health problems might exist in any given group of people. Windsor and colleagues (1994, p. 63) have defined *needs assessment* as "the process by which the program planner identifies and measures gaps between what is and what ought to be." Stated a bit differently, "needs assessment is a planned process that identifies the reported needs of an individual or a group" (Gilmore & Campbell, 1996, p. 5). No matter how it is defined, the concept is the same: identifying the needs of the target population and deciding whether these needs are being met.

Although determining the needs of a target population at first seems a straightforward task, planners must ask, Through whose eyes is the need determined or evaluated? Windsor and colleagues (1994) have applied the vocabulary of marketing to the needs assessment process, identifying two types of health needs. The first type is **service needs.** These are the things that "health professionals believe a given population must have or be able to do in order to resolve a health problem." The other type consists of the things that those in the target population "say they must have or be able to do in order to resolve a health problem" (Windsor et al., 1994, p. 64). These needs are referred to as **service demands.**

Both types of needs are important, and if either is ignored, the true need of a given target population may not be understood. A program that is based entirely on service needs (from the planners' point of view) may not interest or appeal to the target population even though a serious problem exists that the program could help solve. On the other hand, a program that is planned around service demands (from the viewpoint of those being served) may not contribute to solving the real health problem. Therefore, it is important for program planners to identify both types of needs. Once this has been done, planners must blend the two to reflect both perspectives.

In addition to identifying the needs of the target population, a needs assessment can also provide valuable information that can help segment the target population according to demographic variables, such as age, gender, or socioeconomic status; behaviors, such as exercisers versus nonexercisers; and attitudes, for example, those who are for or against permitting smoking in public places. Such **segmenting** allows program planners to design programs for a specific subgroup of the target population and thus increase the program's chance of being effective. This is a key strategy in helping to market a health promotion program; it is discussed in greater detail in Chapter 11.

Acquiring Needs Assessment Data

Program planners can gather needs assessment data in one of two ways. They can use data that are "available from other sources" (Windsor et al., 1994, p. 72), called **secondary data,** or they can collect their own data, thus generating **primary data.**

"The logical first step for acquiring information on any community or other target group is to search for data that already exist in the form of previous structured investigations or routinely gathered records or statistics" (Simons-Morton et al., 1995, p. 134). The advantages of using such data are that (1) they already exist, and thus time to collect them is minimal, and (2) they are usually fairly inexpensive to access. Both of these advantages are important to program planners because programs are often planned when both time and money are limited. However, a drawback of using secondary data is that the information might not identify the true needs of the target population—perhaps because of how the data were collected, when they were collected, what variables were considered, or from whom the data were collected. A good rule is to move cautiously and make sure the secondary data are applicable to the immediate situation before using them.

Primary data have the advantage of directly answering the questions planners want answered by those in the target population. The data are specific to the target population. However, collecting primary data can be expensive and when done correctly can take a great deal of time.

An overview of the means of acquiring primary and secondary data are presented in the following pages. The different sources of data are presented using the classification system presented in Gilmore and Campbell (1996). If you would like a more detailed explanation of the needs assessment process, refer to the text by Gilmore and Campbell (1996).

Sources of Primary Data

Primary data can be divided into two large categories: data gathered from individuals and data gathered from groups.

Gathering Data from Individuals.   Primary data are collected from individuals through the use of a survey. Surveys can take many different forms. One way of classifying surveys is by the number of times those collecting the data ask those in the target population for information. Single-step and multistep surveys are discussed here.

Single-Step or Cross-Sectional Surveys.   Single-step surveys, or as they are often called, *cross-sectional surveys*, are a means of gathering primary data in which the data collectors gather the data from the target population with a single contact—thus, the term *single-step.* Such surveys usually take the form of written questionnaires, telephone interviews, face-to-face interviews, or email interviews (see Chapter 5 for information about conducting such surveys). The resulting data are useful not only for planning an appropriate program but also for providing insight into how best to implement a program (if the surveys include marketing questions, as well). For example, these surveys might include questions that address the best location for a program, the best time of day to offer a program, and how much participants would be willing to pay to take part in the program.

In addition to surveying the target population, there are other groups of individuals who are commonly asked to respond to single-step surveys for the purpose of collecting primary needs assessment data. They include significant others of the target population, community opinion leaders, and key informants. **Significant others** may include family members and friends. Collecting data from the significant others of a group of heart disease patients is a good example. Program planners might find it difficult to persuade the heart disease patients themselves to share information about their outlook on life and living with heart disease. A survey of spouses or other family members might help elicit this information so that the program planners could best meet the needs of the heart disease patients.

Opinion leaders are individuals who are well respected in a community and who have an overall view of its needs. These leaders are:

1. Active users of the media
2. Demographically similar to the target group
3. Knowledgeable about community issues and concerns
4. Early adopters of innovative behavior (see Chapter 11 for an explanation of these terms)
5. Active in persuading others to become involved in innovative behavior

Opinion leaders include political figures, chief executive officers (CEOs) of companies, union leaders, administrators of local school districts, and other highly visible and respected individuals. (See Box 4.1 for a form for tallying opinion leader survey data.)

Key informants are strategically placed individuals who have knowledge and ability to report on the needs of those in the target population (Cleary & Neiger, 1998). They may or may not be in positions with formal authority, but they are often respected by others in the community thus possess informal authority. Because they are important members of the community, "they can can affect the support and buy-in for program changes. They may be biased" (Cleary & Neiger, 1998, p. 26). Therefore, planners need to be careful not to base an entire needs assessment on the data generated from a key informant survey.

Multistep Survey.   As its title might suggest, a multistep survey is one in which those collecting the data contact those who will provide the data on more than one occasion. The technique that uses this process is called the **Delphi technique.** It is a process that generates consensus through a series of questionnaires, which are usually administered via the mail or electronic mail. The process begins with those collecting the data asking the target population to respond to one or two broad questions. The responses are analyzed, and a second questionnaire, with more specific questions, is developed and sent to the target population. The answers to these more specific questions are analyzed again, and a new questionnaire is sent out, requesting additional information. If consensus is reached, the process may end here; if not, it may continue for another round or two (Gilmore & Campbell, 1996). Most often, this process continues for five or fewer rounds.

Gathering Data from Groups.   Several different techniques are available to those collecting primary data from groups. The more commonly used techniques used by health educators include the community forum, the focus group, the nominal group process, and observation.

Community Forum.   Put simply, the community forum approach brings together people from the target population to discuss what they see as their group's problems/needs. It is not uncommon for a community forum to be organized by a group representing the target population, in conjunction with the program planners. Such groups include labor, civic, religious, or service organizations, or groups such as the Parent Teacher Association (PTA) or Parent Teacher Organization (PTO). Once people have arrived, a moderator explains the purpose of the meeting and then asks those from the target population to share their concerns. One or several individuals from the organizing group, called *recorders,* are usually given the responsibility for taking notes or taping the session to ensure that the responses are recorded accurately. However, when moderating a community forum, it is important to be aware that the silent majority may not speak out and/or a vocal minority may speak too loudly. For example, an individual parent's view may be wrongly interpreted to be the view of all parents.

BOX 4.1 • *Form to Tally Opinion Leader Survey Data*

Data collection method   Number of interviewers

                                          From: _____ To: _____
Total number of people interviewed

                                          Date collected _____

Rank Health Problem	Number of Persons Identifying Problem	Percentage of Persons Identifying Problem
1.		
2.		
3.		
4.		
5.		
6.		
7.		
8.		
9.		
10.		

Source:

Source: U.S. Department of Health and Human Services, Centers for Disease Control and Prevention (no date), p. A3–12.

At a community forum, participants may also be asked to respond in writing (1) by answering specific questions or (2) by completing some type of instrument. Figure 4.1 is an example of an instrument that could be used to collect data from a group of people.

Focus Group.   Focus groups are a form of qualitative research that grew out of group therapy. They are used to obtain information about the feelings, opinions, perceptions, insights, beliefs, misconceptions, attitudes, and receptivity of a group of people concerning an idea or issue. Focus groups are rather small, compared to community forums, and usually include only 8 to 12 people. If possible, it is best to have a group of people who do not know one another so that their responses are not inhibited by acquaintance. Participation in the group is by invitation. People are invited about one to three weeks in advance of the session. At the time

FIGURE 4.1   *Instrument for Ranking Program Need*

Directions: Please rank the need for each program in the community by placing a number in the space to the left of the programs. Use 1 to rank the program of greatest need, 2 for the next greatest need, and so forth, until you have ranked all seven programs. The program with the highest number next to it should be the one that, in your opinion, is least needed. If you feel that a program should not be considered for implementation in our community, please place an X in the space to the left of the program instead of a number. Please note that the number you place next to each program represents its need in the community, not necessarily your desire to participate in it. After ranking the program, place an X to the right of the program in the column(s) that represent the age group(s) to which you feel the program should be targeted.

Program	All ages	Children 5–12	Teens 13–19	Adults 20–64	Older adults 65+
_____ Alcohol education:	_____	_____	_____	_____	_____
_____ Exercise/fitness:	_____	_____	_____	_____	_____
_____ Nutrition education:	_____	_____	_____	_____	_____
_____ Safety belt use:	_____	_____	_____	_____	_____
_____ Smoking cessation:	_____	_____	_____	_____	_____
_____ Smoking education:	_____	_____	_____	_____	_____
_____ Weight loss:	_____	_____	_____	_____	_____

Source: Modified from a form developed by Amy L. Bernard, Ph.D., CHES; Assistant Professor, University of Cincinnati. Adapted by permission.

of the invitation, they receive general information about the session but are not given the specifics. This precaution helps ensure that responses will be on target yet spontaneous.

Once assembled, the group is led by a skilled moderator who has the task of obtaining candid responses from the group to a set of predetermined questions. In addition to eliciting responses to the questions, the moderator may ask the group to prioritize the different responses. As in a community forum, the answers to the questions are recorded through either written notes and/or audio or video recordings, so that at a later date the interested parties can review and interpret the results.

For any one project, it may be necessary to hold several different focus groups to collect the needed information. For example, if planners are using focus groups to find out what the people in the community think about a proposed sex education curriculum, it would be helpful to organize focus groups based on the beliefs of certain subsets within the target population. Otherwise, if liberals were brought together with conservatives or prochoice advocates were brought together with prolife people, the focus groups would turn into shouting matches and little would be accomplished. Usually, the more controversial the topic, the greater the need to organize several focus groups with segments of the population.

Focus groups are not easy to conduct. Special care must be given to developing the questions that will be asked. Poorly written questions will yield information that is less than useful. In addition, the facilitator should be one who is skilled in leading a group. As might be surmised, the level of skill needed to conduct a focus group increases as the topic of discussion becomes more controversial.

Although focus groups have been shown to be an effective way of gathering data, they do have one major limitation. Participants in the groups are usually not selected through a random-sampling process. They are generally selected because they possess certain attributes (individuals of low income, city dwellers, parents of disabled children, or chief executive officers of major corporations). Participants are typical, not representative, of the target population. Therefore, the results of the focus group are not generalizable. "Findings [of focus groups] should be interpreted as suggestive and directional rather than as definitive" (Schechter, Vanchieri, & Crofton, 1990, p. 254).

Nominal Group Process.   The nominal group process is a highly structured process in which a few knowledgeable representatives of the target population (five to seven people) are asked to qualify and quantify specific needs. Those invited to participate are asked to record their responses to a question without discussing it among themselves. Once all have recorded a response, each participant shares his or her response in a round-robin fashion. While this is occurring, the facilitator is recording the responses on a chalkboard, paper, or the like, for all to see. The responses are clarified through a discussion. After the discussion, the participants are asked to rank-order the responses by importance to the target population. This ranking may be considered either a preliminary or a final vote. If it is preliminary, it is followed with more discussion and a final vote.

Observation.   Gathering primary needs assessment data via observation can be accomplished in several different ways. It can be done by the planners or their workers, who can become a part of the day-to-day events where the health problems may occur, so that they can observe the actions of the target population. Examples of such fieldwork may include watching the eating patterns of teachers in a school lunchroom, observing workers on an assembly line to see if they are wearing their protective glasses, checking the smoking behavior of employees on break, and observing community members for safety belt use. (See Chapter 5 for more information on observation.)

Self-Directed Assessments.   Data can also be collected by those in the target population through **self-directed assessments.** "Self-directed assessments are personal review procedures. A majority of these approaches address primary prevention issues, such as the assessment of risk factors in one's lifestyle pattern and the secondary prevention process of the early detection of disease symptoms" (Gilmore & Campbell, 1996, p. 109). Examples of such assessments include breast self-examination (BSE), testicular self-examination (TSE), self-monitoring for skin cancer, and **health assessments (HAs).** "Health assessment can be broadly defined as any method that accesses and analyzes data about a person's or populations health" (Hyner et al., 1999, p. xx). "Health assessments include instruments known as health risk appraisals or health risk assessments (HRAs), health status assessments (HSAs), various lifestyle-specific (e.g., nutrition, stress, and physical activity) assessment instruments, wellness and behavioral/habit inventories" (SPM Board of Directors, 1999, p. xxiii), and disease/condition status assessments (e.g., chances of getting heart disease or diabetes).

Of the different self-directed assessments, it is the HAs that have been most useful in the needs assessment process, because from such assessments planners can obtain "group data which summarizes major health problems and risk factors" (Alexander, 1999, p. 5). And of the HAs, it is the HRAs that are most often included in the needs assessment process. HRAs are instruments that estimate "the odds that a person with certain characteristics will die from selected causes within a given time span" (Alexander, 1999, p. 5). Even though HRAs are used as part of needs assessments, it was not their original intent. The original purpose of HRAs was to engage family physicians and their patients in conversation about risks of premature death and preventive health behaviors (Robbins & Hall, 1970).

To use an HRA as part of a needs assessment, planners would have those in the target population complete a questionnaire. The instruments include questions about health behavior (e.g., smoking, exercise), personal or family health history of diseases (e.g., cancer, heart disease), demographics (e.g., age, sex), and usually some physiological data (e.g., height, weight, blood pressure, cholesterol). The resulting risk appraisals, in most cases, are calculated by computers, but there are some HRAs that are hand-scored by the participant or health professional (Alexander, 1999). Most HRAs generate both individual and group reports. Thus, planners can use the individual reports as part of an educational program for the target population and use the group reports as another source of primary needs assessment data.

There are many HA instruments on the market. A wonderful source for examining the different HAs available is the *SPM Handbook of Health Assessment Tools* (Hyner et al., 1999). This volume not only physically presents many of the HAs available today but it also includes information on (1) theoretical models associated with health assessment; (2) the use and selection of health assessment tools, including ethical considerations; (3) specific applications of health assessments; and (4) information on both the historic and forward looks at health assessment. The Society of Prospective Medicine can be contacted at 230 McKee Place, Suite 400, Pittsburgh, PA, 15213 (phone: 412/647-1087, fax: 412/647-1111, email: info@spm.org, website: **<www.spm.org>**).

Although this discussion has revolved around the use of HRAs as means of providing information for a needs assessment, they have also been used in recent years for other purposes: to help motivate people to act on their health, to increase awareness, to serve as cues to action, and to contribute to program evaluation. The expanded use of these instruments has prompted several researchers (Alexy, 1985; Best & Milsum, 1978; Elias & Dunton, 1981; Sachs, Krushat, & Newman, 1980; Smith, McKinlay, & McKinlay, 1989) to question the reliability and validity of HRA data. (See Chapter 5 for a discussion of validity and reliability.)

> When applying the most rigorous scientific criteria, the reliability, validity, and effectiveness of HRAs are minimally acceptable. This is not surprising since many health risk factors likely have not yet been determined, e.g., genetic factors and unknown factors related to future events. These unknowns contribute to a large variance in the various outcome measures, such as mortality, morbidity, and healthcare utilization and costs.... However, if the HRA is to be used as an educational and awareness tool, then the issues of reliability, validity, and effectiveness become less important. (Edington, Yen, & Braunstein, 1999, p. 136)

The following conclusions can be made:

1. The reliability of HRA risk scores can vary greatly from one instrument to another.
2. Reliability scores decrease when users calculate their own score, as opposed to computer scoring.
3. There is a great variance in the self-reporting of specific risk factors and clinical physiologic measurements.
4. Only those HRAs for which reliability can be demonstrated should be used for evaluating the effectiveness of health education.

Sources of Secondary Data

The sources of secondary needs assessment data for program planners are many. The main sources include data collected by governmental agencies at any level (national, regional, state, or local), data available from nongovernmental agencies and organizations, data from existing records, and data that are presented in the literature.

Data Collected by Governmental Agencies. Certain governmental agencies collect data on a regular basis. Some of the data collection is mandated by law (i.e., census, births, deaths, notifiable diseases, etc.), whereas other data are collected voluntarily (i.e., usage rates for safety belts) for use by the public. Since the data are collected by the government, program planners can gain free access to them by contacting the agency that collects the data or by finding them in a library that serves as a United States government depository for government documents. Many college and university libraries and large public libraries serve as such depositories. Presented here is information about some of the more useful sources of data collected by governmental agencies.

From the U.S. Department of Commerce. Within the U.S. Department of Commerce is located the Bureau of Census. The bureau is responsible for taking a census of the United States every 10 years. The first census was ordered by George Washington in 1790 for the purpose of apportioning representation to the House of Representatives. The most recent census, taken in 2000, includes data on number of people, income, employment, family size, education, type of dwelling, and many other social indicators. Census data are important to program planners because they are used in calculating disease and death rates (McKenzie, Pinger, & Kotecki, 1999).

Another Bureau of Census publication is the *Statistical Abstract of the United States (SA)*. This book, published since 1878, provides a summary of statistics on the social, political, and economic organization of the United States. Recent volumes of the book include a selection of data from both government and private statistical publications. Major sections of the book cover population, vital statistics, health and nutrition, education, law enforcement, courts and prisons, and many other areas. A new edition of *SA* is published each January and includes data for years up to two years prior to the publication date. It can be purchased from the U.S. Government Printing Office for approximately $45 and is available in most libraries.

From the Centers for Disease Control and Prevention (CDC) and the National Center for Health Statistics (NCHS). The National Center for Health Statistics (NCHS) is one of the major divisions of the Centers for Disease Control and Prevention (CDC). As the nation's keeper of health data, the NCHS maintains several ongoing data systems. However, "budgetary constraints have caused the center staff to establish priorities for those systems and reduce the frequency of their operation" (Pickett & Hanlon, 1990, p. 138). Though all the data systems are useful, six that have proved very helpful to health promotion program planners have been basic vital statistics, National Health Interview Survey (NHIS), National Health and Examination Survey (NHANES), National Hospital Discharge Survey (NHDS), National Hospital Ambulatory Medical Care Survey (NHAMCS), and the Youth Risk Behavior

Surveillance System (YRBSS). Basic vital statistics are statistical summaries of vital records—that is, records of major life events. Included in the major life events are live births, deaths, marriages, divorces, and infant deaths. These data are published in National Center for Health Statistic's *Monthly Vital Statistic Report: Provisional Data* and in annual volumes making up the *Vital Statistics of the United States.*

The four surveys (NHIS, NHANES, NHDS, and NHAMCS) conducted by the National Center for Health Statistics provide a variety of data that are published *Vital and Health Statistics* series. The NHIS is a telephone-administered survey that collects self-report data about health status and health habits. The NHANES assesses "the health and nutrition status of the general U. S. population. The data are collected, using a mobile examination center, through direct physical examinations, clinical and laboratory testing, and related procedures, on a representative group of Americans. The examinations result in the most authoritative source of standardized clinical, physical, and physiological data on the American people" (McKenzie, Pinger, & Kotecki, 1999, p. 73). The other two surveys conducted by the NCHS provide valuable data related to hospital use. The NHDS provides data on the characteristics of patients discharged from nonfederal short-stay hospitals (Graves & Owings, 1997), whereas the NHAMCS provides data on the health care provided by outpatient and emergency departments to the U.S. population (McCraig, 1997). Of special note to program planners is the availability of the survey questionnaires used in the NHIS, NHANES, NHDS, and NHAMCS. These instruments provide good starting points for program planners who need to collect primary needs assessment data. The instruments are available from the NCHS or government depositories.

The Youth Risk Behavior Surveillance System (YRBSS) can be of special use to those planning programs for adolescents and young adults. The YRBSS monitors six categories of priority health risk behaviors: behaviors that contribute to unintentional and intentional injuries, tobacco use, alcohol and other drug use, sexual behaviors, unhealthy dietary behaviors, and physical inactivity (DASH, 1997). Such data are collected via three surveys: (1) a high school-based survey, (2) a household-based survey of youth (12 to 21 years of age), and (3) a college-based survey. The surveys are conducted by the Division of Adolescent and School Health, National Center for Chronic Disease Prevention and Health Promotion, at the Centers for Disease Control and Prevention (CDC). The results are published as part of the *MMWR's CDC Surveillance Summaries* (McKenzie, Pinger, & Kotecki, 1999).

Other national data that are of use to planners are the data presented in the *Morbidity and Mortality Weekly Report (MMWR)*. Reported cases of specified notifiable diseases are reported weekly in the *MMWR*. The *MMWR* is prepared by the CDC staff, based on reports from state health departments, and published by the Massachusetts Medical Society—publishers of the *New England Journal of Medicine.*

As a final note about sources of data available from national-level governmental agencies, planners should consider contacting the National Health Information Center at P.O. Box 1133, Washington, D.C. 20013-1133 **<www.healthfinder.gov>.**

From State and Local Agencies. Although the discussion to this point has centered on national data, similar data are available from state and local governmental agencies. Program planners should consult with their local and state health departments to see what is available to them. Three sources of data collected at the local and/or state levels that have been especially useful to program planners are (1) vital statistics (e.g., birth and death records), (2) *Behavioral Risk Factor Surveillance System (BRFSS)* data, and (3) data generated from the Assessment Protocol for Excellence in Public Health (APEX/PH). The BRFSS data are collected by a branch of CDC via a state-based telephone survey of the civilian, noninstitutional, adult population. The survey seeks to gather information about such high-risk behaviors as excessive alcohol use, tobacco use, physical inactivity, and the lack of preventive care, such as screening for various cancers. The results of the BRFSS are published periodically as part of *MMWR's CDC Surveillance Summaries* (Powell-Griner, Anderson, & Murphy, 1997). (See the section at the end of this chapter on information about APEX/PH.)

Data Available from Nongovernmental Agencies and Organizations. In addition to the data available from governmental agencies, planners should also consult with nongovernmental agencies and groups for data. Those that often have data are the health care systems, voluntary health agencies, and business, civic, and commerce groups. For example, most of the national voluntary health agencies produce yearly "facts and figures" booklets that include a lot of epidemiological data. In addition, local agencies and organizations often have data they have collected for planning of their own. For example, it is not unusual for a local United Way to have done a needs assessment in the community before distributing funds.

Data from Existing Records. Health data that are often "collected as a by-product of a service effort, such as managing a clinic, an immunization program, or a water pollution control program" (Pickett & Hanlon, 1990, p. 151). These data can also serve as very useful secondary needs assessment data. Clinical indicators—such as blood pressure, height, weight, body composition, or blood analysis—are routinely collected by health care professionals. Also often available are records that deal with the utilization or cost of medical services. These data include such items as health insurance claims paid, hospital utilization rates, visits to a doctor's office, disability benefits and insurance premiums paid, and incidental and disability absenteeism. (See Chapter 5 for more information about data from existing records.)

Data from the Literature. Program planners might also be able to identify the needs of a target population by reviewing any available current literature about that target population. An example would be a planner who is developing a health promotion program for individuals infected by the human immunodeficiency virus (HIV). Because of the relative newness and seriousness of this disease and the number of people who have studied and written about it, there is a good chance that present literature could reflect the need of a certain target population.

The best means of accessing data from the literature is by using the available literature databases. Most literature databases today are available in several different forms, including books and computers, and some are available via the Internet.

Computer access would depend on the capacity of the library or unit housing the databases. Depending on the database used, program planners can expect to find comprehensive listings of citations of journal articles, book chapters, and books, and, in some databases, abstracts of the literature. Within the listings, most databases cite sources by both author and subject/title. Figure 4.2 provides an example of what planners might find when searching a database.

There are many literature databases available to program planners. Next is a short discussion of those databases that have proven helpful to health educators.

PsycLIT.   PsycLIT is a database produced by the American Psychological Association (APA) that includes journal articles, book chapters, and book citations on literature in psychology and related subjects. The database is divided into several major categories, but two of particular interest to health educators are (1) psychological and physical disorders and (2) health and mental health treatment and prevention.

Index Medicus.   Produced monthly by the National Library of Medicine, the *Index Medicus* contains citations to the biomedical journal literature. A companion volume is the annual *Cumulated Index Medicus,* which comprises the contents of the 12 monthly issues (January through December). Indexed in *Index Medicus* are journal articles and those letters, editorials, biographies, and obituaries that have substantive contents (Lindberg, 1995).

Medline.   Medline is an enlarged version of the printed *Index Medicus* (Baumgartner & Strong, 1994). It covers the international literature on biomedicine, including the allied health fields and the biological and physical sciences, humanities, and information science as they relate to medicine and health care. Information is

---

FIGURE 4.2 *Sample Citations*

Author Citation

          Authors   Article title
             ↓   ↓

Kotecki, J. E., & Chamness, B. E., A valid tool for evaluating
health-related www sites. J. of Health Educ. 1999; 30(1):56–59.
                                          ↑

                                       Journal

Subject/Title Citation

          Article Title
             ↓

A valid tool for evaluating health-related www sites. Kotecki,
J. E., & Chamness, B. E., J. of Health Educ. 1999; 30(1):56–59.

---

indexed from approximately 3,600 journals and selected monographs of congresses and symposia.

Education Resources Information Center (ERIC).   ERIC "is a national information system established in 1966 by the federal government to provide ready access to educational literature by and for educational practitioners and scholars" (Houston, 1987, p. x). Today, it is funded by the Office of Educational Research and Improvement in the U.S. Department of Education. ERIC includes all the information from the printed indexes *Current Index to Journals in Education (CIJE)* and *Resources in Education (RIE)*. *CIJE* includes annotated journal articles, whereas *RIE* comprises abstracted citations for nonjournal literature (Baumgartner & Strong, 1994; Houston, 1987).

Cumulative Index to Nursing & Allied Health Literature (CINAHL).   The CINAHL grew out of the work of a hospital librarian in the 1940s who created an index for nursing journals. Demand for this work grew over the years until in 1961 the first volume of *Cumulative Index to Nursing Literature (CINL)* was published. "In order to keep pace with the trend toward a multidisciplinary approach to health care, the scope of coverage was expanded in 1977 to include allied health journals. To reflect this change *CINL* changed its title to *CINAHL*" (Marcarin, 1995, p. 3). This database went online in 1984 and includes references to more than 300 journals.

BIOETHICSLINE.   BIOETHICSLINE is a database that "covers ethical, legal, and policy issues surrounding health care and biomedical research. Citations come from several different bodies of literature including ethics, health sciences, law, philosophy, religion, social sciences, and the popular media" (Cottrell, Girvan, & McKenzie, 1999).

Health Services, Technology, Administration, and Research (Health STAR).   HealthSTAR is a database that was formed by merging two former National Library of Medicine databases: Health and HSTAR. This new database focuses on both clinical (e.g., patient outcomes and effectiveness of procedures, products, and services) and non-clinical aspects (e.g., health care administration, planning, policy) of health care delivery (Faerber, 1999).

Steps for Conducting a Literature Search

General Search Procedures.   The process of searching a database is not difficult, and with the exception of a few individual differences, most indexes are arranged in a similar format. As Figure 4.2 indicated, most indexes include both an author and a subject/title index. An item that is specific to each index is its thesaurus, a listing of the key words the indexes use to index the subject/titles. Program planners can find the thesauri in a separate volume with or near the indexes.

Figure 4.3 provides program planners with a literature search strategy in the form of a flowchart. The chart begins by identifying the need of the target population

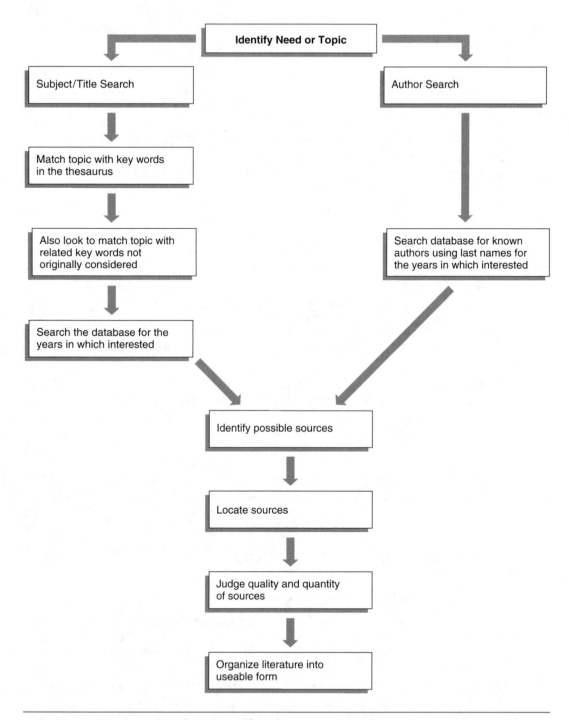

FIGURE 4.3   *Literature Search Strategy Flowchart*

Source: Adapted from Deeds (1992) and Macarin (1995).

or topic to be searched. At this point, planners can search either by subject/title or by author. If planners know of an author who has done work on their topic, they can search the database using the author's last name. If they do not know of any such authors, they will need to match their topic with the key words presented in the thesaurus. Since there are times when a topic is not expressed in the same terms used in the thesaurus, planners will need to look for related terms. Once they have a list of key words, they need to search the database for possible matches. In conducting this search, they need to ensure that they are using the database that covers the years of literature in which they are interested. This search should identify possible sources and citations.

Once the sources are identified, planners will need to locate the sources, judge the quality and quantity of the literature, then organize it in a useful form (Deeds, 1992). One means by which planners can judge the quality and quantity of the literature is to examine the references at the end of the publications. First, this reference list may lead planners to other sources not identified in the original search. But second, if the sources found in the database include all those commonly cited in the literature, this can verify the exhaustiveness of the search.

Searching via the World Wide Web. Through the use of the **World Wide Web (WWW),** program planners can obtain access to a variety of needs assessment data rather easily and quickly. The WWW "is an interactive information delivery service that includes a repository of resources on almost any subject" (Cottrell et al., 1999, p. 229). The WWW, or "the web," "uses a technology called hypertext. A single hypertext document on the WWW is called a web page. Hypertext is a method of transparently linking one information resource to another" (Kotecki & Siegel, 1997, p.117).

A **website** is a collection of WWW "pages, usually consisting of a home page and several other linked pages" (Olpin & Gotthoffer, 2000, p. 155). To search websites for data, planners can enter the WWW through a web browser, such as HotJava, Lynx, Microsoft Internet Explorer, or Netscape Communicator. A **browser** is a special software package that reads the hypertext language and can fetch documents at multiple sites on the web (Daniel & Balog, 1997). On each browser is a field for users to type in the web address of a site, also known as the **Uniform Resource Locator (URL).** The URL is composed of (1) the Internet access protocol (e.g., http://, which stands for hypertext transfer protocol), (2) the location (e.g., www.census, which is the location for the U.S. Census Bureau), and (3) the file name (e.g., stat_abstract, which is the file name for *Statistical Abstract of the United States* mentioned earlier in this chapter) (Cottrell et al., 1999). Entering the specific URL will connect planners with the desired website. Almost all websites contain a **home page** that "acts as a starting point for information about a person or organization" (Olpin & Gotthoffer, 2000, p. 153) and provides a list of what is available at the site. The **home page** can be thought of as "a combination of a cover and a table of contents of a book, in that it names the site and directs the user to a list of information options available at the site" (Cottrell et al., 1999, p. 230). Figure 4.4 presents the home page for the Centers for Disease Control and Prevention **<http:// www.cdc.gov/>.**

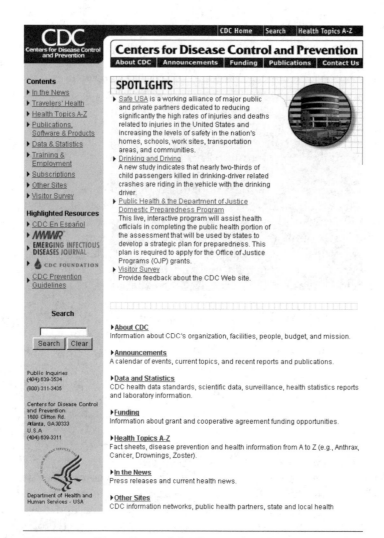

FIGURE 4.4 *Home Page of the Centers for Disease Control and Prevention*

If planners do not know the URL of a specific website, they can search for needed information by using a search archive or a search engine. A number of commercial organizations (e.g., Alta Vista, Excite, Hotbot, and Yahoo!) have categorized websites in these two ways. A **subject archive** organizes information by topic and can be found at these commercial sites (see Figure 4.5). The subject archives presented in Figure 4.5 include Arts and Humanities, Business and Economy, Computers and Internet, and so on. Choosing one of these subject archives categories presents more subcategories, or links, to Internet resources about the

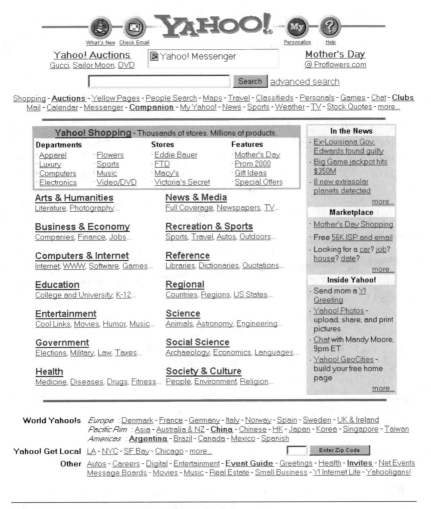

FIGURE 4.5   *Example of a Subject Archive*

subject. For example, say planners wanted information on heart disease. They could select the subject archive of "diseases" under "Health" in Figure 4.5. This will bring up an alphabetized list of diseases from which to choose. Planners would then have many sources from which to choose (Kotecki & Siegel, 1997).

Program planners can also search the web using a search engine. A **search engine**

> is unlike a search archive in that the information is not organized into categories. Instead, a search engine indexes the words in web pages on the Internet. The index created by a search engine is called a catalog and users query the catalog for

keywords that best describes their topic. When using a search engine, a field for typing in keywords is immediately displayed [see topic of Figure 4.5]. After submitting a keyword query, a list of Internet resources is generated. (Kotecki & Siegel, 1997, pp. 118–120)

(See Figure 4.6 for an example from Yahoo!). The planners then can select the sites that best fit their needs. If planners are using a term that has more than one word (i.e., *heart disease*), it is best to use quotation marks around the term when entering it on the search engine. "This will allow the search engine to know that all the words are to be included in the term when the search engine is seeking sites that match. If quotation marks are not used, the search engine may seek sites that match only the first word in the multiword term" (Cottrell et al., 1999, p. 231). In the example used here, it might only search for the word *heart,* and thus locate more sites not of use to the planners. The primary advantage of using a search archive or search engine over a URL (which is specific to one site) is that search archive/engine allows the planners to select a topic (e.g., heart disease) from which several related websites will be identified (Cottrell et al., 1999). Figures 4.5 and 4.6 present an example of a commercial organization's home page (with search archive/engine) and the page that matches the search query for the term *heart disease,* respectfully.

As with any data source, planners need to be aware that not all data found via the WWW are valid and reliable. Thus, planners need to scrutinize sources just as they would data found in hard copies. Several authors (Jadad & Gagliardi, 1998; Kotecki & Chamness, 1999; Pealer & Dorman, 1997; Silberg, Lundberg, & Musacchio, 1997; Tillman, 1997; Venditto, 1997) have published useful guides for evaluating information obtained via the Internet.

Conducting a Needs Assessment

Having explained the general categories of needs assessment data, let's consider how a needs assessment is actually conducted. There are a number of different approaches planners can use to determine the needs of the target population. "Need assessments range from informal approaches, using educated and informed observations to formal, comprehensive research projects. However, the informal approaches are less reliable than a planned and scientifically developed research approach" (Timmreck, 1995, p. 85). Oftentimes, informal approaches are used because of limited time, personnel, and money. However, as noted in the beginning of this chapter, needs assessment may be the most critical step in the planning process and should not be taken lightly. Resources used on need assessments usually pay dividends many times over. Therefore, the authors present a process that is more formal in nature. Because the PRECEDE-PROCEED model is often used in the planning process, the process that will be presented closely aligns with the model. This process includes six steps: (1) determining purpose and defining the scope of the needs assessment, (2) gathering data, (3) analyzing the data, (4) iden-

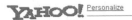

Search Result Found **5** categories and **126** sites for **"heart disease"**

CYMA Systems, Inc.
THE *AFFORDABLE* NONPROFIT ACCOUNTING ALTERNATIVE

CYMA Systems, Inc

Categories	Web Sites	Web Pages	Related News	Net Events

Inside Yahoo! Matches

Health: Find a Cardiologist in your area
Health: Find information about Heart Disease on Yahoo! Health

Search Books!

amazon.com
· "HEART DISEASE"
Buy Books HERE!
· "SEARCH AMAZON

Yahoo! Category Matches (1 - 5 of 5)

Full Coverage > Health

 • Heart Disease

Health > **Disease**s and Conditions

 • Congenital **Heart Disease**

Business and Economy > Shopping and Services > Books > Booksellers > Health > Titles

 • **Heart Disease**

Regional > Countries > New Zealand > Health > **Disease**s and Conditions

 • Congenital **Heart Disease**

Regional > Countries > United Kingdom > Health > **Disease**s and Conditions

 • Congenital **Heart Disease**

Yahoo! Site Matches (1 - 15 of 126)

Health > Nutrition

 • Nutrition, Health and **Heart Disease** - contains information about supplements, foods, **heart disease**, and general health.

Business and Economy > Shopping and Services > Books > Booksellers > Health > Titles > **Heart Disease**

 • Create a Healthy **Heart** - by Narinder Saini, MD, a physician's guide to recovery or prevention of **heart disease**, based on personal experience and medical expertise.

Health > **Disease**s and Conditions > Congenital **Heart Disease**

 • Congenital **Heart Disease** Resources

Health > **Disease**s and Conditions > Heart Failure

 • Cut to the **Heart** - congestive **heart** failure and its treatment, map of **heart** and pumping cycle, pioneers of **heart** surgery and examples of **heart**

FIGURE 4.6 *Example of Internet Resources Generated from a Keyword Query*

tifying the factors linked to the health problem, (5) identifying the program focus, and (6) validating the need before continuing on with the planning process.

Step 1: Determining the Purpose and Scope of the Needs Assessment

The initial step in the needs assessment process is to determine the purpose and the scope of the needs assessment. In other words, what is the goal of the needs assessment? What does the planning committee hope to gain from the needs assessment? How extensive will the needs assessment be? What kind of resources will be available to conduct the needs assessment? Once these questions are answered, the planners are ready to begin collecting the data for the needs assessment.

Step 2: Gathering Data

The second step in the needs assessment process is gathering data. To do this, planners must consider sources of data that reflect needs from the viewpoint of the planners and also needs perceived by those in the target population. This usually means both primary and secondary data need to be collected. Because of the cost and availability, data collection should begin with the collection of relevant secondary data. *Relevant* means that the data apply to the situation for which the planning is taking place. If a national program is being planned, then national secondary data should be sought from appropriate national governmental and non-governmental agencies. If a local program is being planned, then appropriate local data should be sought. When planning a local program, it is not unusual to find that local data do not exist. If that is the case, planners may need to extrapolate from national, regional, and/or state data to create data for local use (Simons-Morton et al., 1995). For example, say diabetes mellitus mortality data are needed for local planning and the only data available are national-level data. Planners could take the national data (e.g., in 1996, 23.2 per 100,000 people had died from diabetes mellitus), and, knowing the population of city X is 250,000, estimate that it would be reasonable to believe that there were approximately 58 (23.2×2.5) diabetes-caused deaths in the city in 1996. Since diabetes deaths are expected more often in an older population, if the average age in the city was higher than the national average, planners should take the 58 deaths as a low estimate. If the average in the city was younger than the national average, the 58 deaths should be seen as a high estimate. Obviously, as noted at the beginning of this chapter, there are disadvantages of using secondary data, but good planners use and interpret them in light of their limitations (McDermott & Sarvela, 1999).

Even though primary data will usually take more resources to collect, they provide valuable information about the specific planning situation not available from secondary data and they provide an opportunity to get those in the target population actively involved in the program planning process. Thus, planners need to decide whom to collect the data from and take the necessary steps to collect the data. (The data collection process is presented at length in Chapter 5.)

As planners conclude the second step in the needs assessment process, they must remember that each planning situation is different. It is desirable to have both primary and secondary needs assessment data in order to gain a clear picture of both service needs and demands; however, depending on the resources and circumstances, planners may have access to only one or the other.

Step 3: Analyzing the Data

At this point in the needs assessment process, the planners must analyze all the data collected, with the goal of identifying and prioritizing the health problems.

The analysis of the data may be formal or informal. The approach used would depend on what data were collected and how exact the planners wanted to be. Formal analysis would consist of some type of statistical analysis. This approach could be used only when appropriate statistical criteria (see any introductory statistics book) have been met. Much of the time, a less formal means of analyzing the data is used. This approach is commonly referred to as **eyeballing the data**—that is, looking at the data for obvious differences between current health status and what could be. As Windsor and colleagues (1994, p. 63) have stated, eyeballing the data means looking for differences between "what is and what ought to be."

Sometimes this step in the needs assessment process is not very complicated because the problem/need is obvious. For example, breast cancer rates may have risen in a given community, the number of breast screenings may be low, and the consumers may recognize this. Or, in another setting, the planners may find a direct correlation between the health status of a community and the lack of health care. However, not all assessments yield an obvious problem. The data may be mixed or confusing. If planners are working with a multicultural target population, data analysis may even be more confusing, because health concepts held by one culture may be very different than the health concepts held by the planners. These cultural differences "often involve family, community, and/or supernatural agents in cause and effect, placation, and treatment rituals to prevent, control, or cure illness. A failure to understand and appreciate these 'differences' can have serious implications for success of any health promotion/disease prevention effort" (Kline & Huff, 1999, p. 106). In such cases, it is probably a good idea to see if additional data might be collected to paint a clearer picture. If obtaining additional data does not help, then leaning on those individuals on the planning committee more familiar with the cultural differences or asking more experienced professionals for their opinions may aid in reaching a conclusion.

In completing this step of the needs assessment process, planners will be working through the first two phases of the PRECEDE-PROCEED model, social assessment, and epidemiological assessment. While analyzing the data, planners may find it helpful to ask the following questions:

1. What is the quality of life of those in the target population?
2. What are social conditions and perceptions shared by those in the target population?
3. What are the social indicators (e.g., absenteeism, crime, discrimination, performance, welfare, etc.) in the target population that reflect the social conditions and perceptions?
4. Can the social conditions and perceptions be linked to health promotion? If so, how?
5. What are the health problems associated with the social problems?
6. Which health problem is most important to change?

The last question in this list is really asking the question, Which health problem/need should get priority? The health problems/needs must be prioritized not because the lowest-priority problems/needs are not important, but because organizations have limited resources. Thus, planners need to see how the health promotion dollars can best be used. Therefore, in setting priorities, the planners should seek answers to these questions:

1. What is the most pressing need?
2. Are there resources adequate to deal with the problem?
3. Can the problem best be solved by a health promotion intervention, or could it be handled better through another means?
4. Can the problem be solved in a reasonable amount of time?

After answering these questions, the planners should be able to prioritize the identified problems/needs.

The actual process of setting priorities can take many different forms and range from basic rank ordering by a group of stakeholders, to use of the nominal group process, to a more complex process called the priority ranking process. The priority ranking process was first presented by Hanlon (1974) (it has been more recently presented in Pickett & Hanlon, 1990) and will be discussed here in greater detail because it can greatly help program planners quantify the subjective process of prioritizing. The process requires program planners to rate four different components of the identified needs and insert the ratings into a formula in order to determine a rating between 0 and 100. The components and their possible scores (in parenthesis) are:

A   size of the problem (0 to 10)
B   seriousness of the problem (0 to 20)
C   effectiveness of the possible interventions (0 to 10)
D   propriety, economics, acceptability, resources, and legality (PEARL) (0 or 1)

The formula in which the scores are placed is:

$$\text{Basic priority rating (BPR)} = \frac{(A + B)C}{3} \times D$$

Component *A*, size of the problem, can be scored by using epidemiological rates or determining the percentage of the target population at risk. The higher the rate or percentage, the greater the score. Pickett and Hanlon (1990) offer the scale noted in Table 4.1 for scoring the size of the problem when using incidence and prevalence rates.

Component *B*, seriousness of the problem, is examined using four factors: economic loss to community, family, or individuals; involvement of other people who were not initially affected by the problem, as with the spread of an infectious disease; the severity of the problem measured in mortality, morbidity, or disability; and the urgency of solving the problem because of additional harm. Although the maximum score for this component is 20, raters can use a 0 to 10 score for each of the factors. If the score for the component adds up to more than 20, a 20 is used.

TABLE 4.1 *Scoring the Size of the Problem*

Incidence or Prevalence per 100,000 Population	Score
50,000 or more	10
5,000 to 49,999	8
500 to 4,999	6
50 to 499	4
5 to 49	2
0.5 to 4.9	0

Source: Public Health: Administration and Practice, G. Pickett and J. J. Hanlon, © 1997, McGraw-Hill. Reproduced with permission of The McGraw-Hill Companies.

Component *C*, effectiveness of the interventions, is often the most difficult of the four components to measure. The efficacy of some interventions is known, such as immunizations (close to 100%) and smoking cessation classes (around 30%), but for many, it is not. Program planners will need to estimate this score based upon the work of others or their own best guess.

Component *D*, PEARL, consists of several factors that determine whether a particular intervention can be carried out at all. The score is 0 or 1; any need that receives a zero will automatically drop to the bottom of the priority list because a score of zero for this component will yield a total score of zero in the formula. Examples of when a zero may result are if an intervention is economically impossible, unacceptable to the target population or planners, or illegal.

Once the score for the four components is determined, an overall priority rating for each need can be calculated, and the prioritizing can take place.

Other means of quantifying the prioritization of the needs may include getting the target population or key people from the community, like opinion leaders, to rank-order the identified needs.

How will planners know when they have completed Step 3 (Analyzing the Data) of the needs assessment process? Planners should be able to list in rank order the health problems/needs of the target population.

Step 4: Identifying the Factors Linked to the Health Problem

Step 4 of the needs assessment process is parallel to the third phase of the PRECEDE-PROCEED model: behavioral and environmental assessment. Planners need to identify and prioritize the behavior and environmental risk factors that are associated with the health problem. Thus, if the health problem is lung cancer, planners should analyze the health behaviors and environment of the target population for known risk factors of lung cancer. For example, higher than expected smoking behavior may be present in the target population, and they may live in a community where smoke-free public environments are not valued. Once these risk factors are identified, they too need to be prioritized (see Figure 2.2 for a means of prioritizing these risk factors).

Step 5: Identifying the Program Focus

The fifth step of the needs assessment process is similar to the fourth phase of the PRECEDE-PROCEED model: educational and ecological assessment. With behavioral and environmental risk factors identified and prioritized, planners need to identify those predisposing, enabling, and reinforcing factors that seem to have a direct impact on the targeted risk factors. In the lung cancer example, those in the target population may not (1) have the skills necessary to stop smoking (predisposing factor), (2) have access to a smoking cessation program (enabling factor), or (3) have people around them who value nonsmokers (reinforcing factor). "Study of the predisposing, enabling, and reinforcing factors automatically helps the planner decide exactly which of the factors making up the three classes deserve the highest priority as the focus of the intervention. The decision is based on their importance and any evidence that change in the factor is possible and cost-effective" (Green & Kreuter, 1999, p. 42)

In addition, when prioritizing needs, planners also need to consider the existing health promotion programs to avoid any duplication with planning efforts. Therefore, program planners should seek to determine the status of existing health promotion programs by trying to answer as many questions as possible from the following list:

1. What health promotion programs are presently available to the target population?
2. Are the programs being utilized? If not, why not?
3. How effective are the programs? Are they meeting their stated goals and objectives?
4. How were the needs for these programs determined?
5. Are the programs accessible to the target population? Where are they located? When are they offered? Are there any qualifying criteria that people must meet to enroll? Can the target population get to the program? Can the target population afford the programs?
6. Are the needs of the target population being met? If not, why not?

There are several ways to seek answers to these questions. Probably the most common way is through **networking** with other people working in health promotion and the health care system—that is, communicating with others who may know about existing programs. (See Chapter 9 for a more detailed discussion of networking.) These people may be located in the local or state health department, in voluntary health agencies, or in health care facilities, such as hospitals, clinics, nursing homes, extended care facilities, or Managed Care Organizations.

Planners might also find information about existing programs by checking with someone in an organization that serves as a clearinghouse for health promotion programs or by using a community resource guide. The local or state health department, a local chamber of commerce, a coalition, the local medical/dental societies, a community task force, or a community health center may serve as a clearinghouse or produce such a guide. Another avenue is to talk with people in the target population. Although they may not know about all existing programs, they may be able to share information on the effectiveness and accessibility of some of the programs. Finally, some of the information could be collected in Step 2 through separate community forums, focus groups, or surveys.

Step 6: *Validating the Prioritized Needs*

The final step in the needs assessment process is to validate the identified need(s). *Validate* means to confirm that the need that was identified is the need that should be addressed. Obviously, if great care was taken in the needs assessment process, validation should be a perfunctory step. However, there have been times when a need was not properly validated; much energy and many resources have thereby been wasted on unnecessary programs.

Validation amounts to "double checking," or making sure that an identified need is the real need. Any means available can be used, such as (1) rechecking the steps followed in the needs assessment to eliminate any bias, (2) conducting a focus group with some individuals from the target population to determine their reaction to the identified need (if a focus group was not used earlier to gather the data), and (3) getting a "second opinion" from other health professionals.

Assessment Protocol for Excellence in Public Health (APEX/PH)

A discussion of the needs assessment process would not be complete without mention of **APEX/PH** (NACHO, 1991), a needs assessment instrument for local health departments. APEX/PH was developed in 1991 by the National Association of County Health Officials (NACHO) and a number of collaborative groups. (*Note:* In July 1994, NACHO combined with the United States Conference of Local Health Officers [USCLHO] to form a new organization called the National Association of County and City Health Officials [NACCHO].) APEX/PH was developed to help local health departments respond to the Institute of Medicine's (IOM) report "The Future of Public Health," in which it was stated every public health agency should regularly and systematically collect, assemble, and analyze information on community health needs (IOM, 1988).

The APEX/PH workbook is divided into two parts: Part I focuses on assessing and improving the organizational capacity of the local health department, and Part II is aimed at identifying and prioritizing the community health needs. Specifically, Part II uses demographic, socioeconomic, and morbidity and mortality data to determine the health status of those in the community. Specific software has been developed for use with this assessment to make the data collection and reporting easier. One criticism early on about Part II of APEX/PH was the lack of attention given to the assessment of environmental health needs (McDonald, Treser, & Hatlen, 1994). However, since that time, NACCHO has developed the Protocol for Assessing Community Excellence in Environmental Health (PACE-EH). Specific to environmental health concerns, PACE-EH includes such steps as identifying community perceptions and issues of concern, selecting standards and indicators, collecting and analyzing data, and developing an action plan.

At the time this book was being written, NACCHO and Centers for Disease Control and Prevention are currently in the process of developing a new planning tool entitled Assessment and Planning Excellence through Community Partners for Health (APEXCPH). This tool will include information on community issues that residents feel are important, assessing the public health system, a community health status assessment (including quality of life; environmental health; socioeconomic, demographic, and behavioral risk factors; infectious disease; sentinel events; social and mental health; maternal and child health; health resource availability; and health status indicators), and identification of forces of change.

These health assessment tools would not be very useful in all needs assessment situations, but they would be when planners are working on community-wide program assessments. Planners should check with their local or state health departments to see if any of these assessment programs are underway in their locale or if they have been completed and the resulting data are available.

Summary

This chapter presented several definitions of needs assessment and a discussion of primary and secondary data. The sources of these data were discussed at length. Also, presented in this chapter was a six-step approach that health planners can follow in conducting a needs assessment on a given group of people. It is by no means the only way of conducting an assessment, but it is workable.

No matter what procedure is used to conduct a needs assessment, the end result should be the same. Planners should finish with a clearly defined program focus.

Questions

1. What does *needs assessment* mean?

2. Why must a needs assessment be viewed through the eyes of both the planners and the consumers?

3. What is the difference between primary and secondary data?

4. Name several different sources of both primary and secondary data.

5. What advice might you give to someone who is interested in using previously collected data (secondary data) for a needs assessment?

6. What is the difference between a single-step (cross-sectional) and a multistep survey?

7. Explain the difference between a community forum and a focus group.

8. What is a health assessment?

9. What are the six steps in the needs assessment process, as identified in the chapter?

10. What is APEX/PH? PACE-EH?

Activities

1. Assume that you have been hired by the board of trustees of your college or university to conduct a needs assessment on the student body for the possibility of developing a health promotion program. Assume that there are few secondary data on this group of people, other than national norms for college students. You could conduct a "university forum" or hold a series of focus groups, but instead you have decided to survey a random sample of the population with a paper-and-pencil instrument. Your task now is to develop a needs assessment instrument. When developing the instrument, use questions that will collect data that are reflective of your target population's awareness of health, attitudes about health, knowledge of health, health behavior, health interests, and demographics, as well as marketing possibilities. After completing the instrument, pilot test it on 10 students (for the purposes of this assignment, this does not need to be a random group). Use the results of the pilot test to complete Steps 2, 3, 4, and 5 in the needs assessment process.

2. Develop a needs assessment instrument for a program you will be planning. Collect the same type of data noted in Activity 1, administer the instrument to a small group of people, then complete Steps 2, 3, 4, and 5 in the needs assessment process.

3. Using secondary data provided by your instructor or obtained from the World Wide Web (such as data from a Behavioral Risk Factor Survey, state or local secondary data, or data from the National Center for Health Statistics), analyze the data and determine the health problems of the target population.

4. Administer an HHA/HRA to a group of 25 to 30 people. Using the data generated, identify and prioritize a collective list of health problems of the group.

5. Plan and conduct a focus group on an identified health problem on your campus. Develop a set of questions to be used, identify and invite people to participate in the group, facilitate the process, and then write up a summary of the results based on your written notes and/or an audiotape of the session.

6. Using the data (paper-and-pencil instruments, clinical tests, and health histories) generated from a local health fair, identify and prioritize a collective list of health problems of those who participated.

Activities on the Web

1. Visit one of the following websites for the specific purpose of using its risk assessment. Complete risk assessments from two different sites and print out the results. Write a paragraph describing how you think each assessment could be used as part of a needs assessment.
   a. Oxygen Media <**http://www.thriveonline. com/cgi-bin/hmi/healthportrait.cgi**>

b. American Heart Association **<http://www.americanheart.org>**

c. Greenstone Healthcare Solution **<http://www.youfirst.com/>**

d. American Diabetes Association **<http://www.diabetes.org/>**

2. Visit the web site of the Association of State and Territorial Health Officials **<http:www.astho.org/>**. Once in the website, select the state and territorial link, then select your state. Print a copy of your state health department home page. Then identify and print out at least five pieces of secondary data that you can use in the program you are planning. Take your printouts to class.

5

Measurement, Measures, Data Collection, and Sampling

After reading this chapter and answering the questions at the end, you should be able to:

- Define measurement and quantitative and qualitative measures.
- Briefly describe the four levels of measurement.
- Describe several methods of data collection.
- Discuss the advantages and disadvantages of data collection from self-report (written surveys, telephone interviews, and face-to-face interviews), direct observation, existing records, and meetings.
- Explain the various types of validity.
- Define *reliability* and explain why it is important.
- Define *bias* in data collection and discuss how it can be reduced.
- Explain why data collection instruments must be culturally appropriate.
- Describe how a sample can be obtained from a population.
- Differentiate between probability and nonprobability samples.
- Describe how a pilot test is used.

Key Terms

anonymous	cultural sensitivity	levels of measurement
bias	direct observation	nominal
census	face validity	nonprobability sample
cluster sample	field study	ordinal
concurrent validity	frame	parallel forms reliability
confidential	indirect observation	parameters
construct validity	internal consistency	pilot test
content validity	interrater reliability	predictive validity
criterion-related validity	interval	preliminary review
cultural competence	intrarater reliability	prepilot

probability sample
proxy measure
qualitative measure
quantitative measure
random-digit dialing
randomization
ratio

reliability
respondents
sample
sampling
self-report data
simple random sample
stability reliability

statistics
stratified random sample
survey population
systematic sample
validity

In Chapter 4, we discussed in detail the needs assessment process, emphasizing the importance of collecting and analyzing appropriate needs assessment data. Later, in Chapters 13 through 15, we will again be concerned about data, but then the discussion will revolve around data and its relationship to program evaluation. In this chapter, we will examine the concepts that are considered when trying to determine the quality of data, whether it is for a needs assessment or a program evaluation. Specifically, we will examine the (1) term *measurement*, (2) types of data generated from measurement, (3) levels of measurement, (4) types of measures, (5) desirable characteristics of measures, (6) methods of data collection, (7) sampling, and (8) the importance of pilot testing data collection processes.

Measurement

Measurement is an integral part of program planning and evaluation. It has been defined as the process of assigning numbers or labels to objects, events, or people according to a particular set of rules (Kerlinger, 1986). For example, planners/evaluators can measure the level of fitness of program participants by asking them a question. Using the numbers *1, 2,* and *3,* planners/evaluators can assign the number *1* to those with poor fitness, 2 to those with average fitness, and 3 to those with good fitness. Further, the planners/evaluators need to specify what constitutes poor, average, and good fitness. In other words, measurement means that the program planners/evaluators need to "clearly specify the objects to be measured, the numbers to use, and the rules by which the numbers are assigned to the objects" (Green & Lewis, 1986, p. 58).

The data generated by measurement can be classified into two different categories, depending on the method by which they are collected. **Quantitative measures** "rely on more standardized data collection and reduction techniques, using predetermined questions or observational indicators and established response items" (Green & Lewis, 1986, p. 151). Quantitative data can be transformed into numerical data. Examples of quantitative data would be the number of participants in a smoking cessation program, the ratings on a patient satisfaction survey, and the pretest and posttest scores on a HIV knowledge test. **Qualitative mea-**

sures "tend to produce data in the language of the subjects, rarely with numerical values attached to observations" (Green & Lewis, 1986, p. 151). Qualitative data are usually assigned labels or categories (Morreale, no date) and often take the form of narrative (Weiss, 1998). Examples include data generated from case studies, interviews, and descriptions and explanations of observations.

Levels of Measurement

A fundamental question of measurement is deciding how something should be measured (McDermott & Sarvela, 1999). What yardstick should be used to measure the object of interest? For example, consider planners/evaluators who need data on the income levels of their program participants. They could ask the participants income level several different ways:

1. Are you on any type of welfare?
2. What income category best describes your family income? $0 to 10,000, $10,001 to 25,000, $25,001 to 40,000, $40,000+
3. What is your family income? _____

Each of these questions gets at one's income level, but each generates a different form of data. Thus, when planners/evaluators begin to think about data collection, they need to consider the form(s) of data they want to use.

There are four **levels of measurement** used to determine how something is to be measured. They are hierarchical in nature, and the form of data collected determines what statistical test can be used to analyze them. The four levels of measurement are:

1. **Nominal** measures, the simplest form, enable planners/evaluators to put data into categories. "The two requirements for nominal measures are that the categories have to be mutually exclusive so that each case fits into one of the categories, and the categories have to be exhaustive so that there is a place for every case" (Weiss, 1998, p. 116). Examples include sex, city of residence, nationality, color of eyes, and participant/nonparticipant.
2. **Ordinal** measures enable planners/evaluators to put data into categories, but also permits them to rank-order the categories. The different categories represent relatively more or less of something. Examples include academic achievement, level of satisfaction with a program, socioeconomic status, and level of health.
3. **Interval** measures enable planners/evaluators to rank the data, but they can also measure the distance separating the points. There is, however, no absolute zero value. Examples include temperature and standardized test scores.
4. **Ratio** measures, the most complex form, enable planners/evaluators to do everything with data that can be done with nominal, ordinal, and interval measures; however, they are done using a scale with an absolute zero. Examples

include height, weight, number of cigarettes smoked, dollars, and ounces of alcohol consumed.

If given the choice, planners/evaluators should strive to collect ratio data. This is the highest level in the hierarchy and allows the planner/evaluators the greatest flexibility in data analysis.

Types of Measures

Many different types of measures are used to conduct needs assessments or evaluate programs. It is important to match the methods of measurement with the focus of the task, whether it be a needs assessments or program evaluation. Typically, health promotion programs focus on one or more of the following areas: awareness, knowledge, attitudes, skills, behavior, health status (i.e., health risks, morbidity, or mortality), and quality of life. In the remaining portions of this chapter, we will discuss methods and techniques for collecting data associated with these areas.

Desirable Characteristics of Data

The results of a needs assessment or program evaluation are only as good as the data that are used to gain the results. If a questionnaire was filled with ambiguous questions and the respondents were not sure how to answer, it is highly likely that the data collected will not be reflective of the true knowledge, attitudes, etc., of those responding. Therefore, it is of vital importance that planners and evaluators make sure that the data they collect are reliable, valid, unbiased, and culturally appropriate.

Reliability

Reliability refers to consistency in the measurement process. A reliable instrument gives the same (or nearly the same) result every time. However, no instrument will ever provide perfect accuracy in measurement. Green and Lewis (1986) illustrate the theory of reliability with an equation, where total score (obtained score) equals the true score (unobservable) plus an error score. The total score represents the individual's score obtained on the measuring instrument. The true score represents the score for the same individual if all conditions and the measuring instrument were perfect. An error score must be included since conditions are never perfect in the real world. Several methods of determining reliability are available.

Internal Consistency.   **Internal consistency** refers to the intercorrelations among the individual items on the instrument, that is, whether all items on the instrument are measuring part of the total area. This can be done by logically examining the instrument to ensure that the items reflect what is to be measured and that the level of difficulty of all items is the same. Statistical methods can also be used to determine internal consistency by correlating the items on the test with the total score.

Stability Reliability. **Stability reliability,** or test-retest reliability, examines whether the results would be the same if the instrument were administered to the same person at a later date. The length of time between test and retest may vary from hours to weeks to years. A maximum amount of time should be allowed so that individuals are not answering on the basis of remembering responses they made on the first test, but it should not be so long that other events could occur in the intervening time to influence their responses. To avoid the problems of retesting, parallel forms (equivalent forms) of the test can be administered to the participants and the results can be correlated.

Rater Reliability. **Rater reliability** focuses on the consistency between individuals who are observing or rating the same event or when one individual is observing or rating a series of events. If two or more raters are involved, it is referred to as **interrater reliability.** If only one individual is observing or rating a series of events, it is referred to as *intrarater reliability.* Both forms are reported as a percentage of agreement between or among raters or within an individual rater. An example of interrater reliability would be the the percent of agreement between two observers who are observing passing drivers in cars for safety belt use. If 10 cars are observed by the raters and they agree 8 out of 10 times on whether the drivers are wearing their safety belts, the interrater reliability would be 80%. **Intrarater reliability** would be the degree to which one rater agrees with himself or herself on the characteristics of an observation over time. For example, when a rater is evaluating the CPR skills of participants in his or her program, the rater should be consistent while observing and evaluating the skills of the participants.

Parallel Forms Reliability. **Parallel forms reliability** determines whether different forms of the same test instrument have equal means, standard deviations, and item intercorrelations. Parallel forms reliability is used to determine if different forms of standardized tests (e.g., college entrance exams) include the same content and are of the same degree of difficulty.

Validity

When designing a data collection instrument, planners/evaluators must ensure that it measures what it is intended to measure. This refers to the **validity** of the measurement—whether it is correctly measuring the concepts under investigation. Using a valid instrument increases the chance that planners/evaluators are measuring what they want to measure, thus ruling out other possible explanations for the results. We will discuss several types of validity.

Face Validity. The lowest level of validity is face validity. A measure is said to have **face validity** if, on the face, the measure appears to measure what it is suppose to measure (McDermott & Sarvela, 1999). It differs from the other forms of validity in that it lacks some form of systematic logical analysis of the content (Hopkins, Stanley, & Hopkins, 1990). An example of face validity might include a planner/evaluator asking a colleague to look over a series of questions to see if the questions seem reasonable to include on a questionnaire about, for example, heart disease.

Content Validity.   *Content validity* refers to the degree to which the items on an instrument are a representative sample of the content and/or behavior of the domain being addressed (Hopkins, Stanley, & Hopkins, 1990). For example, when planning a risk reduction program for cardiovascular disease, the program planner can conduct a review of the literature in the area of cardiovascular risk reduction in order to ensure that all major risk factors, such as smoking, exercise, and diet, are included on a questionnaire.

Content validity is usually established by using a group (jury or panel) of experts to review the instrument. After such a group is identified, they would be asked to review each element of the instrument for its appropriateness to be included. The collective opinion of the experts is then used to determine the content of the instrument. McKenzie and colleagues (1999) present a method of establishing content validity that includes both qualitative and quantitative steps.

Criterion-Related Validity.   **Criterion-related validity** refers to the general category of evidence of the extent to which scores on an instrument are correlated with some measure of an individual's behavior or performance. There are two subtypes of criterion-related validity: predictive and concurrent (McKenzie et al., 1999).

If the measurement used will be correlated with a future measurement of the same phenomenon, as with the use of standardized test scores to predict future college success, the criterion validity is known as **predictive validity. Concurrent validity** is established when a new instrument and an established valid instrument that measure the same characteristics are administered to the same subjects, and the results of the new instrument are compared to the results of the valid instrument. For example, if a planner/evaluator wanted to establish the validity of a new test for breast cancer, he or she administers both the new instrument and another already valid breast cancer instrument to the same subjects and then compares the results. The new instrument would be valid if the results compared favorably with the established instrument. In both subtypes of criterion-related validity, the aim is to legitimize the inferences that can be made by establishing their predictive ability for a related criterion (Borg & Gall, 1989).

Construct Validity.   Another type of validity is *construct validity.* This type of validity has been defined as the extent to which a measure correlates with a psychological characteristic (i.e., construct). "This form of validity is often used when trying to measure a theoretical construct (e.g., locus of control, self-efficacy, or perceived barriers) for which a clear-cut behavioral equivalent does not exist" (McKenzie et al., 1999, p. 312).

Unbiased

Biased data are those data that have been distorted because of the way they have been collected. In order to effectively plan and evaluate health promotion programs, planners/evaluators must work to eliminate bias. Windsor and colleagues (1994) describe ways in which bias can occur in data collection—for example, when participants do not feel comfortable answering a sensitive question, when participants act differently because they know they are being watched, when certain characteristics of the interviewer influence a response, when participants answer questions in a particular way regardless of the questions being asked, or when a bias sample has been selected from the target population (see information later in this chapter on sampling). There are a number of steps planners/evaluators can take to limit bias. For example, if data are being collected via observation, the observation should be as unobtrusive as possible. If sensitive questions are being asked of respondents, then those collecting such data need to ensure that the data are being collected in a confidential way (the identity of the respondent can be determined but not released), and consider collecting the data via an anonymous means (there is no way of identifying the respondent). No matter how data are collected, the reduction of bias techniques will increase the accuracy of the results.

Culturally Appropriate

"Culture shapes the way of life shared by members of a population. It is the sociocultural adaptation or design for living that people have worked out (and continue to work out) in the course of their history" (Ogbu, 1987, 156). Therefore, people from different cultures are likely to possess different values, beliefs, traditions, and perceptions. These cultural values, beliefs, traditions, and perceptions affect nearly all activities of individuals, including their health-related behavior (Kline & Huff, 1999) and responding to questions related to health. "As cultures vary, so do notions of what the human body symbolizes, how it should appear, how it functions most appropriately and why, and when and how it should be treated" (AAHE, 1994, p. 5). Thus, culture influences program participants' ability to understand, internalize, and exercise positive health practices that will enhance the quality of life. For example, if we examine the diet of individuals from different cultures (i.e., religion, race), it is easy to see the impact of culture on what people eat. Some cultures see some foods as an important part of their diet, while others see the same foods as dirty and not to be consumed. Thus, when collecting data from diverse populations, planners/evaluators need to respond appropriately to cultural differences. In other words, planners/evaluators need to be culturally sensitive and work toward being culturally competent. "'**Cultural sensitivity**' implies knowledge that cultural differences (as well as similarities) exist, along with the refusal to assign cultural differences such values as better or worse, more or less intelligent, right or wrong; they are simply differences" (Anderson & Fenichel, 1989, p. 8). **Cultural competence** refers to "a process for effectively working within the cultural context of an individual or community from a diverse cultural or ethnic background" (Campinha-Bacote, 1994, pp. 1–2).

Methods of Data Collection

Self-Report

Written questionnaires, telephone interviews, face-to-face (or in-depth) interviews, and email are methods of collecting self-report data. **Self-report data** refers to data that are generated by having individuals (the **respondents**) report about themselves. Thus, respondents are asked to recall ("When was your last visit to your dentist?") and report accurate ("On average, how many calories do you consume a day?") information. Self-report measures are essential for many needs assessments and evaluations because of the need to obtain subjective assessments of experiences (e.g., feelings about available programs, self-assessments of health status, or health behavior, such as eating patterns) (Bowling, 1997). Self-report measures have broad appeal to those who need to collect data, because "they are often quick to administer and involve little interpretation by the investigator" (Bowling, 1997, p. 12). However, planners/evaluators should be aware that self-report data do have limitations. One such limitation is **bias.** (See the previous section of this chapter for a discussion about bias.) To overcome some of these limitations and to maximize the usefulness of self-report, Baranowski (1985, pp. 181–182) has developed eight steps to increase the accuracy of this method of data collection:

1. Select measures that clearly reflect program outcomes.
2. Select measures that have been designed to anticipate response problems and that have been validated.
3. Conduct a pilot study with the target population.
4. Anticipate and correct major sources of unreliability.
5. Employ quality-control procedures to detect other sources of error.
6. Employ multiple methods.
7. Use multiple measures.
8. Use experimental and control groups with random assignment to control for biases in self-report.

By following these steps, planners/evaluators can enhance the accuracy of self-report, making this a more effective method of data collection.

For a variety of reasons, there are times when those in the target population cannot respond for themselves or do not want to respond. In such situations, planners must collect data from someone other than those in the target population, such as significant others. This is referred to as a **proxy measure.** Stated another way, someone (the significant other) is asked to act for another (the person in the target population) by providing needs assessment data.

Questions Used in Self-Report.   The presentation, wording, and sequence of questions in self-report questionnaires and interviews can be critical in gaining the necessary information. The questionnaire or interview should begin by explaining the purpose of the study and why the individual's responses are important. A cover letter should accompany a mailed questionnaire, explaining the need for the information and including very clear directions for supplying it (see Box 5.1 for an example of a cover letter). The name, address, and telephone number of the planner/ evaluator or another contact person can also be included in case the respondent needs additional information to complete the questionnaire. A stamped, addressed envelope should be enclosed. Figure 5.1 presents a checklist developed by Bourque and Fielder (1995) to use when writing cover letters to potential survey respondents.

With telephone or face-to-face interviews, the interviewer can give information about the study and explain the need for information from the individual contacted. This introduction can be followed by general questions to put the respondent at ease or to develop a rapport between the interviewer and the respondent.

After several general questions come the questions of interest. Any questions that deal with sensitive topics should be posed at the end of the questionnaire or interview. Answers to questions about drug use, sexuality, or even demographic information, such as income level, are more readily answered when the respondents understand the need for the information, are assured of confidentiality or anonymity, and feel comfortable with the interviewer or the questionnaire. If the respondent ends the interview or does not complete the survey when asked sensitive questions, the other information collected can still be used; this is another advantage of putting these questions at the end.

The actual questions should be clear and unbiased. It is important to avoid questions with a specific direction ("How have you enjoyed the class?") that would guide the respondent's answer. Two-part (double-barreled) questions should also be avoided ("Do you brush and floss your teeth?"). Another problem with question design occurs when the question assumes knowledge that individuals may not have or includes terminology that they may not understand ("What cardiovascular benefits do you feel you gain from aerobic exercise?").

The way in which data collection questions are worded is extremely important in gaining the needed information. The result of a poorly worded question was evident to one health promotion planner who was planning a smoking cessation program for employees. When asked, "Do you feel we need a smoking cessation program?" most employees said yes. The planner realized later that he should have also asked the question, "If offered, would you attend a smoking cessation program?" since very few employees participated.

If possible, planners/evaluators should use existing questionnaires. This requires gaining permission from the author if the document is not in the public domain. (Documents in the public domain can be freely used without requesting permission but yet giving credit for the work of others.) The advantages to using questionnaires that have been developed by experts include increased credibility, lower cost, less planning time needed, and more documentation of validity and reliability. The major disadvantage—one that prevents the use of existing questionnaires in many cases—is that the items used to evaluate one program may not all be relevant or appropriate to evaluate a similar program. Adaptations may be needed so that the questionnaire will fit with program objectives or the local target population.

BOX 5.1 • *Example Cover Letter for Data Collection Instrument*

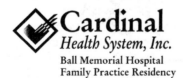

Cardinal
Health System, Inc.
Ball Memorial Hospital
Family Practice Residency

July 15, 2000

Dear Family Physician:

We are conducting a survey to study Indiana family physicians' practices of and preparation for providing patient education.

We are respectfully requesting your response to the enclosed questionnaire at your earliest convenience. The instrument should take you about 10 minutes to complete. There are no right or wrong answers. We recognize that some of the questions are, by necessity, quite personal. Be assured that your individual responses will remain anonymous. Only summarized data will be reported. Your participation in the survey is voluntary.

Since the number of questionnaires being sent out is limited, your participation is important for the success of this project. We therefore request that you complete and return the questionnaire in the enclosed, self addressed, postage paid reply envelope no later than August 4, 2000. If you have any questions about this survey or want to be sent a copy of the results, please contact Jim McKenzie at 765/285-8345 (voice), 765/285-3210 (fax), or 00jfmckenzie@bsu.edu (email).

Thank you in advance for your assistance in completing the enclosed questionnaire.

Sincerely,

Amy Banter, M.D.
Associate Director
Family Practice Residency Program
Ball Memorial Hospital, Inc.

James F. McKenzie, Ph.D., M.P.H.
Professor
Department of Physiology and Health Science
Ball State University

Encl: Questionnaire
         Self-addressed postage paid envelope

2300 W. Gilbert St. • Muncie, IN 47303 • Office: (765) 747-3376 • Toll Free: (800) 279-1666 • Fax: (765) 741-1983
E Mail: jkurtz@iquest.net • Web Site: www.ballhospital.org

FIGURE 5.1 *Checklist for Cover Letter to Survey Respondents*

- Explain the purpose of the study.
- Describe who is sponsoring the study.
- Consider sending an advanced letter.
- Consider using other methods such as newsletters or flyers to publicize the study.
- Include a cover letter with a questionnaire.
  —Use letter head.
  —Date the letter to be consistent with the actual date of the mailing or administration.
  —Provide a name and phone number for the respondent to contact for further information.
  —Personalize the salutation, if feasible.
  —Maximize the attractiveness and readability of the letter.
- Explain how the respondents were chosen and why their participation is important.
- Explain when and how to return the questionnaire.
- Describe incentives, if used.
- Directly or indirectly provide a realistic estimate of the time required by the average respondent to complete the questionnaire.
- Explain how the confidentiality of the respondents' data will be protected.
- Determine whether and how a deadline date will be provided for returning the questionnaires.

Source: L. B. Bourque and E. P. Fielder, *How to Conduct Self-Administered and Mail Surveys,* pp. 121–122, copyright © by Sage Publications. Reprinted by permission of Sage Publications, Inc.

If a questionnaire is not available, one must be developed. When designing a questionnaire (see Figure 5.2 for steps to follow when developing a data collection instrument) to collect self-reported data, evaluators/planners can use several types of questions. The most structured or closed types of questions have yes-no or multiple-choice responses, and are most often used for knowledge questions. These types of responses are the easiest to tabulate but do not allow the individual to elaborate on the answers. They may also force a person into a choice because of the limited number of responses to each question. An "other" category, with space to list the exact nature of the "other" response, may serve to give the respondent another option. However, giving the respondents an opportunity to provide their own answers on multiple-choice questions makes it more difficult to categorize responses when the data are analyzed, thus reducing one of the main benefits of such questions. One way to ensure that the most common responses to questions are included in the multiple choices is to involve several individuals (especially those in the target population) in the formation of the instrument.

Attitude questions generally use less structured forms. Scales, such as Likert or semantic differentials, are often used, with the respondent choosing a response along a continuum, generally ranging from a five- to a seven-point scale. For

FIGURE 5.2   *Steps in the Development of an Instrument*

1. Determine the purpose and objectives of the proposed instrument.
2. Develop instrument specifications.
3. Review existing instruments.
4. Develop new instrument items.
5. Develop directions for administration and examples of how to complete items.
6. Establish procedures used for scoring the instrument.
7. Conduct a preliminary review of the instrument with colleagues.
8. Revise instrument based on review.
9. Pilot test the instrument with twenty to fifty subjects.
10. Conduct item analysis, reliability, and validity studies.
11. Provide instrument specifications and pilot study data to a panel of experts for review.
12. Revise the instrument based on comments from the panel of experts.
13. Determine cut score (for criterion-referenced tests or screening tests).

Source: R. J. McDermott and P. D. Sarvela, *Health Education Evaluation and Measurement: A Practitioner's Perspective,* 2nd ed. (New York: WCB/McGraw-Hill, 1999), p. 96. Reprinted with permission of The McGraw-Hill Companies.

example, responses to the statement, "I feel that it is important to limit my use of salt," might be rated on a five-point scale ranging from "strongly agree" to "strongly disagree" (see examples in Figure 5.3).

Unstructured or open-ended questions—such as essay questions, short-answer questions, journals, or logs—may be used to gain descriptive information about a program, but are generally not used when collecting quantitative data. Such responses are often difficult to summarize or to code for analysis. Figure 5.3 provides examples of structured and unstructured types of questions.

Written Questionnaires.   Probably the most often used method of collecting self-reported data is the written questionnaire. It has several advantages, notably the ability to reach a large number of respondents in a short period of time, even if there is a large geographic area to be covered. This method offers low cost with minimum staff time needed. However, it often has the lowest response rate.

With a written questionnaire, each individual receives the same questions and instructions in the same format, so that the possibility of response bias is less-ened. The corresponding disadvantage, however, is the inability to clarify any questions or confusion on the part of the respondent.

As mentioned, the response rate for mailed questionnaires tends to be low, but there are several ways to overcome this problem. One way is to include with the questionnaire a postcard that identifies the person in some way (such as by name or identification number). The individual is asked to return the questionnaire

FIGURE 5.3 *Examples of Self-Report Questions*

Structured (Closed)

I. *Dichotomous*

    1. What is your gender?

        a. Female   b. Male

    2. A risk factor for heart disease is sedentary lifestyle.

        a. True   b. False

II. *Multiple Choice*

    1. The leading cause of death in the United States for adults is

        a. Cancer   b. Heart disease

        c. Injuries   d. AIDS

    2. What type of computer do you use?

        a. IBM   b. Macintosh

        c. Gateway   d. Other (please specify) _____

III. *Matching*

Vitamin deficiencies

      1. Vitamin A   a. Frequent infection

      2. Vitamin C   b. Slow blood clotting

      3. Vitamin D   c. Night blindness

      4. Vitamin K   d. Bone softening

Grams of saturated fats

      1. Butter, 1 tbsp.   a. 9

      2. Ice cream, 4 oz.   b. 7.1

      3. Chicken, 3 oz.   c. 5

      4. One hot dog   d. 1.2

Less Structured (But Still Closed)

I. *Likert*

	Strongly agree	Agree	Neutral	Disagree	Strongly disagree
1. Women should be able to have an abortion if they choose to do so.	Strongly agree	Agree	Neutral	Disagree	Strongly disagree
2. I feel I can exercise regardless of weather conditions.	Strongly agree	Agree	Neutral	Disagree	Strongly disagree

II. *Semantic Differentials*

    1. Smokeless tobacco is   Good ___ ___ ___ ___ ___ Bad

    2. When taking a test, I feel   Nervous ___ ___ ___ ___ ___ Calm

(continued)

FIGURE 5.3 Continued

III. Rank Order

1. Put the following values in order, from most important in your life to least important:

a. health   _____   d. emotional security   _____

b. love   _____   e. financial security   _____

c. friendship   _____

2. Rank-order the following servings of foods from highest to lowest sources of protein:

a. tuna   _____   d. cottage cheese   _____

b. rice   _____   e. bread   _____

c. sirloin steak   _____   f. broccoli   _____

Unstructured (Open)

I. *Completions*

1. I like to exercise because _____

2. The types of foods I generally eat are _____

II. *Short-answer*

1. List five advantages to conducting a worksite health promotion program.

2. Describe the correct way to lift a heavy object to avoid straining your back.

III. *Essay*

1. Explain the difference between aerobic and anaerobic exercise. Include examples of each type of exercise, and discuss the importance of each in total fitness.

2. Discuss the incidence of tuberculosis in the world today, including who is at risk and the public health measures to reduce the problem.

---

in the envelope provided and to send the postcard back separately. Anonymity is thus maintained, but the planner/evaluator knows who returned a questionnaire. The planner/evaluator can then send a follow-up mailing (including a letter indicating the importance of a response and another copy of the questionnaire with a return envelope) to the individuals who did not return a postcard from the first mailing. The use of incentives also can increase the response rate. For example, some hospitals offer free health risk appraisals to those who return a completed needs assessment instrument.

Another way to overcome the drawback of a low response rate from a mailed questionnaire is to use this method for a homogeneous group (i.e., one composed of similar individuals). The problem of underrepresentation of certain types of individuals may still occur, but if the group is homogeneous in, for example, age or health behaviors, the likelihood that the missing data will be different from the data collected is much less.

The appearance of the questionnaire is extremely important. It should be attractive, be easy to read, and offer ample space for the respondent's answers. It should also be easy to understand and complete, since written questionnaires provide no opportunity to clarify a point while the respondent is completing the questionnaire. All mailed questionnaires should be accompanied by a cover letter, as previously discussed.

Short questionnaires that do not take a long time to complete and questionnaires that clearly explain the need for the information are more likely to be returned. Planners/evaluators should give thought to designing a questionnaire that is as easy to complete and return as possible.

Telephone Interviews.   Compared to mailed surveys or face-to-face interviews, the telephone interview offers a relatively easy method of collecting self-reported data at a moderate cost. The planner/evaluator must choose a way of selecting individuals to participate in this type of data collection; this method will reach only those individuals who have access to a telephone. One possibility is to call a randomly selected group of people who have completed a health promotion program. Another method is to select telephone numbers at random from a telephone directory—for example, a local telephone book, student directory, church directory, or employee directory. This method will not reach all the population, since some people have unlisted telephone numbers. One way to overcome this problem is a method known as **random-digit dialing,** in which telephone number combinations are chosen at random. This method would include businesses as well as residences and nonworking as well as valid numbers, making it more time consuming. The numbers may be obtained from a table of random numbers or generated by a computer. The advantage of random-digit dialing is that it includes all the survey population with a telephone in the area, including people with unlisted numbers. Drawbacks to this method include some people's resistance to answer questions over the telephone or resentment in being interrupted with an unwanted call. This later reason seems to becoming more of a problem with the increase in telemarketing. Those conducting the interviews may also have difficulty reaching individuals because of unanswered phones or answering machines.

Telephone interviewing requires trained interviewers; without proper training and use of a standardized questionnaire, the interviewer may not be consistent during the interview. Explaining a question or offering additional information can cause a respondent to change an initial response, thus creating a chance for interviewer bias. The interviewer does have the opportunity to clarify questions, which is an advantage over the written questionnaire, but does not have the advantage of visual cues that the face-to-face interview offers.

Face-to-Face (or In-Depth) Interviews.   At times, it is advantageous to administer the instrument to the respondents in a face-to-face interview setting. This method is time consuming, since it may require not only time for the actual interview but also travel time to the interview site and/or waiting time between interviews. As with telephone interviews, the interviewer must be carefully trained to conduct the interview in an unbiased manner. It is important to explain the need for the information in order to conduct the evaluation and to accurately record the responses. Methods of probing, or eliciting additional information about an individual's responses, are used in the face-to-face interview, and the interviewer must be skilled at this technique.

This method of self-report allows the interviewer to develop rapport with the respondent. The flexibility of this method, along with the availability of visual cues, has the advantage of gaining more complete evaluation data from respondents. Smaller numbers of respondents are included in this method, but the rate of participation is generally high. It is important to establish and follow procedures for selecting the respondents. There are also several disadvantages to the face-to-face interview. It is more expensive, requiring more staff time and training of interviewers. Variations in the interviews, as well as differences between interviewers, may influence the results.

Email Interviews.   With more and more individuals having access to the Internet, email has been explored (Kittleson, 1995, 1997) as a means of collecting data. Advantages to this type of data collection is that it is low in cost and almost instantaneous (McDermott & Sarvela, 1999). However, it has several drawbacks, including (1) access to a limited population, (2) lack of anonymity for respondents, and (3) and easily ignored (McDermott & Sarvela, 1999). Until the drawbacks are overcome, this means of data collection will be used sparingly.

Group Interviews.   Interviewing individuals in groups provides for economy of scale. That is, data can be collected from several people in a short period of time. But there are some drawbacks of such data collection that primarily revolve around one or more group members influencing the response of others. A specific form of group interview discussed in the previous chapter is focus groups. Focus groups are useful in collecting information for a needs assessment, but can also be used to determine if programs are being implemented effectively or determine program outcomes.

Direct Observation

Observation can be used to obtain information regarding the behavior of participants in a program. The observation can be direct or indirect. *Direct observation* means actually seeing a situation or behavior. For example, planners/evaluators might observe students in the cafeteria to gain information about actual food choices and consumption. This method is somewhat time consuming, but it seldom encounters the problem of people refusing to participate in the data collection, resulting in a high response rate.

Observation is generally more accurate than self-report, but the presence of the observer may alter the behavior of the people being observed. For example, having someone observe smoking behavior may cause smokers to smoke less out of self-consciousness due to their being under observation, not as a result of the program. Observers must be unobtrusive; conspicuous note taking or recording behavior may bias a needs assessment or evaluation.

Differences among observers may also bias the results, since different observers may not observe and report behaviors in the same manner. Some behaviors, such as safety belt use, are very easy to observe accurately. Others, such as degree of tension, are more difficult to observe. This method of data collection requires a clear definition of the exact behavior to observe and how to record it, in order to avoid subjective observations. Observer bias can be reduced by providing training and by determining rater reliability. If the observers are skilled, observation can provide accurate evaluation data at a moderate cost.

Indirect observation methods or proxy measures can also be used to determine whether a behavior has occurred. Examples of indirect methods include measuring weight loss (indirect measure of dieting and exercise) and monitoring blood pressure (indirect measure of medication compliance). These measures can be used to verify self-reports when observations of the actual changes in behavior cannot be observed.

Existing Records

Using existing records may be an efficient way to obtain the necessary information for a needs assessment or evaluation without the need for additional data collection. The advantages include low cost, minimum staff needed, and ease in randomization. The disadvantages to using this method of data collection include difficulty in gaining access to necessary records and the possible lack of availability of all the information needed for program evaluation.

Examples of the use of existing records include checking physician records to monitor blood pressure and cholesterol levels of participants in an exercise program, reviewing insurance usage of employees enrolled in an employee health promotion program, and comparing the academic records of students engaging in an after-school weight loss program. In these situations, as with all needs assessments or evaluations using existing records, the cooperation of the agencies that hold the records is essential. At times, agencies may be willing to collect additional information to aid in the needs assessment for or an evaluation of a health promotion program. Keepers of records are concerned about confidentiality and the release of private information. Planners/evaluators can deal with this by getting permission from all participants in the evaluation to use their records or by using only anonymous data.

Meetings

Meetings are a good source of information for a preliminary needs assessment or various aspects of evaluation. For example, if a fitness program is being evaluated, the evaluators, staff, and some participants may meet early in the planning and implementation stages to discuss the status of the program.

The meeting structure can be flexible to avoid limiting the scope of the information gained. The cost of this form of data collection is minimal. Possible biases may occur when meetings are used as the sole source of data collection. Those involved may give "socially acceptable" responses to questions rather than discussing actual concerns. There also may be limited input if relatively few participants are included, or if one or two participants dominate the discussion.

Summarized in Table 5.1 are the advantages and disadvantages of the various methods of data collection. As discussed in Chapter 14, it may be beneficial to combine methods of data collection as well as to incorporate quantitative and qualitative data.

Sampling

The need to select participants from whom data will be collected can occur at several times during the processes of program planning or evaluation. Depending on the size of the target population, planners/evaluators may want to collect data from all participants **(census)** or from only some of the participants **(sample).**

Figure 5.4 illustrates the relationship between groups of individuals. All individuals, unspecified by time or place, constitute the universe—for example, all U.S. citizens, regardless of where they reside in the world. Within the universe is a population of individuals specified by time or place, such as all U.S. residents in the 50 United States on January 1, 2001. Within this population is a **survey population,** composed of all individuals who can be contacted. The key term here is *accessible.* For example, all U.S. citizens who are accessible and can be reached by telephone would be a survey population. Obviously, this would not include those without telephones, such as those who chose not to own them, those institutionalized, and the homeless.

A survey population may still be too large to include in its entirety. For this reason, a sample is chosen from the survey population, a process called **sampling.** These are the individuals who will be included in the data collection process. Using a sample rather than an entire survey population helps contain costs. For example, using a sample reduces the amount of staff time needed to conduct interviews, the cost of postage for written questionnaires, and the time and cost of travel to conduct observations.

How the sample is chosen is critical to the result of the needs assessment or evaluation: Does the information gained from the sample reflect the knowledge, attitudes, and behaviors of the population? According to Green and Lewis (1986), the sampling bias is the difference between the sampling estimate and the actual population value. The sampling bias can be controlled by controlling the sampling procedure—that is, how the sample is chosen. The ability to generalize the results to the population is greater when the sampling bias is reduced.

Probability Sample

Increasing the chance that the sample is representative of the population is achieved by **randomization.** This assures that each person in the survey population has an equal chance and known probability of being selected, thus creating a **probability sample.** A **simple random sample** can be obtained by taking a list of all participants **(frame)** and choosing the sample by following a table of random numbers (see Table 5.2), giving each individual an equal chance of being selected.

TABLE 5.1 *Methods of Data Collection*

Method	Advantages	Disadvantages
Self-Report		
Written questionnaire via mail	Large outreach	Possible low response rate
	No interviewer bias	Possible unrepresentation
	Convenient	No clarification of questions
	Low cost	Need homogeneous group if response is low
	Minimum staff time required	
	Easy to administer	No assurance addressee was respondent
	Quick	
	Standardized	
Telephone interview	Moderate cost	Possible problem of representation
	Relatively easy to administer	Possible interviewer bias
	Permits unlimited callbacks	Requires trained interviewers
	Can cover wide geographic area	
Face-to-face interview	High response rate	Expensive
	Flexibility	Requires trained interviewers
	Gain in-depth data	Possible interviewer bias
	Develop rapport	Limits sample size
		Time consuming
*Electronic mail**	Low cost	Must have email access
	Ease and convenience	Self-selection
	Almost instantaneous	Lacks anonymity
		Risk of being "purged"
		Lack of "cueing"
		Must be short
		Noninvasive items only
Group interview	High response rate	May intimidate and suppress individual differences
	Efficient and economical	Fosters conformity
	Can stimulate productivity of others	Group pressure may influence responses
Observation	Accurate behavioral data	Requires trained observers
	Can be unobtrusive	May bias behavior
	Moderate cost	Possible observer bias
		May be time consuming

(continued)

TABLE 5.1   Continued

Method	Advantages	Disadvantages
Existing Records	Low cost	May need agency cooperation
	Easy to randomize	Certain data may be unavailable
	Avoid data collection	Often incomplete
	Minimum staff needed	Confidential restrictions
Meetings	Good for formative evaluation	Possible result bias
	Low cost	Limited input from participants
	Flexible	

*From McDermott and Sarvela (1999).

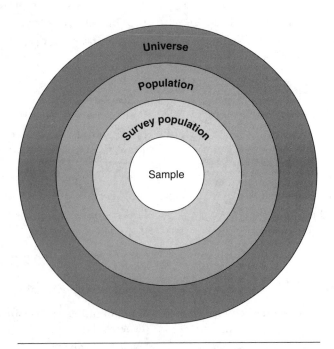

FIGURE 5.4   *Relationship of Groups of Individuals*

A **systematic sample** also uses a list of participants and takes every Nth person (determined by dividing the population size by the sample size, N/n), beginning with a randomly selected individual. For example, suppose that we want to choose a sample of 10 people from a survey population of 100. We start by randomly choosing a number between 001 and 100, such as 026, using a table of random numbers. We then choose every tenth ($N/n = 100/10 = 10$) person (036,

TABLE 5.2   *Abbreviated Table of Random Numbers*

Row/Column	A	B	C	D	E
1	75 51	02 17	71 04	33 93	36 60
2	42 75	76 22	23 87	56 54	84 68
3	00 47	37 59	08 56	23 81	22 42
4	74 01	23 19	55 59	79 09	69 82
5	66 22	42 40	15 96	74 90	75 89
6	09 24	34 42	00 68	72 10	71 37
7	89 22	10 23	62 65	78 77	47 33
8	51 27	23 02	13 92	44 13	96 51
9	17 18	01 34	10 98	37 48	93 86
10	02 28	54 60	01 11	28 35	54 32

046, 056, 076, 086, 096, 006, 016) until we have the 10 subjects for the sample. In this way, everyone in the survey population has an equal chance of being selected. A simple random sample or systematic sample can also be used to select groups instead of individuals. When this occurs, it is called **cluster sampling.**

If it is important that certain groups should all be represented in a sample, a **stratified random sample** can be obtained. For example, if representatives from all age groups are needed, a predetermined number from each age group would be randomly chosen. The predetermined number is based on representation. For example, if the evaluator is selecting 100 out of a population of 1,000 college students (1 in 10), it may be important to ensure that all class ranks are represented. If 400 of the students are freshmen, 300 sophomores, 200 juniors, and 100 seniors, then the representative sample would contain 1 in 10 of each of those subgroups: 40 freshmen, 30 sophomores, 20 juniors, and 10 seniors. Within each class rank, the appropriate number of students would be randomly selected. (See Figure 5.5 for a summary of probability sampling procedures.)

Nonprobability Sample

There are times when a probability sample cannot be obtained or is not needed. In such cases, planners/evaluators can take **nonprobability samples,** samples in which all individuals in the survey population did not have an equal chance and a known probability of being selected to participate in the needs assessment or evaluation. Participants can be included on the basis of convenience (because they have volunteered or because they are available or can be easily contacted) or because they have a certain characteristic.

Nonprobability samples have limitations in the extent to which the results can be generalized to the total survey population. Bias may also occur since those

FIGURE 5.5   *Summary of Probability Sampling Procedures*

Sample	Primary Descriptive Elements
Simple Random	Each subject has an equal chance of being selected if table of random numbers is used.
"Fishbowl" (or "Out of a Hat")	Approximates simple random sampling, but not as precise. Can be done with or without replacement.
Systematic	Using a list (e.g., membership list or telephone book), subjects are selected at a constant interval (N/n) after a random start.
Nonproportional Stratified	The population is divided into subgroups based on key characteristics (strata), and subjects are selected from the subgroups at random to ensure representation of the characteristic.
Proportional Stratified	Like the stratified random sample, but subjects are selected in proportion to the numerical strength of strata in the population.
Cluster or Area	Random sampling of groups (e.g., teachers' classes) or areas (e.g., city blocks) instead of individuals.
Matrix	The responses of several randomly selected subjects to different items are combined to form the response of one.

Source: Adapted from E. R. Babbie, *The Practice of Social Research,* 6th ed. (Belmont, CA: Wadsworth, 1992); P. C. Cozby, *Methods in Behavioral Research,* 3rd ed. (Palo Alto, CA: Mayfield, 1985); P. D. Leedy, *Practical Research: Planning and Design,* 5th ed. (New York: Macmillan, 1993); and R. J. McDermott and P. D. Sarvela, *Health Education Evaluation and Measurement: A Practitioner's Perspective,* 2nd ed. (New York: McGraw-Hill, 1999).

who are not included in the sample may differ in some way from those who are included. For example, including only the individuals who complete a health promotion program may bias the results; the findings might be different if all participants, including those who attended but did not complete the program, were surveyed.

Nonprobability samples can be used when planners/evaluators are unable to identify or contact all those in the survey population. These samples can also be used when resources are limited and a probability sample is too costly or time-consuming. It is important that planners/evaluators understand the limitations of this type of sample when reporting the results. (See Figure 5.6 for a summary of nonprobability sampling procedures.)

Sample Size

How many individuals to include in the sample is difficult to determine. Green and Lewis (1986) give guidelines for determining the sample size, with the objective being to obtain the highest level of precision for a given cost. *Precision* refers to

FIGURE 5.6 *Summary of Nonprobability Sampling Procedures*

Sample	Primary Descriptive Elements
Convenience	Includes any available subject meeting some minimum criterion usually being part of an accessible intact group.
Volunteer	Includes any subject motivated enough to self-select for a study.
Grab	Includes whomever investigators can access through direct contact, usually for interviews.
Homogeneous	Includes individuals chosen because of a unique trait or factor they possess.
Judgmental	Includes subjects whom the investigator judges to be "typical" of individuals possessing a given trait.
Snowball	Includes subjects identified by investigators, and any other persons referred by initial subjects.
Quota	Includes subjects chosen in approximate proportion to the population traits they are to "represent."

Source: R. J. McDermott & P. D. Sarvela, *Health Education Evaluation and Measurement: A Practitioner's Perspective,* 2nd ed. (New York: McGraw-Hill, 1999). Reprinted with permission of The McGraw-Hill Companies.

how accurately the sample values **(statistics)** reflect the actual values **(parameters)** in the population. Another consideration is variability in the survey population: The greater the differences among the survey population, the larger the sample size needed.

Additional guidelines refer to the sampling method selected, with stratified random sampling offering the greatest level of precision for a given cost. The cost of the evaluation is also a consideration in determining whether a desired sample size is affordable. Planners/evaluators can choose actual numbers of participants with the help of statistics textbooks, giving consideration to statistical power and level of statistical significance.

Pilot Test

A **pilot test** (sometimes referred to as *piloting* or a *pilot study*) is a set of procedures used by planners/evaluators to try out various processes during program development on a small group of subjects prior to actual implementation. In other words, a pilot test can be thought of as a dress rehearsal for planners/evaluators (McDermott & Sarvela, 1999). The purpose of using pilot tests is to identify and, if necessary, correct any problems prior to implementation with the target population.

Thus, pilot tests permit a thorough check of all planned processes to help increase the chances of having a successful program. Throughout the program development process, planners/evaluators may use pilot tests to detect any problems with sampling, data collection instruments, data collection procedures, data analysis procedures, interventions, curricula, and program evaluation (McDermott & Sarvela, 1999). Since this chapter has focused on data collection, the remaining portions of this discussion will focus on the pilot testing of data collection. Pilot testing will also be discussed in Chapter 12, as it relates to the implementation of a program.

Once the data collection method has been determined and the data collection instrument has been selected or created, a trial run of the instrument, data collection procedures, and analyses should be conducted. During the piloting process, it would not be uncommon for the planners/evaluators to find problems, such as ambiguous questions, difficulty with code sheets, and misunderstood directions. Further, the data collected in the pilot test should be statistically analyzed or compiled to make sure that there is no difficulty with this step in the data collection process. Revising the data collection process using the information gained from the pilot test helps ensure that the actual data collection will proceed smoothly.

Several authors (Borg & Gall, 1989; McDermott & Sarvela, 1999; Parkinson and Associates, 1982; Stacy, 1987) have suggested processes for pilot testing. They have been combined here into a single process. Several of the preceding authors have presented hierarchies for pilot testing: preliminary review, prepilot, pilot tests, and field tests. The first, and lowest, level in the piloting hierarchy is a preliminary review. A **preliminary review** is conducted when those responsible for the data collection process ask colleagues, not people from the target population, to review the data collection instrument. At a minimum, all data collection instruments should be subjected to this type of review. Specifically, in a preliminary review, colleagues would be asked to complete the instrument as if they were subjects in hopes of identifying problems, and also respond to several other questions about the instrument, such as the appropriateness of (1) the instrument's title, (2) the introductory statement explaining the purpose of the data collection, (3) the directions, (4) the order or grouping of the questions, (5) the questions (unclear or too personal), (6) the length of the instrument, and (7) the method of returning the instrument, to name a few. **Prepilots** (or **mini-pilots**) are used by planners/evaluators with five or six target subjects to assess the quality of materials, instruments, and data collection techniques. Methods used to collect this information include observations, interviews, and focus groups. The **pilot test** requires the actual implementation of the instrument. A representative sample of the target population is used to determine the quality of the instrument. A **field study** is a final pilot test, combining all materials previously tested separately (e.g., instrument, curriculum materials) into a complete program. If enough subjects are used during the field study, it may be possible to check the validity and reliability of the instrument. If at all possible, the use of this sequence of piloting techniques is desirable, but planners/evaluators are often limited by time and resources, and so not all the steps can be completed.

Ethical Issues Associated with Data Collection

Several ethical issues should be considered when collecting data. Weiss (1998) begins a discussion of these issues with the need for voluntary participation by the respondents. Planners/evaluators should make it clear to the respondents that they have the opportunity to decline to participate without penalty. A second issue is that of private and/or sensitive data. If planners/evaluators need to ask questions that reveal private and sensitive data, they need to ensure anonymity or not report results that could identify a given individual. During data collection, planners/evaluators may hear about illegal acts, such as drug use or other crimes, or the data collectors may be provided with access to confidential data. The planners/evaluators must consider the ethical issues and the legal ramifications of such issues. Weiss (1998) advises checking out state and national laws, and discussing these ethical situations with knowledgeable colleagues.

Summary

This chapter focused on helping you understand the terms measurement, measures, data collection, and sampling. A brief overview of measurement and measures was provided, along with the four levels of measurement: nominal, ordinal, interval, and ratio. Several different examples of questions used at each of the levels were also presented. Next, four desirable characteristics of data were discussed, including reliability, validity, unbiased, and culturally appropriate. With this background information, you were introduced to the primary means of data collection, mainly self-report, observation, existing records, and meetings. This was followed by a discussion of techniques used to draw the various probability and nonprobability samples, and when the various sampling techniques might be most useful. The chapter concluded with a short presentation on the importance of using a pilot test and ethical issues associated with data collection.

Questions

1. What is meant by *measurement,* and *qualitative and quantitative measures?*

2. Describe each method of data collection (self-report, direct observation, existing data, and meetings), and list two advantages and disadvantages of each.

3. Name and give an example of each of the four levels of measurement.

4. What are the advantages and disadvantages of using an existing data collection instrument?

5. What is validity? What is reliability? Why are they so important?

6. What is bias in data collection? Name three ways in which it can be reduced.

7. Why must data collection instruments be culturally appropriate?

8. How does an evaluator determine who will participate in the data collection?

9. Describe three types of probability samples.

10. When, if ever, should nonprobability samples be used?

11. What is the purpose of a preliminary review, a prepilot (or mini-pilot), a pilot test, and a field study? How is each conducted?

12. What ethical issues should be considered when collecting data?

Activities

1. Construct a three-page written questionnaire on a health promotion topic of your choice that could be administered to a group of college students.

2. Conduct a prepilot test on your written questionnaire developed in activity number 1 on five or six of your friends, colleagues, or classmates. After the pilot test, identify any flaws you see in the questionnaire or data collection process.

3. Assume that you are charged with the responsibility of collecting data from all the students on your campus who have enrolled in a fitness course. Assume also that this group of students is too large to collect data from everyone. Explain how you would obtain a representative sample from this population.

4. Visit a survey research center on your campus or in your community. Ask about the methods of data collection, and if possible arrange to observe a face-to-face or telephone interview. Write a two-page paper describing your reaction to this experience.

5. Review a needs assessment or evaluation instrument. Identify the level of measurement for the questions, types of measurement, and the types of question.

6. Photocopy a page from a local telephone book. Let's assume that this page represents a sampling frame for your target population. Go through the frame and divide it into groups of 10 by using the first 10 numbers as group 1, the second 10 as group 2, and so on, until all the numbers are used. Be sure you do not use fax or business numbers. If you have an odd number of telephone numbers (not an even 10), do not use that group. With this information, explain how you would select a simple random sample of 20 numbers, a systematic sample of 10 numbers, a stratified sample of 40 numbers stratified on the first 3 numbers of the telephone numbers, and a cluster sample of 10 groups, assuming that the groups of 10s you formed are your clusters.

Activities on the Web

1. Visit the website for the Association of State and Territorial Health Officials that link to the state/territorial page <**http://www. astho.org/state.html**>. Select the state or territory of your choice. Once you are in the state health department's home page, select the health data and statistics link. Then locate data from a statewide survey (e.g., BRFSS). Identify what data collection and sampling methods were used in the survey. Print out the pages with the information on them and take them to class.

2. Visit the website for the Division of Adolescent and School Health (DASH) of the Centers for Disease Control and Prevention (CDC) that links to the Youth Risk Behavior Surveillance System (YRBSS) page <**http://**

www.cdc.gov/nccdphp/dash/yrbs/index. htm>. Once there, locate a copy of the most recent YRBS questionnaire. Try to find and print out four questions that are examples of the four levels of measurement: nominal, ordinal, interval, and ratio. Which of the four levels was most difficult to find? Take your work to class.

6

Mission Statement, Goals, and Objectives

After reading this chapter and answering the questions at the end, you should be able to:

- Explain what is meant by the term *mission statement*.
- Define *goals* and *objectives*, and distinguish between the two.
- Identify the different levels of objectives as presented in the chapter.
- State the necessary elements of an objective as presented in the chapter.
- Specify an appropriate criterion for objectives.
- Write program goals and objectives.
- Describe the use for *Healthy People 2010*.

Key Terms

conditions
criterion
goal

mission statement
objectives
outcomes

target population

To plan, implement, and evaluate effective health promotion programs, planners must have a solid foundation in place to guide them through their work. The mission statement, goals, and objectives of a program can provide such a foundation. If prepared properly, a mission statement, goals, and objectives should not only give the necessary direction to a program but also provide the groundwork for the eventual program evaluation. There are two old sayings that help express the need for a mission statement, goals, and objectives. The first is: If you do not know where you are going, then any road will do—and you may end up someplace where you do not want to be, or you may eventually end up where you want to be, but after wasted time and effort. The second is: If you do not know where you are going, how will you know when you have arrived? Without a mission statement, goals, and objectives, a program may lack direction, and at best it will be difficult to evaluate. Figure 6.1 shows the relationship between a mission statement, goals, and objectives.

Mission Statement

Sometimes referred to as a program overview or program aim, a **mission statement** is a short narrative that describes the general focus of the program. The statement not only describes the intent of a program but also may reflect the philosophy behind it. The mission statement also helps to guide program planners in the development of program goals and objectives. Figure 6.2 presents examples of mission statements for several different settings.

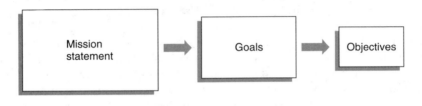

FIGURE 6.1 *Relationship of Mission Statement, Goals, and Objectives*

FIGURE 6.2 *Examples of Mission Statements*

Setting	Mission Statement
Community Setting	The mission of the Walkup Health Promotion Program is to provide a wide variety of primary prevention activities for residents of the community.
Medical Care Setting	This program is aimed at helping patients and their families to understand and cope with physical and emotional changes associated with recovery following cancer surgery.
School Setting	School District #77 wants happy and healthy students. To that end, the district's personnel strives, through a coordinated school health program, to provide students with experiences that are designed to motivate and enable them to maintain and improve their health.
Worksite Setting	The purpose of the employee health promotion program is to develop high employee morale. This is to be accomplished by providing employees with a working environment that is conducive to good health and by providing an opportunity for employees and their families to engage in behavior that will improve and maintain good health.

Program Goals

Although some individuals use the terms *goals* and *objectives* synonymously, they are not the same: There are important differences between them. Ross and Mico (1980, p. 219) have stated that "a goal is a future event toward which a committed endeavor is directed; objectives are the steps to be taken in pursuit of a goal." Deeds (1992, p. 36) defines a goal as a "broad timeless statement of a long-range program purpose," whereas Neiger (1998) defines goals as general statements of intent. In comparison to objectives, a **goal** is an expectation that:

1. Is much more encompassing, or global
2. Is written to include all aspects or components of a program
3. Provides overall direction for a program
4. Is more general in nature
5. Usually takes longer to complete
6. Usually is not observed, but rather must be inferred because it includes words like *evaluate, know, improve,* and *understand* (Jacobsen, Eggen & Kauchak, 1989)
7. Is often not measurable in exact terms

Program goals are not difficult to write and need not be written as complete sentences. They should, however, be simple and concise, and should include two basic components: who will be affected, and what will change as a result of the program. A program need not have a set number of stated goals. It is not uncommon for some programs to have a single goal while others have several. Figure 6.3 presents some examples of goals for health promotion programs.

Objectives

As Ross and Mico (1980) have indicated, **objectives** are more precise and represent smaller steps than program goals—steps that, if completed, will lead to reaching the program goal(s). Objectives outline in measurable terms the specific

FIGURE 6.3 Examples of Program Goals

- To reduce the incidence of cardiovascular disease in the employees of the Smith Company.
- All cases of measles in the City of Kenzington will be eliminated.
- To stop the spread of HIV in the youth of Indiana.
- To reduce the cases of lung cancer caused by exposure to secondhand smoke in Yorktown, IN.
- To reduce the incidence of influenza in the residents of the Delaware County Home.
- The survival rate of breast cancer patients will be raised through the optimal use of community resources.

changes that will occur in the target population at a given point in time as a result of exposure to the program. "Objectives are crucial. They form a fulcrum, converting diagnostic data into program direction" (Green & Kreuter, 1999, p. 106). Objectives can be thought of as the bridge between needs assessment and a planned intervention. Knowing how to construct objectives for a program is a most important skill for program planners.

Different Levels of Objectives

There are several different levels of objectives associated with program planning. The different levels are sequenced or placed in a hierarchical order to allow for more effective planning (Cleary & Neiger, 1988; Deeds, 1992; Parkinson & Associates, 1982). Objectives are created at each level in order to help attain the program goal. The "objectives should also be *coherent* across levels, with objectives becoming successively more refined and more explicit, level by level" (Green & Kreuter, 1999, p. 107). Achievement of the lower-level objectives will contribute to the achievement of the higher-level objectives and goals. Table 6.1 presents the hierarchy of objectives and indicates their relationship to program outcomes and evaluation.

Process/Administrative Objectives. The process/administrative objectives are the daily tasks, activities, and work plans that lead to the accomplishment of all other levels of objectives (Deeds, 1992). They help shape or form the program and thus focus on all program inputs (all that are needed to carry out a program), implementation activities (actual presentation of the program), and stakeholder reactions. More specifically, these objectives would focus on such things as program resources (materials, funds, space); appropriateness of intervention activities; target population exposure, attendance, participation, and feedback; feedback from other stakeholders such as the funding and sponsoring agencies; and data collection techniques, to name a few.

Learning Objectives. The second level of objectives in the hierarchy comprises learning objectives. (*Note:* Cleary and Neiger (1998) have also referred to these objectives as *process/learning objectives.* The authors have chosen to not include the word process, since it may be confused with process/administrative objectives.) They are the educational or learning tools that are needed in order to achieve the desired behavior change. They are based upon the analysis of educational and organizational assessment of the PRECEDE-PROCEED model. They address the predisposing, reinforcing, and enabling factors (Deeds, 1992).

Within this level of objectives, there is another hierarchy (Parkinson & Associates, 1982). This hierarchy includes four types of objectives, beginning with the least complex and moving toward the most complex. Complexity is defined in terms of the time, effort, and resources necessary to accomplish the objective. The learning objectives hierarchy begins with awareness objectives and moves through knowledge, attitude, and skill development or acquisition objectives. This hierarchy indicates that if those in the target population are going to adopt and maintain

TABLE 6.1   *Hierarchy of Objectives and Their Relation to Evaluation*

Type of Objective	Program Outcomes	Possible Evaluation Measures	Type of Evaluation
Process/ Administrative objectives	Activities presented and tasks completed	Number of sessions held, exposure, attendance, participation, staff performance, appropriate materials, adequacy of resources, tasks on schedule	Process (form of formative)
Learning Objectives	Change in awareness, knowledge, attitudes, and skills	Increase in awareness, knowledge, attitudes, and skill development/ acquisition	Impact (form of summative)
Action/Behavioral and Environmental Objectives	Behavior adoption, change in environment	Change in behavior, hazards or barriers removed from the environment	Impact (form of summative)
Program Objectives	Change in quality of life (QOL), health status, or risk, and social benefits	QOL measures, morbidity data, mortality data, measures of risk (i.e., HRA), physiological measures, signs and symptoms.	Outcome (form of summative)

Source: Adapted from Deeds (1992) and Cleary and Neiger (1998).

a health-enhancing behavior to alleviate a health concern or problem, they must first be aware of the health concern. Second, they must expand their knowledge and understanding of the concern. Third, they must attain and maintain an attitude that enables them to deal with the concern. And fourth, they need to possess the necessary skills to engage in the health-enhancing behavior.

Action/Behavioral and Environmental Objectives.   Action/behavioral objectives describe the behaviors or actions in which the target population will engage that will resolve the health problem and move you toward achieving the program goal (Deeds, 1992). Environmental objectives outline the nonbehavioral causes of a health problem that are present in the social, physical, or psychological environment. These objectives are based on the results of the behavioral and environmental assessment of the PRECEDE-PROCEED model or the behavior and environmental changes indicated by the needs assessment of another planning model. Action/behavioral objectives are commonly written about adherence (e.g., regular exercise), compliance (e.g., taking medication as prescribed), consumption patterns (e.g., diet), coping (e.g., stress-reduction activities), preventive actions (e.g., brushing and flossing teeth), self-care (e.g., first aid), and utilization (e.g, appropriate use of the emergency room). Environmental objectives are written about such things as the state of the physical environment (e.g., clean air or water), the social environment (e.g., access to health care), or the psychological environment (e.g., the emotional learning climate).

Program Objectives.   Program objectives are the ultimate objectives of a program and are aimed at changes in health status, social benefits, or quality of life. "They are outcome or future oriented" (Deeds, 1992, p. 36). If these objectives are achieved, then the program goal will be achieved. These objectives are commonly written in terms of reduction of risk, physiologic indicators, sign and symptoms, morbidity, disability, mortality, or quality of life measures.

Developing Objectives

Does every program require objectives from each of the levels just described? The answer is yes! Too often, health promotion programs have too few objectives, all of which fall into one or two levels. Many planners have developed programs hoping solely to change the health behavior of a target population. For example, a smoking cessation program may have an objective of getting 30% of the participants to stop smoking. Perhaps this program is offered, and only 10% of the participants quit smoking. Is the program a failure? If the program has a single objective of changing behavior, its sponsors would have a good case for saying that the program was not effective. However, it is quite possible that as a result of participating in the smoking cessation program, the participants increased their awareness of the dangers of smoking. They probably also increased their knowledge, changed their attitudes, and developed skills for quitting or cutting back on the number of cigarettes they smoke each day. These are all very positive outcomes—and they could be overlooked when the program is evaluated, if the planner did not write objectives that cover a variety of levels.

Criteria for Developing Objectives

In addition to making sure that the objectives are written in an appropriate manner, planners also need to be realistic with regard to the other parameters of the program. These are some of the questions that program planners should consider when writing objectives:

1. Can the objective be realized during the life of the program or within a reasonable time thereafter? It would be quite realistic to assume that a certain number of people will not be smoking one year after they have completed a smoking cessation program, but it would not be realistic to assume that a group of elementary school students could be followed for life to determine how many of them die prematurely due to inactivity.

2. Can the objective realistically be achieved? It is probably realistic to assume that 30% of any smoking cessation class will stop smoking within one year after the program has ended, but it is not realistic to assume that 100% of the employees of a company will participate in its fitness program.
3. Does the program have enough resources (personnel, money, and space) to obtain a specific objective? It would be ideal to be able to reach all individuals in the target population, but generally there are not sufficient resources to do so.
4. Are the objectives consistent with the policies and procedures of the sponsoring agency? It would not be realistic to expect to incorporate a no-smoking policy in a tobacco company.
5. Do the objectives violate any of the rights of those who are involved (participants or planners)? Right-to-know laws make it illegal to withhold information that could cause harm to a target population.
6. If a program is targeted at a particular ethnic/cultural population, do the objectives reflect the relationship between the cultural characteristics of the target group and the changes sought?

Elements of an Objective

For an objective to provide direction and to be useful in the evaluation process, it must be written in such a way that it can be clearly understood, states what is to be accomplished, and is measurable. To ensure that an objective is indeed useful, it should include the following elements:

1. The outcome to be achieved, or what will change.
2. The conditions under which the outcome will be observed, or when the change will occur.
3. The criterion for deciding whether the outcome has been achieved, or how much change.
4. The target population, or who will change.

The first element, the **outcome,** is defined as the action, behavior, or something else that will change as a result of the program. In a written objective, the outcome is usually identified as the verb of the sentence. Thus, words such as *apply, argue, build, compare, demonstrate, evaluate, exhibit, judge, perform, reduce, spend, state,* and *test* would be considered outcomes (see Figure 6.4 for a more comprehensive listing of appropriate outcome words). It should be noted that not all verbs would be considered appropriate outcomes for an objective; the verb must refer to something measurable and observable. Words such as *appreciate, know, internalize,* and *understand* by themselves do not refer to something measurable and observable, and therefore they are not good choices for outcomes.

The second element of an objective is the **conditions** under which the outcome will be observed, or when it will be observed. "Typical" conditions found in

FIGURE 6.4 *Outcome Verbs for Objectives*

abstract	copy	gather (information)	organize	seek
accept	count	generalize	pair	select
adjust	create	generate	participate	separate
adopt	criticize	group	partition	share
advocate	deduce	guess	perform	show
analyze	defend	hypothesize	persist	simplicity
annotate	define	identify	plan	simulate
apply	delay (response)	illustrate	practice	solve
approximate	demonstrate	imitate	praise	sort
argue	derive	improve	predict	spend (money)
(a position)	describe	infer	prepare	state
ask	design	initiate	preserve	structure
associate	determine	inquire	produce	submit
attempt	develop	integrate	propose	subscribe
balance	differentiate	interpolate	prove	substitute
build	discover	interpret	qualify	suggest
calculate	discriminate	invent	query	summarize
categorize	dispute	investigate	question	supply
cause	distinguish	join	recall	support
challenge	effect	judge	recite	symbolize
change	eliminate	justify	recognize	synthesize
choose	enumerate	keep	recommend	tabulate
clarify	estimate	label	record	tally
classify	evaluate	list	reduce	test
collect	examine	locate	regulate	theorize
combine	exemplify	manipulate	reject	translate
compare	exhibit	map	relate	try
complete	experiment	match	reorganize	unite
compute	explain	measure	repeat	visit
conceptualize	express	name	replace	volunteer
connect	extend	obey	represent	weigh
construct	extract	object (to an idea)	reproduce	write
consult	extrapolate	observe	restructure	
contrast	find	offer	round	
convert	form	order	score	

objectives might be "upon completion of the exercise class," "as a result of partici-pation," "by the year 2010," "after reading the pamphlets and brochures," "orally in class," "when asked to respond by the facilitator," "one year after the program," "by May 15th," or "during the class session."

The third element of an objective is the **criterion** for deciding when the outcome has been achieved, or how much change will occur. The purpose of this element is to provide a standard by which the program planners/evaluators can determine if an outcome has been performed in an appropriate and/or successful manner. Examples might include "to no more than 105 per 1,000," "with 100% accuracy," "as presented in the lecture," "300 pamphlets," "according to the criteria developed by the American Heart Association," "95% of the motor vehicle occupants," or "using the technique outlined in the American Cancer Society's pamphlet."

The last element that needs to be included in an objective is mention of the **target population,** or who will change. Examples are "1,000 teachers," "all employees of the company," and "those residing in the Muncie and Bowling Green areas." Figure 6.5 summarizes the key elements in an objective. (See Box 6.1 for examples of objects that would include the four primary components.)

Goals and Objectives for the Nation

A chapter on goals and objectives would not be complete without at least a short discussion of the health goals and objectives of the nation. These goals and objectives have been most helpful to program planners throughout the United States.

The U.S. government is very interested in improving the health status of Americans. It is concerned about individuals and the population as a whole. The country is facing many problems and issues that revolve around health; the cost of ill health is the most obvious. Therefore, for at least some parts of the federal government, there is a goal to improve the health status of the public. Objectives have been developed to guide the work of reaching this goal. Some people have referred to these statements of objectives as the *health plan* or *blueprint of health* for the United States.

The first set of objectives was developed by many health professionals throughout the country; it was published in 1980 under the title *Promoting Health/ Preventing Disease: Objectives for the Nation* (USDHHS, 1980). This volume was divided into three main areas: preventive services, health protection, and health promotion. Each of these contained 5 focus areas, or 15 in all. From these 15 areas came a total of 226 objectives. These objectives, which were based on the data collected for the U.S. Surgeon General's report *Healthy People* (1979), were the basis for health promotion and disease prevention planning during the 1980s.

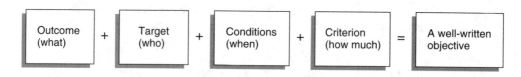

FIGURE 6.5 *Elements of a Well-Written Objective*

BOX 6.1 • *Examples of Objectives to Support the Program Goal "To reduce the amount of heart disease in the residents of Franklin County"*

Process/Administrative Objectives

A. During the next six months, 300 community residents will participate in one of the health department's health promotion activities.
   Outcome (what): Will participate in an activity.
   Target population (who): Community residents.
   Conditions (when): During the next six months.
   Criterion (how much): 300 residents.

B. By August 4, two different heart disease brochures will be distributed to all residences in the county.
   Outcome (what): Will be distributed.
   Target population (who): To all residences.
   Conditions (when): By August 4.
   Criterion (how much): Two different.

C. During the pilot testing, the program facilitators will receive a "good" rating from the program participants.
   Outcome (what): Will receive.
   Target population (who): Program facilitators.
   Conditions (when): During the pilot testing.
   Criterion (how much): "Good" rating.

D. The reading materials will be made available to the program participants 10 days prior to the start of the activity.
   Outcome (what): Materials made available.
   Target population (who): Program participants.
   Conditions (when): Prior to the start.
   Criterion (how much): 10 days prior.

Learning Objectives

A. Awareness level: After the American Heart Association's pamphlet on cardiovascular health risk factors has been placed in grocery bags, at least 20% of the shoppers will be able to identify two of their own risks.
   Outcome (what): Identify their own risks.
   Target population (who): Shoppers.
   Conditions (when): After distribution of the pamphlet.
   Criterion (how much): Two risks.

B. Knowledge level: When asked over the telephone, one out of three viewers of the heart special television show will be able to explain with 100% accuracy the four principles of cardiovascular conditioning.
   Outcome (what): Able to explain.
   Target population (who): Television viewers.
   Conditions (when): When asked over the telephone.
   Criterion (how much): 100% accuracy.

C. Attitude level: During one of the class sessions, the participants will defend two of their reasons for regular exercise.
   Outcome (what): Defend their reasons.
   Target population (who): Class participants.
   Conditions (when): During one of the class sessions.
   Criterion (how much): Two of their reasons.

D. Skill development/acquisition level: After viewing the video "How to Exercise," those participating will be able to locate their pulse and count it every time they are asked to do it.
   Outcome (what): Locate their pulse and count it.
   Target population (who): Those participating.
   Conditions (when): After viewing the video.
   Criterion (how much): Every time.

(continued)

BOX 6.1   Continued

Action/Behavioral and Environmental Objectives

A. One year after the formal exercise classes have been completed, 40% of those who completed 80% of the classes will still be involved in a regular aerobic exercise program.
  Outcome (what): Will still be involved.
  Target population (who): Those who completed 80% of the classes.
  Conditions (when): One year after the classes.
  Criterion (how much): 40%.

B. During the telephone interview follow-up, 50% of the residents will report having had their blood pressure taken during the previous six months.
  Outcome (what): Will report.
  Target population (who): Residents.
  Conditions (when): During the telephone interview follow-up.
  Criterion (how much): 50%.

C. The percentage of household wells checked by the Franklin County Health Department will increase to 95% by the year 2010.
  Outcome (what): Wells checked.
  Target population (who): Household wells.
  Conditions (when): By the year 2010.
  Criterion (how much): 95%.

D. By the end of the year, all senior citizens will be provided transportation to the congregate meals.
  Outcome (what): Provided transportation.
  Target population (who): Senior citizens.
  Conditions (when): By end of year.
  Criterion (how much): All.

Program Objectives

A. By the year 2010, heart disease deaths will be reduced to no more than 100 per 100,000 in the residents of Franklin County.
  Outcome (what): Reduce heart disease deaths.
  Target population (who): Residents of Franklin County.
  Conditions (when): By the year 2010.
  Criterion (how much): To no more than 100 per 100,000.

B. By 2010, increase to at least 25% the proportion of men in Franklin County with hypertension whose blood pressure is under control.
  Outcome (what): Blood pressure under control.
  Target population (who): Men in Franklin County.
  Conditions (when): By 2010.
  Criterion (how much): To at least 25%.

C. Half of all those in the county who complete a regular, aerobic, 12-month exercise program will reduce their "risk age" on their follow-up health risk appraisal by a minimum of two years compared to their preprogram results.
  Outcome (what): Will reduce their "risk age."
  Target population (who): Those who complete an exercise program.
  Conditions (when): After the 12-month exercise program.
  Criterion (how much): Half.

D. Those who participate in a formal exercise and fitness program will use 10% fewer sick days during the life of the program than those who do not participate.
  Outcome (what): Use fewer sick days.
  Target population (who): Those who participate.
  Conditions (when): During the life of the program.
  Criterion (how much): 10% fewer sick days.

Data for 1987 give evidence that nearly half of those objectives had been achieved or were likely to be achieved by 1990, while about a quarter were unlikely to be achieved; the status of the remaining quarter was in doubt because tracking data were not available. Progress was slow for some of the 15 priorities identified in 1980, such as pregnancy and infant health, nutrition, physical fitness and exercise, family planning, sexually transmitted diseases, and occupational safety and health. Substantial progress was made, however, in high blood pressure control, immunization, unintentional injury prevention and control, control of infectious diseases, smoking, and alcohol and drugs (Mason & McGinnis, 1990, p. 442).

As the 1980s came to a close, it was obvious from the evaluation conducted on these national goals and objectives (USDHHS, 1986b) that there was a need to develop new goals and objectives to guide the country through the 1990s. Therefore, a second set of goals and objectives called *Healthy People 2000: National Health Promotion and Disease Prevention Objectives* was developed (USDHHS, 1990a). That set was much more detailed than the first and was much more useful to all program planners. It included fewer goals and more objectives. In addition, subobjectives were established for people with low incomes, people who are members of some racial and ethnic minority groups, and people with disabilities to help meet their unique needs and health problems (USDHHS, 1994).

Just as the 1990 objectives were not all met, neither were the Healthy People 2000 objectives. In the mid-1990s, the U.S. government published *Healthy People 2000: Midcourse and 1995 Revisions* (USDHHS, 1995). That document served as a self-study of progress toward the year 2000 objectives and the beginning point for planning the year 2010 objectives. The context in which the *Healthy People 2010* was framed differed from the 2000 objectives in that planners were working with a broaden scientific base, improved surveillance and data systems, and the knowledge that the public had a heightened awareness and demand for preventive services and quality health care (USDHHS, 1997). In January 2000, the latest version of the objectives for the nation, *Healthy People 2010,* was released (see Figure 6.6). As with previous editions of this work, program planners should become very familiar with this document and consider aligning the goals and objectives of the programs they are planning with the national and spinoff state and territorial documents.

Documents Related to Healthy People 2000 *and* 2010

The importance of the national health promotion disease prevention goals and objectives serving as a blueprint for the health promotion programs of the nation is evidenced by their widespread use. Since the development of *Healthy People* goals and objectives, there have been a number of other documents created that can help planners develop or adopt appropriate objectives for their programs. The

FIGURE 6.6 Healthy People 2010 *Goals and Objectives*

Goals

   I. Increase Quality and Years of Healthy Life

  II. Eliminate Health Disparities

Objectives

   I. Promote Healthy Behaviors

     1. Physical Activity and Fitness

     2. Nutrition/Overweight

     3. Tobacco Use

  II. Promote Healthy Communities

     4. Educational and Community-Based Programs

     5. Environmental Health

     6. Food Safety

     7. Injury/Violence Prevention

     8. Occupational Safety and Health

     9. Oral Health

 III. Improve Systems for Personal and Public Health

    10. Access to Quality Health Services

    11. Family Planning

    12. Maternal, Infant, and Child Health

    13. *Medical Product Safety

    14. Public Health Infrastructure

    15. *Health Communication

 IV. Prevent and Reduce Diseases and Disorders

    16. *Arthritis, Osteoporosis, and Chronic Back Conditions

    17. Cancer

    18. *Chronic Kidney Disease

    19. Diabetes

    20. *Disability and Secondary Conditions

    21. Heart Disease and Stroke

    22. HIV

    23. Immunization and Infectious Disease

    24. Mental Health and Mental Disorders

    25.* Respiratory Diseases

    26. Sexually Transmitted Diseases

    27. Substance Abuse

    28. *Vision and Hearing

---

*New focus areas

Source: Handout from the Office of Disease Prevention and Health Promotion, U.S. Department of Health and Human Services, Room 738G, Hubert Humphrey Building, 200 Independence Avenue, Washington, DC, 1999.

most notable is *Healthy Communities 2000: Model Standards.* It was jointly prepared by the American Public Health Association, American Society of State and Territorial Health Officers, National Association of County Health Officers, U.S. Conference of Local Health Officers, and the Association of Schools of Public Health (1991), in conjunction with the Centers for Disease Control and Prevention, to assist states and localities in putting the year 2000 objectives into practice. Specifically, this document provided "skeleton" objectives for each of the priority areas in which state and local agencies can create target population specific objectives based on the framework of *Healthy People 2000.* It is assumed a similar document will be developed for *Healthy People 2010.*

The spin-off of the *Healthy People 2000* goals and objectives is apparent in several other documents, as well. Individual states have taken the national objectives and created similar documents specific to their own residents. As of July 1997, 44 states, the District of Columbia, and Guam had all developed their own *Healthy People* plans. In addition, a 1993 survey by the National Association of County and City Health Officials showed that 70% of the local health departments used *Healthy People 2000* objectives in their local planning (USDHHS, 1997). Other organizations have taken similar steps to make the national objectives appropriate for their target populations, including the American Association of School Administrators (AASA, 1990), the American College Health Association (ACHA, no date), the American Indian Health Care Association (AIHCA, no date), and the National Dairy Council (NDC, 1992).

The national goals and objectives have been important components in the process of health promotion planning since 1980. It is highly recommended that planners review these objectives before developing goals and objectives for programs. The national objectives may be helpful in providing a rationale for a program and in focusing program goals and objectives toward the areas of greatest need, as planners work toward the year 2010.

Summary

The mission statement provides an overview of a program and is most useful in the development of goals and objectives. The terms *goals* and *objectives* are sometimes used synonymously, but they are quite different. Together, the two provide a foundation for program planning and evaluation. Goals are more global in nature and often are not measurable in exact terms, whereas objectives are more specific and consist of the steps used to reach the program goals. Program objectives can and should be written for several different levels. For objectives to be useful, they should be written so as to be observable and measurable. At a minimum, an objective should include the following elements: a stated outcome (what), conditions under which the outcome will be observed (when), a criterion for considering that the outcome has been achieved (how much), and mention of the target population (who). As planners develop their goals and objectives for their programs, they should find the *Healthy People 2010* objectives very useful.

Questions

1. Why is a mission statement important?

2. What is (are) the difference(s) between a goal and an objective?

3. What is the purpose of program goals and objectives?

4. What are the different levels of objectives?

5. What are the necessary elements of an objective?

6. What are the goals and objectives for the nation? How can they be used by program planners?

Activities

1. Write a mission statement, a goal, and supporting objectives (one at each level) for a program you are planning.

2. Identify which of the following objectives include all four elements necessary for a complete objective; revise those objectives that do not include all the elements:
   a. After the class on objective writing, the students will know the difference between a goal and an objective.
   b. The students know how a skinfold caliper works.
   c. After completing this chapter, the students will be able to write objectives for each of the levels based on the four elements outlined in the chapter.
   d. Given appropriate instruction, the employees will be able to accurately take blood pressure readings of fellow employees.
   e. Program participants will be able to list the reasons why people do not exercise.

3. Write a mission statement, a goal, and supporting objectives (one at each level) for a workshop on responsible use of alcohol by college students.

Activities on the Web

1. Visit the website for the *Healthy People 2010* **<http://web.health.gov/healthypeople>.** Once at the site, try to identify and print out at least one objective for each of the levels (eight in all) mentioned in this chapter. Take the printout to class.

2. Visit the website for the state or territorial health department where you live. Search the site to determine if your state/territory has a complementary document *Healty People 2010.* If so, download the information about the document and take it to class for discussion.

3. Visit the website for at least one of the following volunteer health organizations. Once at the site, examine the health promotion programs offered by the organization for the purpose of identifying the mission, goal(s), and objectives of the program. Print out this information and take it to class to share:
   American Cancer Society **<http://www.cancer.org/>**
   American Diabetes Association **<http://www.diabetes.org/>**
   American Heart Association **<http://www.americanheart.org/>**
   American Lung Association **<http://www.lungusa.org/>**

7

Theories and Models Commonly Used for Health Promotion Interventions

After reading this chapter and answering the questions at the end, you should be able to:

- Define *theory, model, constructs, concepts,* and *variables.*
- Explain why health promotion interventions should be planned using theoretical frameworks.
- Briefly explain the theories and models identified in the chapter.

Key Terms

action stage
aversive stimulus
behavioral capability
concepts
construct
contemplation
decisional balance
direct reinforcement
ecological perspective
efficacy expectations
emotional-coping responses
expectancies
expectations
field test
health belief model
likelihood of action

locus of control
maintenance
model
negative punishment
negative reinforcement
outcome expectations
perceived barriers
perceived benefits
perceived seriousness
perceived susceptibility
perceived threat
positive punishment
positive reinforcement
precontemplation stage
preparation
process of change

punishment
recidivism
reciprocal determinism
reinforcement
relapse
relapse prevention
self-control
self-efficacy
self-management
self-regulation
stage
temptation
theory
variable
vicarious reinforcement

Whenever there is a discussion about the theoretical bases for health education and health promotion, we often find the terms *theory* and *model* used. Some use the terms correctly, while others either use them synonymously or confuse their meaning. We begin this chapter with a brief explanation of these terms, to establish a common understanding of their meaning.

One of the most frequently quoted definitions of **theory** is one in which Glanz, Lewis, and Rimer (1997) modified an earlier definition written by Kerlinger (1986). It states, "A *theory* is a set of interrelated concepts, definitions, and propositions that presents a *systematic* view of events or situations by specifying relations among variables in order to *explain* and *predict* the events of the situations" (Glanz, Lewis, & Rimer, 1997, p. 21). Green and colleagues (1994, p. 398) have stated, "The role of theory is to untangle and simplify for human comprehension the complexities of nature." In other words, a theory is a systematic arrangement of fundamental principles that provide a basis for explaining certain happenings of life. Hochbaum, Sorenson, and Lorig (1992, p. 298) defined theories in relationship to health education as "tools to help health educators better understand what influences health—relevant individuals, group, and institutional behaviors—and to thereupon plan effective interventions directed at health-beneficial results."

The primary elements of theories are known as **concepts** (Glanz, Lewis, & Rimer, 1997). When a concept has been developed, created, or adopted for use with a specific theory, it is referred to as a **construct** (Kerlinger, 1986). "In other words, constructs are synthesized thoughts of key concepts or specific theories" (Cottrell, Girvan, & McKenzie, 1999, p. 91). The operational (practical use) form of a construct is known as a **variable.** Variables "specify how a construct is to be measured in a specific situation" (Glanz & Rimer, 1995, p. 11).

In comparison, a **model** is a subclass of a theory. "Models draw on a number of theories to help people understand a specific problem in a particular setting or context" (Glanz, Lewis, & Rimer, 1997, p. 24). Unlike theories, models do "not attempt to explain the processes underlying learning, but only to represent them" (Chaplin & Krawiec, 1979, p. 68).

Now consider how these terms are used in practical application. A personal belief is a *concept* that has been shown to relate to various health behaviors. Using a *theory* that includes the concept of personal beliefs helps explain why people fear being trapped in a burning vehicle if they use their safety belts. This personal belief of fear acts as a perceived barrier to safety belt use. Perceived barrier is a part of a specific theory and is referred to here as a *construct.* If a health educator develops a program around a theory to help people overcome this barrier and wear their safety belts, then safety belt use is the *variable* being studied. The health educator realizes that this theory, which emphasizes personal beliefs, will not explain all the reasons why people do not wear safety belts. Thus other theories, which emphasize other concepts (i.e., knowledge, environment, incentives, comfort, convenience, etc.) need to be considered.

Eventually, all of these theories may be combined into a *model* that will explain, at least in part, why people wear safety belts. If a model were a perfect model, it would predict with 100% accuracy who would wear safety belts. Unfortunately, behavior is very complex and there are no perfect models in health education. It is therefore important for health educators to keep revising their models to improve their understanding of health behavior. (Cottrell et al., 1999, p. 91)

Based on these descriptions, it seems logical to think of theories as the backbone of the processes used to plan, implement, and evaluate health promotion interventions. "A theory based approach provides direction and justification for program activities and serves as a basis for processes that are to be incorporated into the health promotion program" (Cowdery et al., 1995, p. 248). For example, developmental theories can be used to ensure that the goals and objectives of programs are consistent with the participants' developmental stages and abilities. Theories also can guide program planners in selecting the types of interventions that are needed to accomplish the stated goals and objectives. Appropriate use of learning and behavioral theories can help to ensure congruence between the planned interventions and expected outcomes. Stated a bit differently, "Theories can provide answers to program developers' questions regarding *why* people aren't already engaging in a desirable behavior of interest, *how* to go about changing their behaviors, and *what* factors to look at when evaluating a program's focus" (van Ryn & Heaney, 1992, p. 326). In addition, theoretical frameworks can alert planners to consider important influences outside the teaching-learning process, such as social support and environment, that have an impact on targeted program outcomes (Parcel, 1983). Models provide the vehicle for applying the theories.

All health promotion interventions should be planned and evaluated based on proven theories. "Theory is not a substitute for professional judgment, but it can assist health educators in professional decision making. Insofar as the application of theory to practice strengthens program justification, promotes the effective and efficient use of resources, and improves accountability, it also assists in establishing professional credibility" (D'Onofrio, 1992, p. 394). However, this is not to say that a theory cannot be modified or expanded to include a logically valid idea or parts of other theories. "In fact, it is well understood that working with a theory has certain disadvantages; one of which is leaving out or ignoring factors that happen not to be theoretically relevant, even though they may be empirically significant" (Jessor & Jessor, 1977).

The importance of theory in planning health promotion interventions is best shown by the large number of health promotion programs that are designed to help facilitate health behavior change in the target population. Getting people to engage in health behavior change is a complicated process that is very difficult under the best of conditions. Without the direction that theories provide, planners can easily waste valuable resources in trying to achieve the desired behavior change. Therefore, program planners should ground their programming process in the theories that have been the foundation of other successful health promotion efforts. An article by Shea and Basch (1990) provides a good review and rationale of the theories behind and the models used in some of the most successful health promotion programs: the North Karelia Project, the Stanford Three Community Study, the Stanford Five-City Project, the Minnesota Heart Health Program, and the Pawtucket Heart Health Program. Table 7.1 summarizes the theories and models used in these programs, based on the information provided by Shea and Basch (1990). As can be

TABLE 7.1   *Theories and Models Used in Five Community-Based Cardiovascular Disease Prevention Programs*

Program	Year Begun	Theories and Models Used
Minnesota Heart Health Program	1980	• Social learning theory[a] • Communication-persuasion model[b] • Model of innovation diffusion[d] • Community development[c] • Problem-behavior theory[a]
North Karelia Project	Late 1950s	• Social learning theory[a] • Theory of reasoned action[a] • Communication-persuasion model[b] • Model of innovation diffusion[d] • Community organization model[c]
Pawtucket Heart Health Program	1980	• Community organization model[c] • Social behavioral community psychology theory[a]
Stanford Five-City Project	1978	• Social learning theory[a] • Theory of reasoned action[a] • Communication-persuasion model[b] • Model of innovation diffusion[d]
Stanford Three Community Study	1972	• Social learning theory[a]

[a] = Discussed in Chapter 7.
[b] = Discussed in Chapter 8.
[c] = Discussed in Chapter 9.
[d] = Discussed in Chapter 11.

seen by the information presented in the table, each of these programs is well grounded in theory.

Essentially, the principles and practices of health education are "derived from the egalitarian spirit and progressive theories of education and the fundamental theories of the behavioral sciences" (National Task Force, 1985, p. vii). The remaining sections of this chapter present an overview of the theories and models that are most often used in planning and evaluating health promotion interventions. As you read about and study the various models and theories, you will find that some express the same general ideas, but employ "a unique vocabulary to articulate the specific factors considered to be important" (Glanz, Lewis, & Rimer, 1997, p. 23).

Behavior Change Theories

Stimulus Response (SR) Theory

One of the theories used to explain and modify behavior today is the stimulus response, or SR, theory (Thorndike, 1898; Watson, 1925; Hall, 1943). This theory reflects the combination of classical conditioning (Pavlov, 1927) and instrumental conditioning (Thorndike, 1898) theories. These early conditioning theories explain learning based on the associations among stimulus, response, and reinforcement (Parcel & Baranowski, 1981; Parcel, 1983). "In simplest terms, the SR theorists believe that learning results from events (termed 'reinforcements') which reduce physiological drives that activate behavior" (Rosenstock, Strecher, & Becker, 1988, p. 175). The behaviorist B. F. Skinner believed that the frequency of a behavior was determined by the reinforcements that followed that behavior.

In Skinner's view, the mere temporal association between a behavior and an immediately following reward is sufficient to increase the probability that the behavior will be repeated. Such behaviors are called *operants*; they operate on the environment to bring about changes resulting in reward or reinforcement (Rosenstock et al., 1988, p. 176). Stated another way, operant behaviors are behaviors that act on the environment to produce consequences. These consequences, in turn, either reinforce or do not reinforce the behavior that preceded.

The consequences of a behavior can come as either **reinforcement** or **punishment.** Individuals can learn from both. Reinforcement has been defined by Skinner (1953) as any event that follows a behavior, which in turn increases the probability that the same behavior will be repeated in the future. Stated differently, reinforcement has "a *strengthening effect* that occurs when operant behaviors have certain consequences" (Nye, 1992, p. 16). Behavior has a greater probability of occurring in the future (1) if reinforcement is frequent and (2) if reinforcement is provided soon after the desired behavior. This immediacy clarifies the relationship between the reinforcement and appropriate behavior (Skinner, 1953). If a behavior is complex in nature, smaller steps working toward the desired behavior with appropriate reinforcement will help to shape the desired behavior. This was found to be true in getting pigeons to play Ping-Pong, and it can be useful in trying to change a complex health behavior like smoking or exercise. While reinforcement will increase the frequency of a behavior, punishment will decrease the frequency of a behavior. However, both reinforcement and punishment can be either positive or negative. The terms *positive* and *negative* in this context do not mean good and bad; rather, *positive* means adding something (effects of the stimulus) to a situation, whereas *negative* means taking something away (removal or reduction of the effects of the stimulus) from the situation.

If individuals act in a certain way to produce a consequence that makes them feel good or that is enjoyable, it is labeled **positive reinforcement.** Examples of this would be an individual who is involved in an exercise program and "feels good" at the end of the workout, or one who participates in a weight loss program and receives verbal encouragement from the facilitator, again making that person "feel good." Stimulus response theorists would note that in both of these situations, the pleasant experiences (internal feelings and verbal encouragement, respectively) occur right after the behavior, which in turn increases the chances that the frequency of the behavior will increase.

While positive reinforcement helps individuals learn by shaping behavior, behavior that avoids punishment is also learned because it reduces the tension that precedes the punishment (Rosenstock et al., 1988). "When this happens, we are being conditioned by *negative reinforcement:* A response is strengthened by the *removal* of something from the situation. In such cases, the 'something' that is removed is referred to as a *negative reinforcer* or *aversive stimulus* (these two phrases are synonymous)" (Nye, 1979, p. 33). A good example of **negative reinforcement** is a weight loss program that requires weekly dues. When participants stop paying dues because they have met their goal weight, this removal of an obligation should increase frequency of the desired behavior (weight maintenance).

Some people think of negative reinforcement as a form of punishment, but it is not. While negative reinforcement increases the likelihood that a behavior will be repeated, punishment typically suppresses behavior. "Skinner suggests two ways in which a response can be punished: by *removing a positive reinforcer* or by *presenting a negative reinforcer* (aversive stimulus) as a consequence of the response" (Nye, 1979, p. 43). Punishment is usually linked to some uncomfortable (physical, mental, or otherwise) experience and decreases the frequency of a behavior. An aversive smoking cessation program that circulates cigarette smoke around those enrolled in the program as they smoke is an example of **positive punishment.** It decreases the frequency of smoking by presenting (adding) a negative reinforcer or **aversive stimulus** (smoke) as a consequence of the response. Examples of **negative punishment** (removing a positive reinforcer) would include not allowing teachers to use the teacher's lounge if they continue to smoke while using it or reducing the health insurance benefits of employees who continue to participate in health-harming behavior such as not wearing a safety belt. Stimulus response theorists would note that taking away the privilege of using the teacher's lounge or enhanced health insurance benefits would cause a decrease in frequency of smoking among the teachers and an increase in the wearing of safety belts, respectively. Figure 7.1 illustrates the relationship between reinforcement and punishment.

Finally, if reinforcement is withheld—or, stating it another way, if the behavior is ignored—the behavior will become less frequent and eventually will not be repeated. Skinner (1953) refers to this as extinction. Teachers frequently use this technique with disruptive children in the classroom. If a child is acting up in class,

		Consequences	
		Positive (adding to)	Negative (taking away)
Behavior	Increase in frequency	Positive reinforcement	Negative reinforcement
	Decrease in frequency	Positive punishment	Negative punishment

FIGURE 7.1   *2 × 2 Table of the Stimulus Response Theory*

the teacher may choose to ignore the behavior in hopes that the nonreinforced behavior will go away.

Social Cognitive Theory (SCT)

The social learning theories (SLT) of Rotter (1954) and Bandura (1977b)—or, as Bandura (1986) relabeled them, the *social cognitive theory (SCT)*—combine SR theory and cognitive theories. Stimulus response theorists emphasize the role of reinforcement in shaping behavior and believe that no "thinking" or "reasoning" is needed to explain behavior. Those who espouse SCT believe that reinforcement is an integral part of learning, but emphasize the role of subjective hypotheses or expectations held by the individual (Rosenstock et al., 1988). In other words, reinforcement contributes to learning, but reinforcement along with an individual's expectations of the consequences of behavior determine the behavior. "Behavior, in this perspective, is a function of the subjective value of an outcome and the subjective probability (or 'expectation') that a particular action will achieve that outcome. Such formulations are generally termed 'value-expectancy' theories" (Rosenstock et al., 1988, p. 176). In brief, SCT describes learning as a reciprocal interaction between the individual's environment, cognitive processes, and behavior (Parcel, 1983). The constructs of the SCT that have been most often used in designing health education/promotion interventions will be presented here.

Parcel and Baranowski (1981) have provided an explanation of several constructs of SCT and health education, starting with reinforcement. As already noted, reinforcement is an important component of SCT. According to SCT, reinforcement can be accomplished in one of three ways: directly, vicariously, or through self-management. An example of **direct reinforcement** is a group facilitator who provides verbal feedback to participants for a job well done. **Vicarious reinforcement** is having the participants observe someone else being reinforced for behaving in an appropriate manner. This is often referred to as *social modeling*. In a system of reinforcement by **self-management,** the participants would keep records of their own behavior, and when the behavior was performed in an appropriate manner, they would reinforce or reward themselves.

In addition to the constructs dealing with reinforcement, SCT has other constructs applicable to health promotion. Although there may be some situations in which more than one construct will be applicable to a learning situation, program planners will find that certain constructs will be more useful than others, depending on the type of learning taking place. Those constructs identified by Parcel and Baranowski (1981) include behavioral capability, expectations, expectancies, self-control, self-efficacy, emotional-coping responses, and reciprocal determinism.

If individuals are to perform specific behaviors, they must know first what the behaviors are and then how to perform them. This is referred to as **behavioral capability.** For example, if people are to exercise aerobically, first they must know that aerobic exercise exists, and second they need to know how to do it properly. Many people begin exercise programs, only to quit within the first six months (Dishman, Sallis, & Orenstein, 1985), and some of those people quit because they do not know how to exercise properly. They know they should exercise, so they decide to run a few miles, have sore muscles the next day, and quit. Skill mastery is very important. The construct of **expectations** refers to the ability of human beings to think and thus to expect certain things to happen in certain situations. For example, if people are enrolled in a weight loss program and follow the directions of the group facilitator, they will expect to lose weight. **Expectancies,** not to be confused with expectations, are the values that individuals place on an expected outcome. If people value an expected outcome, they are more likely to perform the necessary behavior to yield the outcome. Someone who enjoys the feeling of not smoking more than that of smoking is more likely to try to do the things necessary to stop. The construct of **self-control** or **self-regulation** states that individuals may gain control of their own behavior through monitoring and adjusting it (Clark et al., 1992). When helping individuals to change their behavior, it is a common practice to have them monitor their behavior over a period of time, through 24-hour diet or smoking records or exercise diaries, and then to have them reward (reinforce) themselves based upon their monitored performance.

One construct of SCT that has received special attention in health promotion programs is **self-efficacy** (Strecher et al., 1986), which refers to the internal state that individuals experience as "competence" to perform certain desired tasks or behavior. This state is situation specific; that is, someone may be self-efficacious when it comes to aerobic exercise but not so when faced with reducing the amount of fat in her diet. People's competency feelings have been referred to as **efficacy expectations.** Thus, someone who thinks he can exercise on a regular basis no matter what the circumstances has efficacy expectations. Even though people have efficacy expectations, they still may not want to engage in a behavior because they may not think the outcomes of that behavior would be beneficial to them. Stated another way, they may not feel that the reward (reinforcement) of performing the behavior is great enough for them. These beliefs are called **outcome expectations.** For example, in order for a person to quit smoking for health reasons (behavior), she must believe both that she is capable of quitting (efficacy expectation) and that cessation will benefit her health (outcome expectation) (I. M. Rosenstock, personal communication, April 1986). Figure 7.2 (Bandura, 1977b) illustrates efficacy and outcome expectations.

Individuals become self-efficacious in four main ways:

1. Through performance attainments (personal mastery of a task)
2. Through vicarious experience (observing the performance of others)
3. As a result of verbal persuasion (receiving suggestions from others)
4. Through emotional arousal (interpreting one's emotional state)

The construct of **emotional-coping responses** states that for a person to learn, he must be able to deal with the sources of anxiety that may surround a behavior. For example, fear is an emotion that can be involved in learning; according to this construct, participants would have to deal with the fear before they could learn the behavior.

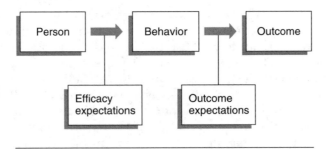

FIGURE 7.2   *Diagrammatic Representation of the Difference between Efficacy and Outcome Expectations*

Source: *Social Learning Theory* by Bandura, Albert, © 1977. Reprinted by permission of Prentice-Hall, Inc., Upper Saddle River, NJ.

The construct of **reciprocal determinism** states, unlike SR theory, that there is an interaction among the person, the behavior, and the environment, and that the person can shape the environment as well as the environment shaping the person. All these relationships are dynamic. Glanz and Rimer (1995, p. 15) provide a good example of this construct:

> A man with high cholesterol might have a hard time following his prescribed low-fat diet because his company cafeteria doesn't offer low-fat food choices that he likes. He can try to change the environment by talking with the cafeteria manager or the company medical or health department staff, and asking that healthy food choices be added to the menu. Or, if employees start to dine elsewhere in order to eat low-fat lunches, the cafeteria may change its menu to maintain its lunch business.

Finally, there is one other construct that grew out of the social learning theory of Rotter (1954) that needs to be mentioned because of its association with health behavior. "Rotter posited that a person's history of positive or negative reinforcement across a variety of situations shapes a belief as to whether or not a person's own actions lead to those reinforcements" (Wallston, 1994, p. 187). Rotter referred to this construct as **locus of control.** Thus, he felt that people with internal locus of control perceived that reinforcement was under their control, whereas those with external locus of control perceived reinforcement to be under the control of some external force. In the 1970s, Wallston and his colleagues at Vanderbilt University began testing the usefulness of this construct in predicting health behavior (Wallston, 1994). They explored the concept of whether individuals with internal locus of control were more likely to participate in health-enhancing behavior than those with external locus of control. They began their work by examining locus of control as a two-dimensional construct (internal vs. external), then moved to a multidimensional construct when they split the external dimension into "powerful others" and "chance" (Wallston, Wallston, & DeVellis, 1978). After a number of years of work by many different researchers, Wallston has come to the conclusion that locus of control accounts for only a small amount of the variability in health behavior (Wallston, 1992). The internal locus of control belief about one's own health status is a necessary but not sufficient determinate of health-enhancing behavior (Wallston, 1994). Since the rise of the construct of self-efficacy, Wallston (1994) feels that self-efficacy is a better predictor of health-promoting behavior than locus of control. This not to say that locus of control is not a useful construct in developing health promotion programs. Knowing the locus of control orientation of those in the target population can provide planners with valuable information when considering social support as part of a planned intervention. Table 7.2 provides a summary of the constructs of the SCT and an example of how each construct might be operationalized.

Theory of Reasoned Action (TRA)

Another theory that has received considerable attention in the literature of health behavior change is Fishbein's *theory of reasoned action (TRA)* (Fishbein & Ajzen, 1975). Like the theories already discussed, this theory was developed to explain not just health behavior but all volitional behaviors. The theories discussed earlier in this chapter were directly concerned with behavior; however, this one provides a framework to study attitudes toward behaviors.

Fishbein and Ajzen distinguish among *attitude, belief, behavioral intention,* and *behavior,* and they present a conceptual framework for the study of the relationship among these four constructs. According to the model, an individual's intention to perform a given behavior is a function of her attitude toward performing the behavior and normative beliefs about what relevant others think she should do, weighted by motivation to comply with those others. Behavioral intention is viewed as a special type of belief and is indicated by the person's subjective perception and report of the probability that she will perform the behavior (Parcel, 1983, p. 41).

In our opinion, this theory has one element that distinguishes it from other theories that try to explain human behavior: This is the construct that deals with the normative beliefs about what relevant others think the person should do. This construct states that individuals' intent to perform a given behavior is dependent partly on their belief that others (individuals or groups) think they should do so, and partly on the fact that they care about what these others think. This construct is often referred to as the *subjective norm.* An example of this construct applied to health promotion is the employee who intends to participate in the company's exercise program because he believes his boss thinks he should engage in exercise. For many behaviors, the relevant others may include a person's parents, spouse, close friends, and coworkers, as well as experts or professionals like physicians or lawyers.

Theory of Planned Behavior (TPB)

The theory of reasoned action has proved to be most successful when dealing with purely volitional behaviors, but complications are encountered when the theory is

TABLE 7.2 *Often-Used Constructs of the Social Cognitive Theory and Examples of Their Application*

Construct	Definition	Example
Behavioral Capability	Knowledge and skills necessary to perform a behavior	If people are going to exercise to perform aerobically, they need to know what it is and how to do it.
Expectations	Beliefs about the likely outcomes of certain behaviors	If people enroll in a weight-loss program, they expect to lose weight.
Expectancies	Values people place on expected outcomes	How important is it to people that they become physically fit?
Locus of Control	Perception of the center of control over reinforcement	Those who feel they have control over reinforcement are said to have internal locus of control. Those who perceive reinforcement under the control of some external force are said to have external locus of control.
Reciprocal Determinism	Behavior changes result from an interaction between the person and the environment; change is bidirectional (Glanz & Rimer, 1995)	Lack of use of vending machines could be a result of the choices within the machine. Notes about the selections from the nonusing consumers to the machine's owners could change the selections and change the behavior of the consumers to that of users.
Reinforcement (directly, vicariously, self-management)	Responses to behaviors that increase the chances of recurrence	Giving verbal encouragement to those who have acted in a healthy manner.
Self-Control or *Self Regulation*	Gaining control over own behavior through monitoring and adjusting it	If clients want to change their eating habits, have them monitor their current eating habits for seven days.
Self-Efficacy	People's confidence in their ability to perform a certain desired task or function	If people are going to engage in a regular exercise program, they must feel they can do it.
Emotional-Coping Response	For people to learn, they must be able to deal with the sources of anxiety that surround a behavior	Fear is an emotion that can be involved in learning, and people would have to deal with it before they could learn a behavior.

Source: Cottrell, Girvan, and McKenzie (1999), p. 109. Reprinted by permission.

applied to behaviors that are not fully under volitional control. A good example of this is a smoker who intends to quit but fails to do so. Even though intent is high, nonmotivational factors—such as lack of requisite opportunities, skills, and resources—could prevent success (Ajzen, 1988).

The *theory of planned behavior (TPB)* (see Figure 7.3) is an extension of the theory of reasoned action that addresses the problem of incomplete volitional control. The major difference between TPB and TRA is the addition of a third, conceptually independent determinant of intention. Like TRA, TPB includes attitude toward the behavior and subjective norm, but it has added the concept of perceived behavioral control. This refers to the perceived ease or difficulty of performing the behavior and is assumed to reflect past experience as well as anticipated impediments and obstacles. As a general rule, the more favorable the attitude and subjective norm with respect to a behavior, and the greater the perceived behavioral control, the stronger should be the individual's intentions to perform the behavior under consideration (Ajzen, 1988, pp. 132–133).

Figure 7.3 illustrates two important features of this theory. First, perceived behavioral control has motivational implications for intentions. That is, without perceived control, intentions could be minimal even if attitudes toward the behav-

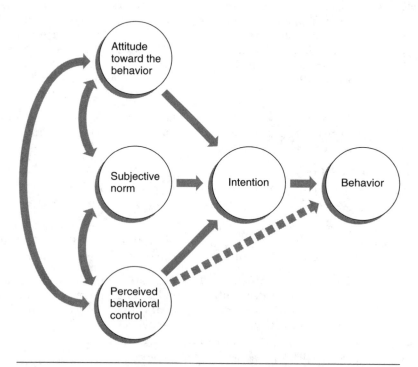

FIGURE 7.3   *Diagram of the Theory of Planned Behavior*

Source: I. Ajzen, *Attitudes, Personality, and Behavior* (Chicago: Dorsey Press, 1988), p. 118. Reprinted by permission.

ior and subjective norm were strong. Second, there may be a direct link between perceived behavioral control and behavior. Behavior depends not only on motivation but also on adequate control. Thus, it stands to reason that perceived behavioral control can help predict goal attainment independent of behavioral intention (Ajzen, 1988). To use the example of smoking once again as a behavior not fully under volitional control, TPB predicts that a person will give up smoking if she:

1. Has a positive attitude toward quitting
2. Thinks others whom she values believe it would be good for her to quit
3. Perceives that she has control over whether she quits

Because the TPB is comparatively new, evidence about its usefulness is just now becoming more common. Godin and Kok (1996) presented a review of 58 studies where the theory was applied to health-related behaviors. They found that the efficiency of the theory seemed "to be quite good for explaining intention, perceived behavioral control being as important as attitude across behavioral categories. The efficiency of the theory, however, varied between health-related behavior categories" (Godin & Kok, 1996, p. 87).

Theory of Freeing (TF)

A theory that takes a much different approach from the other theories presented is the *theory of freeing (TF)* (Freire, 1973, 1974). Like the others, it is not specific to health promotion, but it does have application to health promotion. It is a theory aimed at empowering education. Wallerstein and Bernstein (1988, p. 380) define *empowerment* as "a social action process that promotes participation of people, organizations, and communities in gaining control over their lives in their community and larger society. With this perspective, empowerment is not characterized as achieving power to dominate others, but rather power to act with others to effect change."

The theory was first used in the late 1950s when Paulo Freire, a Brazilian educator, initiated a successful literacy and political consciousness program for shantytown dwellers and peasants in Brazil (Freire, 1973). Since that time, the theory has been applied to many other problems.

One of the first to apply this theory to health promotion was Greenberg. He stated (1978, p. 20) that the task of health education should be to "free people so they may make health-related decisions based upon their needs and interests as long as these needs and interests do not adversely affect others." In essence, Freire's concept of freeing contrasts "being free with being oppressed" (Walker & Bibeau, 1985/1986, p. 5). People become free by being critically conscious.

The underlying concept of this theory is that critical consciousness is determined by the interaction with culture. Consciousness is influenced by and influences the culture. Oppressed people are "of the world," and their consciousness is a product of the culture. Being "of the world" is defined by the lack of the person's ability to perceive, respond, and act with power to change concrete reality (Walker

& Bibeau, 1985/1986). Free people are "in the world," and their consciousness is a producer of culture.

Education is the key to becoming critically conscious. However, the education that is meant here is not education in the traditional sense. Education occurs through dialogue, not through lecture. People who use dialogue are teachers, whereas those who just talk are lecturers. And in this type of education, participants replace pupils. All those involved in the educational process learn from one another.

A very useful summary of the applications of Freire's work to health promotion has been presented by Wallerstein and Bernstein (1988) and Wallerstein (1994). They state that Freire's theory includes three stages. Stage 1 is the listening stage, in which those in the target population have the opportunity to share their thoughts, identify the problems, and set the priorities. Unlike in a more traditional planning process, the program planners do not collect data and determine the needs. Instead, the target population is identifying the issues and prioritizing the needs.

Stage 2 is a dialogue process. The dialogue revolves around a *code.*"A 'code' is a concrete physical representation of an identified community issue in any form: role plays, stories, slides, photographs, songs, etc." (Wallerstein & Bernstein, 1988, p. 383). After experiencing a code, group facilitators lead the target population through a discussion that helps the people move from a personal to a social analysis and action level. They do this by asking the target population to respond to these five statements (Wallerstein & Bernstein, 1988):

1. Describe what you see and feel.
2. As a group, define the many levels of the problem.
3. Share similar experiences from your lives.
4. Question why this problem exists.
5. Develop action plans to address the problem.

Stage 3 of this theory is the action stage, in which those in the target population try out the plans that came from the listening and dialogue stages. As the people put their plans into action, they reflect on their new experiences and create a thinking-acting cycle. "This recurrent spiral of action-reflection-action enables people to learn from their collective attempts at change and to become more deeply involved to surmount the cultural, social, or historic barriers" (Wallerstein & Bernstein, 1988, p. 383).

Problem-Behavior Theory (PBT)

Because many health promotion programs focus on problem behaviors, program planners have found *problem-behavior theory (PBT)* to be a useful framework for guiding program development. This theory rests on the social-psychological relationships that occur within and among the three major systems of personality, perceived environment, and behavior. Each of these systems includes a variety of variables that are interrelated and organized in such a manner as to generate a greater or lesser likelihood of occurrence of problem behavior (Jessor & Jessor, 1977).

The logic and rationale of the original formulation of PBT were presented by Jessor and colleagues (1968), and the present content and structure of the framework were presented in detail by Jessor and Jessor (1977). This later presentation of the theory was based on the study of adolescence and youth in U.S. society in the late 1960s and early 1970s. As such, the theory is designed to account for problem behaviors that organize the daily lives of young people (Jessor & Jessor, 1977). A schematic representation of this theory is presented in Figure 7.4.

The personality system, found in box A of the schematic diagram in Figure 7.4, contains three major structures: motivational-instigation, personal belief, and personal control. The interaction of these three structures determines a person's personality as it relates to a problem behavior. The motivational-instigation structure is concerned with the directional orientation of the action or goals (not directly related to problem behavior) toward which the individual strives and the motivation to begin behaviors to work toward the goals. The greater the value placed on a goal, the greater the likelihood of action directed toward the goal. The personal belief structure deals with the cognitive controls exerted against the occurrence of a problem behavior. There are four variables in this structure: social criticism, alienation, self-esteem, and locus of control. The third structure in this system, personal control, includes variables that are directly linked to the problem behaviors.

The second system in this theory is the perceived environment system (box B), which Jessor and Jessor describe as "the environment that is contributed by the actor from his experience with it" (1977, p. 27). This structure includes both distal variables (those that are remote from the causal chain) and proximal variables (those obviously related to the occurrence of problem behavior). Both types of variables deal with the individual's interactions with friends and parents/family. The distal variables can be thought of as the social content in which a person is located, while the proximal variables determine the degree to which the person is located in the social content.

The third system of the theory is the behavior system, represented by box C. This component contains two major areas: problem behavior and conventional behavior. *Problem behavior* refers to behavior that is undesirable by the norms of society and needs some type of social control, whereas *conventional behavior* includes what are seen as desirable behaviors by society.

Two other boxes (D and E) shown in Figure 7.4 contain antecedent and background variables, mainly demography—social structure and socialization. These variables affect both the personality and perceived environment systems, but the amount of impact is hard to measure.

In applying this theory to health promotion programs, we would refer to a problem behavior as one that is detrimental to good health. This detrimental health behavior is thus related to the personality and perceived environment systems, which in turn are affected by the social structure and socialization of a person. In other words, if a person is an overeater or a nonexerciser, there are many variables that could lead to this behavior and would need to be examined if the behavior is to be changed.

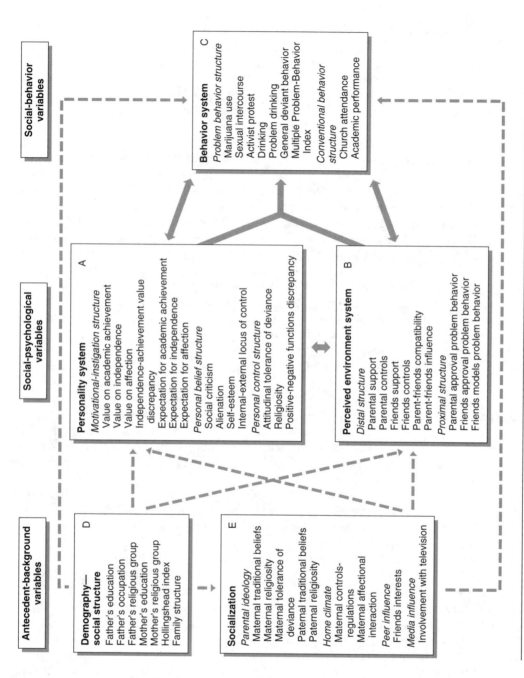

FIGURE 7.4 *Conceptual Structure of Problem-Behavior Theory*

Source: Jessor and Jessor (1977). Reprinted by permission.

Health Behavior Models

Several models have been developed (Becker & Maiman, 1983) to explain the various types of health behavior. Several of these models are based upon parts of theories that have been discussed earlier in this chapter. This section presents the best known of these models, the health belief model and the transtheoretical model. It also presents the cognitive-behavioral model of the relapse process.

Health Belief Model (HBM)

The **health belief model (HBM),** which is the one most frequently used in health behavior applications, was developed in the 1950s by a group of psychologists to help explain why people would or would not use health services (Rosenstock, 1966). The HBM is based on Lewin's decision-making model (Lewin, 1935, 1936; Lewin et al., 1944). Since its creation, the HBM has been used to help explain a variety of health behaviors (Becker, 1974; Janz & Becker, 1984).

The HBM hypothesizes that health-related action depends on the simultaneous occurrence of three classes of factors:

1. The existence of sufficient motivation (or health concern) to make health issues salient or relevant.
2. The belief that one is susceptible (vulnerable) to a serious health problem or to the sequelae of that illness or condition. This is often termed **perceived threat.**
3. The belief that following a particular health recommendation would be beneficial in reducing the perceived threat, and at a subjectively acceptable cost. Cost refers to the **perceived barriers** that must be overcome in order to follow the health recommendation; it includes, but is not restricted to, financial outlays (Rosenstock et al., 1988, p. 177). In fact, the lack of self-efficacy is also seen as a perceived barrier to taking a recommended health action (Strecher & Rosenstock, 1997).

Figure 7.5 provides a diagram of the HBM as presented by Becker, Drachman, and Kirscht (1974).

As noted, the HBM has been applied to all types of health behavior. Here is an example of the HBM applied to exercise. Someone watching television sees an advertisement about exercise. This is a cue to action that starts her thinking about her own need to exercise. There may be some variables (demographic, sociopsychological, and structural) that cause her to think about it a bit more. She remembers her college health course that included information about heart disease and the importance of staying active. She knows she has a higher than normal risk for heart disease because of family history, poor diet, and slightly elevated blood pressure. Therefore, she comes to the conclusion that she is susceptible to heart disease **(perceived susceptibility).** She also knows that if she develops heart disease, it can be very serious **(perceived seriousness**/severity). Based on these factors, the individual thinks that there is reason to be concerned about heart disease

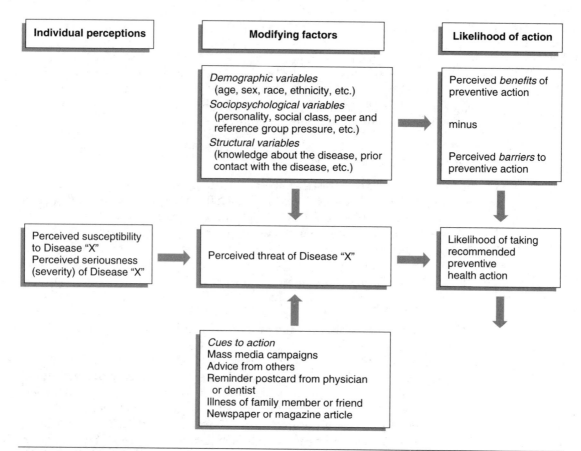

FIGURE 7.5   *The HBM as a Predictor of Preventive Health Behavior*

Source: M. H. Becker, R. H. Drachman, and J. P. Kirscht, "A New Approach to Explaining Sick-Role Behavior in Low Income Populations," *American Journal of Public Health, 64* (March 1974): 205–216. © 1974 American Public Health Association. Reprinted by permission.

(perceived threat). She knows that exercise can help delay the onset of heart disease and can increase the chances of surviving a heart attack if one should occur **(perceived benefits).** But exercise takes time from an already busy day, and it is not easy to exercise in the variety of settings in which she typically finds herself, especially during bad weather **(perceived barriers)**. She must now weigh the threat of the disease against the difference between benefits and barriers. This decision will then result in a likelihood of exercising or not exercising **(likelihood of taking recommended preventive health action).**

The Transtheoretical Model (TTM)

"The Transtheoretical Model is an integrative framework for understanding how individuals and populations progress toward adopting and maintaining health behavior change for optimal health. The Transtheoretical Model uses stages of change to integrate processes and principles of change from across major theories of intervention, hence the name 'Transtheoretical'" (Prochaska, Johnson, & Lee, 1998, p. 59). The model has its roots in psychotherapy and was developed by Prochaska (1979) after he completed a comparative analysis of 18 therapy systems and a critical review of three hundred therapy outcome studies. From the analysis and review, Prochaska found that some common processes were involved in change.

As this model has evolved, researchers have applied it to many different types of health behavior change, including but not limited to contraceptive use (Grimley et al., 1993, 1995), addictive behaviors (Prochaska, DiClemente, & Norcross, 1992), smoking cessation (DiClemente et al., 1991; DiClemente & Prochaska, 1982; Prochaska & DiClemente, 1983; Prochaska et al., 1985; Snow, Prochaska, & Rossi, 1992; Velicer et al., 1995), condom use (Prochaska et al., 1990), alcohol abuse (Norcross, Prochaska, & Hambrecht, 1991), HIV prevention (Prochaska et al., 1994), weight control (Prochaska et al., 1992; Prochaska & DiClemente, 1985), exercise (Cardinal, 1995; Laforge et al., 1999; Marcus et al., 1992; Pinto & Marcus, 1995), stress (Velicer et al., 1998), and dietary fat (Greene et al., 1994).

The core constructs of the transtheoretical model include the stages of change, the processes of change, the pros and cons of changing, self-efficacy, and temptation (see Table 7.3). In addition, this model is "based on critical assumptions about the nature of behavior change and interventions that can best facilitate change" (Prochaska et al., 1998, p. 60). These constructs and assumptions will be discussed next.

Behavioral change does not occur overnight. A person does not go to bed at night as a nonexerciser and wake up the next morning as an exerciser. Behavior change occurs over a period of time. Thus, the **stage** construct is an important part of the transtheoretical model because it represents the temporal dimension of change (Prochaska et al., 1998). The model suggests that "people move from *precontemplation*, not intending to change, to *contemplation*, intending to change within 6 months, to *preparation*, actively planning change, to *action*, overtly making changes, and into *maintenance*, taking steps to sustain change and resist temptation to relapse" (Prochaska et al., 1994). The **precontemplation stage** is defined as a time when people are not seriously thinking about changing their behavior during the next six months. "Many individuals in this stage are unaware or underaware of their problems" (Prochaska, DiClemente, & Norcross, 1992, p. 1103). People in this stage "tend to avoid reading, talking, or thinking about their high-risk behaviors" (Prochaska et al., 1998). The second stage, **contemplation** occurs when people are aware that a problem exists and are seriously thinking about a behavior change but have not yet made a commitment to take action. They are more open to feedback and information about the problem behavior than those in the precontemplation stage (Redding et al., 1999). For example, most smokers know that smoking is bad for them and consider quitting, but are not quite ready to do so. The third stage is called **preparation** and combines intention and behavioral criteria. "Individuals in this stage are intending to take action in the next month and have unsuccessfully taken action in the past year" (Prochaska, DiClemente, & Norcross, 1992, p. 1104). In this stage, they may have taken some

TABLE 7.3   *Transtheoretical Model Constructs*

Constructs	Description
Stages of Change	
Precontemplation	No intention to take action within the next 6 months
Contemplation	Intends to take action within the next 6 months
Preparation	Intends to take action within the next 30 days and has taken some behavioral steps in this direction
Action	Has changed overt behavior for less than 6 months
Maintenance	Has changed overt behavior for more than 6 months
Decisional Balance	
Pros	The benefits of changing
Cons	The costs of changing
Self-Efficacy	
Confidence	Confidence that one can engage in the healthy behavior across different challenging situations
Temptation	Temptation to engage in the unhealthy behavior across different challenging situations
Processes of Change	
Consciousness Raising	Finding and learning new facts, ideas, and tips that support the healthy behavior change.
Dramatic Relief	Experiencing the negative emotions (fear, anxiety, worry) that go with unhealthy behavioral risks
Self-Reevaluation	Realizing that the behavior change is an important part of one's identity as a person
Environmental Reevaluation	Realizing the negative impact of the unhealthy behavior, or the positive impact of the healthy behavior, on one's proximal social and/or physical environment
Self-Liberation	Making a firm commitment to change
Helping Relationships	Seeking and using social support for the healthy behavior change
Counterconditioning	Substitution of healthier alternative behaviors and/or cognitions for the unhealthy behavior
Reinforcement Management	Increasing the rewards for the positive behavior change and/or decreasing the rewards of the unhealthy behavior
Stimulus Control	Removing reminders or cues to engage in the unhealthy behavior and/or adding cues to reminders to engage in the healthy behavior
Social Liberation	Realizing that social norms are changing in the direction of supporting the healthy behavior change.

Source: Redding et al. (1999). Reprinted by permission.

small steps toward action, such as buying the necessary clothes for exercising or cutting back on the fat grams they consume or the cigarettes they smoke, but they have not reached an effective criterion for effective action (Prochaska et al., 1992). "These are the people we should recruit for such action-oriented programs as smoking cessation, weight loss, or exercise" (Prochaska et al., 1998, p. 61).

People are in the fourth stage, the **action stage,** when they are overtly making changes in their behavior, experiences, or environment in order to overcome their problems. This stage of change reflects a consistent behavior pattern, is usually the most visible, and receives the greatest external recognition (Prochaska, DiClemente, & Norcross, 1992). Since the behavior change is very new in this stage and the chance of relapse is high, considerable attention still must be given to relapse prevention (Redding et al., 1999). Also, "not all modifications of behavior count as action in this model. People must attain a criterion that scientists and professionals agree is sufficient to reduce risks of disease" (Prochaska et al., 1998, p. 61). For example, in smoking, reduction in the number of cigarettes smoked does not count, only total abstinence (Prochaska et al., 1998). If those making changes continue with their new pattern of behavior, they will move into the fifth stage, maintenance.

Working to prevent relapse is the focus of the **maintenance stage.** People in this stage have changed their problem behavior for at least six months and are increasingly more confident that they can continue their changes (Prochaska et al., 1998; Redding et al., 1999). The person's change has become more of a habit and the chance of relapse is lower, but it still requires some attention (Redding et al., 1999).

The final stage is **termination.** This stage is defined as the time when the individuals who have changed have zero temptation to return to their old behavior and they have 100% self-efficacy—that is, a lifetime of maintenance. No matter what their mood, they will not return to their old behavior (Prochaska et al., 1998). This is a stage that few people reach with certain behaviors (i.e., alcoholics). Since this may not be a practical goal for the majority of people, it has been given less attention in the research (Prochaska et al., 1998). Figure 7.6 provides a summary of the stages of change.

The second major construct of the transtheoretical model is the **processes of change** (see Table 7.3 for an explanation of the 10 processes). "These are the covert and overt activities that people use to progress through the stages" (Prochaska et al., 1998, p. 62). Study over the years has indicated that some of the processes are more useful at specific stages of change. The experimental set of processes (consciousness raising, dramatic relief, self-reevaluation, environmental reevaluation, and social liberation) are most often emphasized in earlier stages (precontemplation, contemplation, and preparation) to increase intention and motivation, whereas the behavioral set of processes (helping relationships, counterconditioning, reinforcement management, stimulus control, and self-liberation) are most often utilized in the later stages (preparation, action, maintenance) as observable behavior change efforts get underway and need to be maintained (Redding et al., 1999) (see Table 7.4).

The construct of **decisional balance** refers to the pros and cons of the behavioral change. That is, individuals' decisions to move from one stage to the next is based on the relative importance (pro), or the lack thereof (con), of the behavior

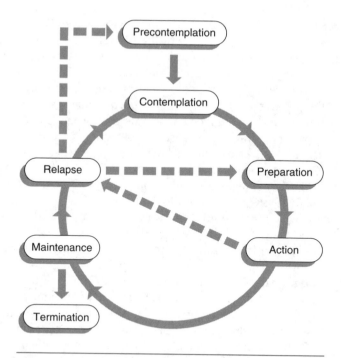

FIGURE 7.6   *The Stages of Change*

Source: M. G. Goldstein, J. DePue, A. Kazura, and R. Niaura, "Models for Provider-Patient Interaction: Applications to Health Behavior Change," in S. A. Shumaker, E. B. Schron, J. K. Ockene, and W. L. McBee (Eds.), *The Handbook of Health Behavior Change* (2nd ed.) (New York: Springer, 1998), p. 98. Springer Publishing Company, Inc., New York 10012. Used by permission.

change for the individuals. "Characteristically, the pros of healthy behavior are low in the early stages and increase across the stages of change, and the cons of the healthy behavior are high in the early stages and decrease across the stages of change" (Redding et al., 1999, p. 90).

The fourth construct of the transtheoretical model is **self-efficacy.** The developers of this model see self-efficacy as it was defined by Bandura (1977b) earlier in this chapter.

The final core construct of the transtheoretical model is temptation. **Temptation** refers to the situational temptation of those making change to engage in the unhealthy behavior. As one might guess, temptation decreases as one moves through the stages; however, even in the maintenance stage temptation is still present.

As noted at the beginning of this discussion, the transtheoretical model not only includes the five core constructs but it is also based on seven critical assumptions. The assumptions (Prochaska et al., 1998) include:

TABLE 7.4 *Stages of Change in Which Processes Are Most Emphasized*

	Stages of Changes				
Processes	*Precontemplation*	*Contemplation*	*Preparation*	*Action*	*Maintenance*
	Consciousness raising				
	Dramatic relief				
	Environmental reevaluation				
		Self-reevaluation	Self-liberation		
				Contingency managment	
				Helping relationship	
				Counterconditioning	
				Stimulus control	

Source: O. J. Prochaska, S. Johnson, and P. Lee, "The Transtheoretical Model of Behavior Change," in S. A. Shumaker, E. B. Schron, J. K. Ockene, and W. L. McBee (Eds.), *The Handbook of Health Behavior Change* (2nd ed.) (New York: Springer, 1998), p. 70. Springer Publishing Company, Inc., New York 10012. Used by permission.

1. No single theory can account for all the complexities of behavior change. Therefore, a more comprehensive model will most likely emerge from an integration across major theories.
2. Behavior change is a process that unfolds over time through a sequence of events.
3. Stages are both stable and open to change, just as chronic behavioral risk factors are stable and open to change.
4. Without planned interventions, populations will remain stuck in the early stages. There is no inherent motivation to progress through the stages of intentional change as there seems to be stages of physical and psychological development.
5. The majority of at-risk populations are not prepared for action and will not be served by traditional action-oriented prevention programs. Health promotion can have much greater impacts if it shifts from an action paradigm to a stage paradigm.
6. Specific processes and principles of change need to be applied at specific stages if progress through the stages is to occur. In the stages of change, paradigm intervention programs must be matched to each individual's stage of change.
7. Chronic behavior patterns usually are under some combination of biological, social, and self-control. Staged-matched interventions have been primarily designed to enhance self-controls. (p. 64)

Since its development, the Transtheoretical Model has been useful in several different ways. The first is that it makes program planners aware that not everyone is ready for change "right now," even though there is a program that can help them modify their behavior. People proceed through behavior change at different paces. Second, if individuals are not ready for action right now, then other programs can be developed to help them become ready for action. This second aspect fits in nicely with the effort to market a program and is discussed further in Chapter 11.

Cognitive-Behavioral Model of the Relapse Process

For most people, relapse is a part of change. **Relapse** "refers to the breakdown or failure in a person's attempt to change or modify a particular habit pattern, such as stopping 'bad habits' or developing new, optimal health behaviors" (Marlatt & George, 1998, p. 33). Marlatt and George (1998) differentiate between relapse (an indication of total failure) and a **lapse** (a single slip or mistake). The first drink or cigarette following a period of abstinence would be consider a lapse. It has been said that getting people to change behavior is hard, but having them maintain the behavior is much harder. This is nicely illustrated by the old saying "Giving up smoking is easy; I've done it a hundred times." At one time, it was enough for health promotion program planners just to get people to change their behavior; now they need to do more. Because of the difficulty of maintaining a new behavior, program planners need to give special attention to helping those in the target population avoid slipping back to their previous behaviors.

Although much of the early research dealing with this concept of slipping back was conducted using addictive behaviors, such as substance abuse and gambling, the concept applies to all behavior change, including preventive health behaviors. Marlatt (1982) indicates that a high percentage of individuals who enter programs for health behavior change relapse to their former behaviors within one year. More specifically, researchers have warned program planners of **recidivism** problems with participants in exercise (Dishman, Sallis, & Orenstein, 1985; Horne, 1975; Simkin & Gross, 1994), oral health care treatment (McCaul et al., 1990), weight loss (Stunkard & Braunwell, 1980), and smoking cessation (Leventhal & Cleary, 1980) programs. Therefore, planners need to make sure that program interventions include the skills necessary for dealing with those difficult times during behavior change.

Marlatt (1982) refers to the process of trying to prevent slipping back as relapse prevention. **Relapse prevention (RP),** which is based on the social cognitive theory, combines behavioral skill-training procedures, cognitive therapy, and lifestyle rebalancing (Marlatt & George, 1998). Relapse prevention is "a self-control program designed to help individuals to anticipate and cope with the problem of relapse in the habit-changing process" (Marlatt & George, 1998, p. 33). Relapse is triggered by *high-risk situations.* "A high-risk situation is defined broadly as any situation (including emotional reactions to the situation) that poses a threat to the individual's sense of control and increases the risk of potential relapse" (Marlatt & George, 1998, p. 38). Cummings, Gordon, and Marlatt (1980), in a study of clients with a variety of problem behaviors (drinking, smoking, heroin addiction, gambling, and overeating), found high-risk situations to fall into two major categories: intrapersonal and interpersonal determinants. They found that 56% of the relapse situations were caused by intrapersonal determinants, such as negative emotional states (35%), negative physical states (3%), positive emotional states (4%), testing personal control (5%), and urges and temptations (9%). The 44% of the situations represented by interpersonal determinants included interpersonal conflicts (16%), social pressure (20%), and positive emotional states (8%). These determinants can be referred to as the *covert antecedents* of relapse. That is to say, these high-risk situations do not just happen; instead, they are created by what Marlatt (1982) calls *lifestyle imbalances.*

People who have the coping skills to deal with a high-risk situation have a much greater chance of preventing relapse than those who do not. Figure 7.7 illustrates the possible paths one may take in a high-risk situation (Marlatt, 1982).

Marlatt has developed both global (Figure 7.8) and specific (Figure 7.9) self-control strategies for relapse intervention. Specific intervention procedures are designed to help participants anticipate and cope with the relapse episode itself, whereas the global intervention procedures are designed to modify the early antecedents of relapse, including restructuring of the participant's general style of life. A complete application of the relapse prevention model would include both specific and global interventions (Marlatt, 1982).

Applying Theory to Practice

Learning and understanding the theories presented in this chapter are manageable tasks. However, learning "how to apply given theories to 'real life' projects where theories usually have to be bent and twisted and adapted to uncontrollable conditions" (Hochbaum et al., 1992, p. 311) is a much more difficult task. Several

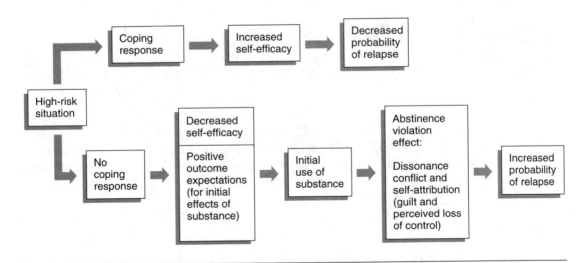

FIGURE 7.7 *Cognitive-Behavioral Model of the Relapse Process*

Source: "Relapse Prevention: Theoretical Rationale and Overview of the Model," by G. A. Marlatt, in G. A. Marlatt and J. R. Gordon (Eds.), *Relapse Prevention* (p. 38), 1985, New York: Guilford Press. Reprinted by permission of Guilford Press.

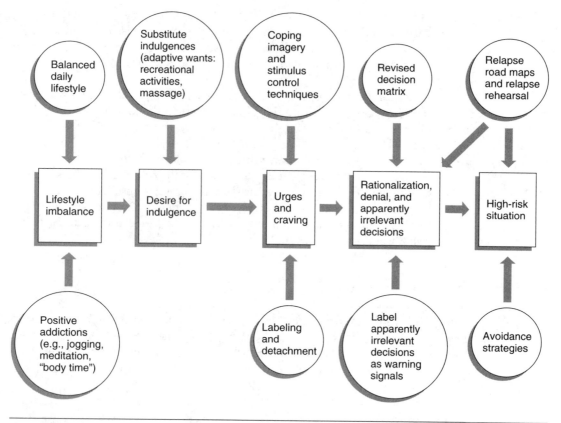

FIGURE 7.8 *Relapse Prevention: Global Self-Control Strategies*

Source: "Relapse Prevention: Theoretical Rationale and Overview of the Model," by G. A. Marlatt, in G. A. Marlatt and J. R. Gordon (Eds.), *Relapse Prevention* (p. 61), 1985, New York: Guilford Press. Reprinted by permission of Guilford Press.

authors (Burdine & McLeroy, 1992; D'Onofrio, 1992; Glanz, Lewis, Rimer, 1997; Hochbaum et al., 1992; McLeroy, 1993; van Ryn and Heaney, 1992) have reported the difficulties practitioners have had in applying theory. In the sections below, we will discuss the reported barriers to applying theory in the field and provide suggestions for choosing and applying theory.

Barriers to Applying Theory

Burdine and McLeroy (1992) have reported on semistructured interviews with health professionals on the use of theory in practice. Though the group was not randomly selected—it was part of a workgroup in eastern Pennsylvania—it was thought to be broadly representative of "practicing health educators." From these interviews came three primary reasons why practitioners were not using theory

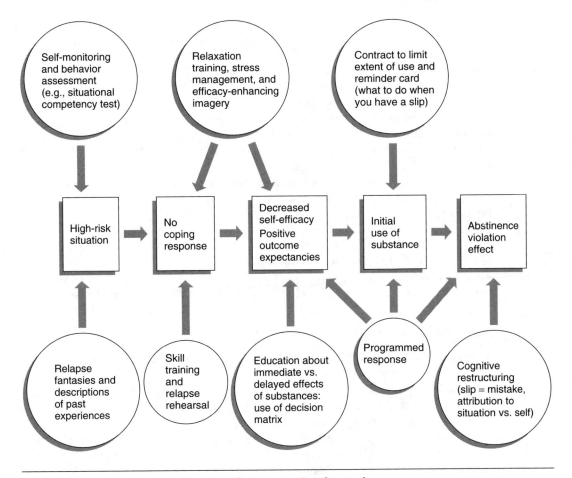

FIGURE 7.9 *Relapse Prevention: Specific Intervention Strategies*

Source: "Relapse Prevention: Theoretical Rationale and Overview of the Model," by G. A. Marlatt, in G. A. Marlatt and J. R. Gordon (Eds.), *Relapse Prevention* (p. 54), 1985, New York: Guilford Press. Reprinted by permission of Guilford Press.

learned in their professional preparation courses in college. They included "(1) the failure of theory to adequately guide practice in specific settings or contexts; (2) the lack of appropriate theories to guide community-oriented interventions; and (3) difficulties in transferring theories from the academic training context to the practice environment" (Burdine & McLeroy, 1992, p. 336).

The concern about the failure of theory to adequately guide practice in specific settings or contexts stems from the fact that the theory on which the health education discipline was built is borrowed from the social and behavioral sciences. It primarily revolves around individual behavior change. Even though behavior change is an important part of the work of health educators, the theories do not match well with the expanded role of health educators when they address problems such as controlling environmental health hazards, increasing access to and utilization of health care facilities, limiting the commercial promotion of alcohol and tobacco (D'Onofrio, 1992), and organizing committees to deal with these problems (Burdine & McLeroy, 1992).

The issue of the lack of appropriate theory to guide community-oriented interventions speaks to the fact that the discipline lacks process or practical guide theory. The discipline needs a theory to take one from the social science theory to creating appropriate interventions for a specific target population (Burdine & McLeroy, 1992).

The third reason shared by Burdine and McLeroy (1992) for practitioners not using theory in practice is the means by which theory is taught by academicians. Instead of presenting the theories and asking how they apply to a problem, it is suggested (Burdine & McLeroy, 1992; D'Onofrio, 1992) that academicians should be teaching theory by starting with a specific health problem and asking how each of the theories helps one understand the problem.

Now that you know a bit about what appears to be some of the reasons for not using theory in practice, let's look at how it can be implemented.

Suggestions for Applying Theory to Practice

Several authors (D'Onofrio, 1992; Hochbaum et al., 1992; van Ryn & Heaney, 1992) have suggested ideas for applying theory to practice. Following is a summary compilation of their ideas.

The first step is having a basic grasp of the theories—old and new (D'Onofrio, 1992). Practitioners should take the time to review the theories and not depend on memory. Theories, like most other knowledge, are forgotten over time if they are not used. Also, the very nature of theory suggests that it can change and be updated. The theory of reasoned action and the theory of planned behavior are good examples. Practitioners also need to become familiar with new theories and models.

Once practitioners feel comfortable with the theories and models, they should examine the applicability of these theories and models to the problem they are addressing (D'Onofrio, 1992; van Ryn & Heaney, 1992). This can be done by taking the goals of a proposed program and matching them with the most applicable theories. For example, some theories were developed to help explain behavior change of individuals, whereas others were developed to help explain change at the community level. Thus, some theories and models work better in some situations than others, depending on which level of influence the program is being planned. The concept of the level of influence is included in the ecological perspective (McLeroy et al., 1988). The **ecological perspective** "recognizes that health behaviors are part of the larger social system (or ecology) of behaviors and social influences, much like a river, forest or desert is part of a larger biological system (or ecosystem), and that lasting changes in health behaviors require supportive changes in the whole system, just as the addition of a power plant, the flooding of a reservoir, or the growth of a city in a desert produce changes in the whole eco-system" (O'Donnell, 1996, p. 244). The ecological perspective includes five levels of influence on health-related behaviors and conditions:

1. Intrapersonal (or individual) factors
2. Interpersonal factors
3. Institutional (or organizational) factors
4. Community factors
5. Public policy factors

Here is how the levels of influence might be applied to assisting individuals in starting an exercise program. At the *intrapersonal (or individual) level,* a health educa-tion class could be planned for the target population to present the knowledge and skills necessary to begin an exercise program. Going beyond the individual level, program planners could consider setting up social support networks of family and friends to help encourage those in the target population. Such an approach would be at the *interpersonal level.* If planners worked with and through the institutions in which the members of the target population were associated (e.g., churches and worksites) to get the target population exercising, they would be working at the *in-stitutional (or organizational) level* of influence. Creating a *community culture* that favors active community members would be a strategy for influencing at the next level. And finally, planners can work to influence *public policy* that encourages phys-ically active community members. This may take the form of getting the city council to pass an ordinance that would establish bike lanes in the roads.

To assist program planners with matching theories and models with the ap-propriate level of influence, Glanz and Rimer (1995) modified the five levels of in-fluence into three. They have done this by using the first two levels, intrapersonal and interpersonal, and combining institutional, community, and public policy into one level called *community.* Table 7.5 categorizes, by level of influence, the theories and models commonly used in developing health promotion programs. (*Note:* Some of the theories and models included in Table 7.5 are not presented in this text; refer to Glanz, Lewis, and Rimer [1997].)

Knowing that several theories or models are applicable to the problem they are addressing, planners should look for evidence that the theories or models will work in their particular situation. Have others used theories or models with suc-cess with the same or a similar problem or target population (van Ryn & Heaney, 1992)? Some theories or models may have to be adjusted or modified to be appli-cable to certain target populations. For example, can the same theory apply to people from different cultural backgrounds within the United States? Or, what is the applicability of behavioral theories based on Western thought to people from non-Western cultures (D'Onofrio, 1992)?

It is also important to remember that seldom does a single theory or model address all the complexities of a problem. Planners will more than likely have to use more than one theory or model to adequately address all the components of the problem. To do so, planners will need to synthesize and integrate the theories

TABLE 7.5   *Theories and Models Categorized by Level of Influence*

Level of Influence	Theory/Model	Where Discussed in This Book
Intrapersonal	Stimulus Response Theory	Chapter 7
	Theory of Planned Behavior	Chapter 7
	Health Belief Model	Chapter 7
	Transtheoretical Model	Chapter 7
Interpersonal	Social Cognitive Theory	Chapter 7
	Social Support/Networks	Chapter 8
	Patient-Provider Communication	*
Community	Community Organization	Chapter 9
	Diffusion Theory	Chapter 11
	Organizational Change	*
	Theory of Freeing	Chapter 7

* = Not presented in this text

and models to fit their particular situation (D'Onofrio, 1992). In bringing theories or models together, planners are warned against using only selected parts of a theory or model. Theories are based on the interaction of several variables. When some of those variables are removed, the theory or model is not the same. For example, if cues to action or motivation are removed from the health belief model, planners will not know the true effectiveness of the model. Thus, the most effective use of a theory or model is to use it in total (Hochbaum et al., 1992).

In the final step in choosing a theory, planners need to select "a theory that makes sense to them, given their experience and what they know and believe about the world" (van Ryn & Heaney, 1992, p. 320). This is not to say that planners should not consider theories and models that may be different from their own views, but it "does not make sense to base a program on theoretical ideas that are at odds with one's own philosophy or belief system" (van Ryn & Heaney, 1992, p. 320).

Summary

This chapter presented an overview of several theories and three models that underlie the interventions used in many of today's health promotion programs. These theories and models are important components for planning and evaluating health promotion programs because they provide planners with ideas that have been tried and tested. They provide the framework on which to build. The theories and models reviewed include stimulus response theory, the social cognitive theory, the theory of reasoned action, the theory of planned behavior, problem-behavior theory, the theory of freeing, the health belief model, the transtheoretical model, and the cognitive-behavioral model of the relapse process (see Table 7.6 for a summary of the major components).

TABLE 7.6 Major Components of the Theories and Models That Underlie Health Promotion Interventions

Stimulus Response Theory	Social Cognitive Theory	Theory of Reasoned Action	Theory of Planned Behavior	Problem-Behavior Theory	Theory of Freeing	Health Belief Model	Transtheoretical Model	Cognitive-Behavior Model of the Relapse Process
Operant behavior	Reinforcement 1. Direct 2. Vicarious 3. Self-management	Attitude toward behavior	Attitude toward behavior	Personality system	Free	Perceived susceptibility	Stages of change	Global self-control strategies
Consequences	Behavioral capability	Subjective norm	Subjective norm	Perceived environment system	Oppressed	Perceived seriousness	Decisional balance	High-risk situation
Positive reinforcement	Expectations	Intentions	Perceived behavioral control	Behavior system	Critical consciousness	Perceived benefits	Processes of change	Specific intervention strategies
Negative reinforcement	Expectancies	Behavior	Intentions	Antecedent variables	Education	Perceived barriers	Self-efficacy	
Positive punishment	Self-control		Behavior	Background variables		Motivation (cues to action)	Temptation	
Negative punishment	Self-efficacy					Self-efficacy		
	Emotional coping response							
	Reciprocal determinism							

Finally, the chapter provides a discussion of some of the roadblocks to using theory, suggestions for applying theory to practice, and an example of how theory can be applied to practice.

Questions

1. Define *theory,* using your own words.

2. How is a theory different from a model?

3. How do concepts, constructs, and variables relate to theories and models?

4. Why is it important to use theories when planning and evaluating health promotion programs?

5. What is the underlying concept for each of the following theories?
   a. Stimulus response theory
   b. Social cognitive theory
   c. Theory of reasoned action
   d. Theory of planned behavior
   e. Theory of freeing
   f. Problem-behavior theory

6. What are the major components of the Health Belief Model? Explain each.

7. What are the constructs of the transtheoretical model? Why is it important to understand this model?

8. How can program planners help to prepare those in the target population for relapse prevention?

9. What are the major barriers to using theories and models in practice?

10. How can the ecological perspective be used in applying theories and models?

Activities

1. Assume that you have identified a need (health problem) for a given target population. In a two-page paper:
   a. State who the target population is and what the need is.
   b. Select a theory or model to use as a guide in developing an intervention to address the problem.
   c. Explain why you chose the theory or model that you did.
   d. Defend why you think this is the best theory or model to use.
   e. Show how the problem "fits into" the theory or model.

2. In a two-page paper, identify a theory or model that you plan to use in developing the intervention for the program you are planning. Explain why you chose the theory or model, and why you think it is a good fit for the problem you are addressing.

3. Write a paragraph on each of the following:
   a. Using the stimulus response theory, explain why a person might smoke.
   b. Using the social cognitive theory, explain how you could help people change their diets.
   c. Explain how the SCT construct of behavioral capability applies to managing stress.
   d. Explain the differences between and the relationship of the SCT constructs of expectations and expectancies.
   e. Explain what would have to take place for a person to be self-efficacious with regard to being able to take her insulin.
   f. According to the theory of reasoned action, what would increase intent to exercise?
   g. Use the theory of planned behavior to explain how a smoker stops smoking.

h. Using the theory of freeing, describe an ideal teacher.

i. Apply the health belief model to getting a person to take a "flu shot."

j. Apply the transtheoretical model to getting a person to change any health behavior.

Activities on the Web

1. Using a search engine (i.e., Excite, GoTo.com, Snap, or Lycos), enter the name of one of the theories or models presented in this chapter. Identify at least three websites that contain information about the theory/model. Visit each of the three websites and obtain the following information:

   a. Website URL

   b. Purpose of the site

   c. At least two items of interest about the theory/model that you did not already know before visiting the site

   d. The health behaviors in which the theory/model has been most used

2. Visit the website for the University of Rhode Island that presents measures for the transtheoretical model <**http://uri.edu/research/cprc/measures.htm**>. In searching this site, find at least 10 questions that can be used to help determine at which stage people are in for various health behaviors. Download the questions and take them to class for discussion.

8

Interventions

After reading this chapter and answering the questions at the end, you should be able to:

- Define the word *intervention* and apply it to a health promotion setting.
- Provide a rationale for selecting an intervention strategy.
- Explain the advantages of using a combination of several intervention activities rather than a single intervention activity.
- Explain the difference between micro and macro interventions.
- List and explain the different categories of intervention activities.
- List some of the documents that provide guidelines or criteria for developing health promotion programs and interventions.
- Discuss the ethical concerns related to intervention development.
- Create an intervention for a health promotion program.

Key Terms

codes of practice	intervention	risk reduction
disincentive	intervention activity	segmenting
ethics	penetration rate	tailoring
incentives	risk appraisal	treatment

Once the goals and objectives have been developed, program planners need to decide on the most appropriate means of reaching, or attaining, the goals and objectives. The planners must design an activity or set of activities that would permit the most *effective* (leads to desired outcome) and *efficient* (uses resources in a responsible manner) achievement of the outcomes stated in the goals and objectives.

These planned activities make up the **intervention,** or what some refer to as **treatment.** The intervention is the activity or experience to which those in the target population will be exposed or in which they will take part. In the strictest sense, *intervention* means "to occur, fall, or come between points of time or events" (Woolf, 1979, p. 600). When applied to the planning of health promotion programs, it is usually thought of as something that occurs between the beginning and the end of a program or between pre- and postprogram measurements. For example, let's say that you want the employees of Company S to increase their use of safety belts while riding in company-owned vehicles. You can measure their safety belt use before doing anything else, by observing them driving out of the motor pool; this would be a preprogram measure. Then you can intervene in a variety of ways. For example, you could provide an incentive by stating that all employees seen wearing their safety belts would receive a $10 bonus in their next paycheck. Or you could put in each employee's pay envelope a pamphlet on the importance of wearing safety belts. You could institute a company policy requiring all employees to wear safety belts while driving company-owned vehicles. Each of these activities for getting employees to increase their use of safety belts would be considered part of an intervention. After the intervention, you would complete a postprogram measurement of safety belt use to determine the success of the program.

The term *intervention* is used to describe all the activities that occur between the two measurement points. Thus, an intervention may be a single activity, or it may be a combination of two or more activities. In the case of the example just given, you could use an incentive by itself and call it an intervention, or you could use an incentive, pamphlets, and a company policy all at the same time to increase safety belt use and refer to the combination as an intervention.

With regard to the number of activities that should be included in an intervention, research (Erfurt et al., 1990; Kline & Huff, 1999; Shea & Basch, 1990) shows that interventions that include several activities are more likely to have an effect on the target population than are those that consist of only a single activity. In other words, "dosage" is important in health promotion. Few people change their behavior based on a single exposure (or dose); instead, multiple exposures (doses) are generally needed to change most behaviors. It stands to reason that "hitting" the target population from several angles or through multiple channels should increase the chances of making an impact. Although research has shown that several activities are better than one, it has not identified an exact number of activities or a specific combination of activities that will ensure the most effective results (Kline & Huff, 1999). It is still a best guess situation.

Selecting Appropriate Intervention Activities

Selection of intervention activities for a health promotion program should be based on a sound rationale as opposed to chance; an activity should not be selected just because the planners think it "sounds good" or because they have a "feeling" that it will work. As mentioned earlier, planners should choose an intervention that will be both effective and efficient. Although no prescription for an appropriate intervention has been developed, experience has indicated that the results of some interventions are more predictable than others. In this section, we present seven major questions that planners need to consider when creating health promotion interventions. Figure 8.1 summarizes these major considerations.

1. Do the intervention activities fit the goals and objectives of the program? It is important that there be a good fit between the goals and objectives of a program and the intervention activities used to reach the desired outcomes. If the single purpose of a program was to increase the awareness of the target population, the intervention would be very different from what it would be if the pur-

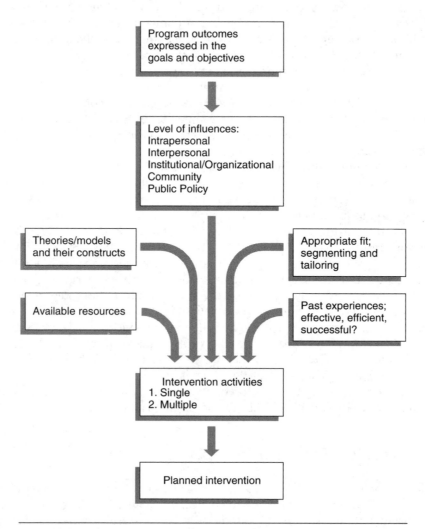

FIGURE 8.1 *Items to Consider when Creating a Health Promotion Intervention*

pose was to change behavior. Matching goals and objectives sounds easy enough, but creating such a match is a bit more difficult because of the "gray areas" created by the lack of empirical data to support such claims. Anderson and O'Donnell (1994) created such an intervention-outcome matrix based upon work presented in the *American Journal of Health Promotion*. Figure 8.2 presents a similar matrix using the terminology presented in this textbook.

2. At what level(s) of influence will the intervention be focused? Planners need to decide at what level or levels of influence they can best obtain the goals and objectives of the program. For example, if the goal of the program is to increase safety belt use, can that best be accomplished by trying to intervene at an intrapersonal level with an individual education program, at the institutional level with a company policy, or at the public policy level with a enhanced state safety belt law?

3. Are the activities based on an appropriate theory? Interventions have a much greater chance of reaching the desired outcome if they are planned using sound learning and educational theories and models that have proved their worth

Type of objective	Program outcome	Intervention activities										
		Educational	Behavior modification	Environmental	Regulatory	Community advocacy	Organizational culture	Communication	Incentives	Social	Health status evaluation	Technology-delivered
Process/ Administrative	1. Activities presented	X	X	X	X	X	X	X	X	X	X	X
	2. Tasks completed	X	X	X	X	X	X	X	X	X	X	X
Learning	1. Awareness	X	X	?	X	X	?	X	?	X	X	X
	2. Knowledge	X	?	?	?	X	?	X	?	X	X	X
	3. Attitudes	X	?	?	?	X	?	X	?	X	X	X
	4. Skills	X	X	X	X	?	?	X	X	X	?	X
Action/ Behavioral and Environmental	1. Behavior change	?	X	X	X	?	X	X	X	X	X	?
	2. Environmental change	?	X	X	X	X	X	X	?	?	?	?
Program	1. Quality of life	?	?	?	?	?	?	X	?	X	?	?
	2. Health status	?	X	X	X	?	?	X	X	X	?	?
	3. Health risks	?	X	X	X	?	?	X	X	X	?	?
	4. Social benefits	?	?	?	?	X	X	X	X	X	?	?

FIGURE 8.2 *Matrix of Intervention Activities, Objectives, and Program Outcomes*

through experience and social science research. Interventions should not be without a solid basis in theory. Refer to Chapter 7 to review (1) the relationship between the levels of influence and the theories and models and (2) Table 7.6 for a listing of the constructs of the various theories and models.

4. Is the intervention an appropriate fit for the target population? Intervention activities need to be designed to "fit" the target population. Each target population has certain characteristics that impact how it will receive an intervention. It is important for planners to try to identify these characteristics in order to segment a target population. **Segmenting** is the process of dividing a broader population into smaller groups with similar characteristics that are likely to exhibit similar behavior/reaction to an intervention (Wright, 1997) (see Figure 11.5 for ways by which planners can segment the target population). Segmentation allows planners to create an intervention to "fit the needs and characteristics of a target audience" (Pasick, D'Onofrio, & Otero-Sabogal, 1996, p. S145). Following are a few examples of how target population segmentation can be applied. If program planners are developing written materials as part of their intervention, they need to make sure that the materials are written at an acceptable reading level for the target population. From a developmental stage perspective, it is not reasonable to expect kindergartners to sit still for a one-hour lesson. Interventions also need to "fit" culturally with the target population (Huff & Kline, 1999; Pahnos, 1992; LeMaster & Connell, 1994) and be culturally sensitive. Cultural-sensitive interventions are those "that are relevant and acceptable within the cultural framework of the population to be reached" (Frankish, Lovato, & Shannon, 1998).

If an intervention activity is created specifically for an individual's needs, it is referred to as a **tailored** activity. The rationale for tailoring an intervention activity is based on research that shows people pay more attention to information that is personally relevant to them. Tailored intervention activities have been used with cancer screening (Skinner, Strecher, & Hospers, 1994), exercise (Marcus et al., 1998), immunizations (Kreuter, Vehige, & McGuire, 1996), nutrition (Campbell et al., 1994), and smoking cessation (Strecher et al., 1994).

5. Are the necessary resources available to implement the intervention selected? Obviously, some intervention activities require more money, time, personnel, or space to implement than others. For example, it may be prudent to provide each person in the target population with $100 for participating in the health promotion program, but it may not be possible because of budget limitations.

6. What types of intervention activities are known to be effective (i.e., have been successfully used in previous programs) in dealing with the program focus? By networking with other health educators and by reviewing the literature, planners can find out what interventions have been effective with certain target populations or in dealing with specific health problems.

7. Would it be better to use an intervention that consists of a single activity or one that is made up of multiple activities? A single-activity intervention would most likely be easier and less expensive to implement and easier to evaluate.

There are, however, some real advantages to using several activities. These advantages include: (1) "hitting" the target population with a message in a variety of ways; (2) appealing to the variety of learning styles within any target population; (3) keeping the health message constantly before the target population; (4) hoping that at least one activity appeals enough to the target population to help bring about the expected outcome; and (5) appealing to the various senses (such as sight, hearing, or touch) of each individual in the target population. Probably the biggest drawback to using multiple activities is the difficulty of separating the effects of one activity from the effects of others in evaluating the impact of the total program and of individual components (Ad Hoc Work Group, 1987). However, Glasgow, Vogt, and Boles (1999) have proposed an evaluation model titled RE-AIM (acronym for reach, efficacy, adoption, implementation, and maintenance) for use with multiple activity interventions.

Types of Intervention Activities

As mentioned earlier, there are many different types of activities that planners can use as part of an intervention. We present here several categories covering the more common activities, but in actuality the variety of activities is limited only by the planner's imagination. Note that the categories we have created are not always independent of each other—that is, some of the examples that we use to help explain the activities could be used in more than one category. Even with this limitation, we have categorized activities into the following groups:

1. Communication activities
2. Educational activities
3. Behavior modification activities
4. Environmental change activities
5. Regulatory activities
6. Community advocacy activities
7. Organizational culture activities
8. Incentives and disincentives
9. Health status evaluation activities
10. Social activities
11. Technology-delivered activities

Communication Activities

We present communication activities first for several different reasons. First, almost all interventions include some form of communication, whether it be as simple as just speaking, reading, or writing, or more complex, such as the production of small media (i.e., handouts, brochures, etc.), or very complex in the development of mass media (i.e., radio, TV, or newspaper) campaigns. Second, communication activities are very useful in helping reach so many of the goals and objectives of health promotion programs, such as the following:

1. Increase awareness.
2. Increase knowledge.
3. Change attitudes (for example, about blood pressure, cancer screenings, and the ills of smoking).
4. Reinforce attitudes (for example, about smoking in public places).
5. Maintain interest (for example, for those contemplating a behavior change).
6. Provide cues for action.
7. Demonstrate simple skills (as in self-screening) (Bellicha & McGrath, 1990; Erickson, McKenna, & Romano, 1990).

Third, communication activities probably have the highest **penetration rate** (number in the target population exposed or reached) of any of the intervention activities. And fourth, they are also much more cost effective and less threatening than many other types of intervention activities.

Probably the most visible forms of communication activities are those in the mass media (both electronic and print), which include daily newspapers with national or local circulation; local weekly newspapers; local, public, and network television, including cable television; public and commercial radio stations; and magazines with either a broad readership or a narrow focus. There are many ways to convey a message using the mass media. These include news coverage (see Appendix A for an example of a news release and copy for a newspaper column), public affairs coverage, talk shows, public service roundtables, entertainment, public service announcements (PSAs) (see Appendix B for an example of a radio PSA and a TV PSA), paid advertisements, editorials, letters to the editor, comic strips, and columnists' commentaries (Arkin, 1990). But communication activities are not limited to mass media; they can take many other forms. Information can be presented on billboards, in booklets, on bulletin boards, in church bulletins, in fliers, through direct mail (such as the mailing on the subject of AIDS sent by the Public Health Service to every U.S. household), on product labels (for alcohol, foods, and tobacco), in newsletters, in pamphlets, on posters (Miller, 1992), and through self-help materials in print or on audio and video, and, of course, through interpersonal communication, primarily involving health professional/client interactions (Clift & Freimuth, 1995). The cost of communication activities can range from almost nothing (e.g., elementary school children making posters for a health awareness campaign) to moderately priced (e.g., production of a brochure) to expensive (e.g., personal counseling) to very expensive (e.g., a prime-time television commercial). However, no matter what form the communication activities take or their cost, to be effective, they need to be carefully planned.

The knowledge and skills for planning effective communication activities vary from novice to expert. It is not the purpose of this book to make health educators communication experts; the experts are those with college degrees in the field of communication. Instead, we present here the procedures recommended by two different authors (McGuire, 1981; USDHHS, 1989) for planning effective communication activities, and we present guidelines (Meyer & Rainey, 1994; USDHHS, 1989) for skills often used by health educators: preparing print communications.

One of the most often used procedures for developing communication activities for health educators was developed by McGuire (1981). McGuire set out a seven-step approach for designing a public health communications campaign. The first step involves analyzing the situation to determine if the health problem of concern is sufficiently severe, if corrective behaviors for the problem are available, and if such behaviors can be effectively promoted through communication activities. The second step determines whether the communication activity is cost beneficial compared to other means of dealing with the problem. The third step examines the sociocultural factors of the target population to determine which could facilitate or impede the campaign's effectiveness. In the fourth step, planners seek to find out the psychological matrix of thoughts, feelings, and behaviors that instigate and sustain undesirable health behavior. For example, do those in the target population not eat properly because they do not know any better, cannot afford it, or do not care? The fifth step consists of analyzing the data collected in the first four steps to select the most promising target groups and techniques for the communication activities. The sixth step includes the construction of the persuasive communication by choosing the source, message, channel, receiver, and destination variables that have the greatest promise for changing the undesirable behavior. The seventh and last step, as with many planning procedures, is to evaluate the effectiveness of the campaign by monitoring each of the previous six steps and examining the end results.

The National Cancer Institute compiled a book (USDHHS, 1989) that is most useful for developing communication activities in both mass media and printed materials (other than newspapers). The book is organized around six stages in health communication. Figure 8.3 graphically represents these stages. Stage 1 is planning and strategy selection. This includes studying the health problem and the target population, deciding what objectives are to be accomplished, and deciding what the target population should be told. Stage 2 deals with selecting the appropriate communication channels (e.g., face-to-face, like provider to patient; group delivery, like at a worksite or in a classroom; organizational, such as to members of an association; mass media, such as television, radio, and newspapers; community presentations, such as in libraries, malls, or government agencies; or any combination of these) to be used and deciding which format (booklets, videotapes, newsletters) will best suit the channels and messages. Stage 3 consists of developing materials that are appropriate for the target population (See Box 8.1 for items to consider when producing materials for special populations.) Also in Stage 3, planners need to pretest the materials. Feedback from the target population is most important at this stage. Stage 4 is the implementation of the activity. During this stage, the effect of the activity is tracked to determine if any alterations are needed. Stage 5 is evaluation, which should be based on the objectives identified in Stage 1. Stage 6, which loops right back to Stage 1, incorporates feedback gained in the other stages to prepare for a new cycle of the communication. This

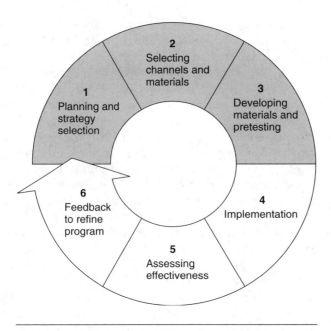

FIGURE 8.3   *Stages in Health Communication*

Source: U.S. Department of Health and Human Services (1989).

method answers many key questions: What worked and did not work? How can it be improved the next time? Knowing the answers to these questions will lead to improved future interventions.

Most health education materials are written at a reading level too difficult for many people in the general public to understand. That holds for both printed materials (Buxton, 1999; Davis et al., 1994; Dollahite, Thomson, & McNew, 1996) and those on the World Wide Web (Graber, Roller, & Kaeble, 1999). Meyer and Rainey (1994) created a set of guidelines for health educators to follow when creating health education materials for low-literacy populations. We found their guidelines to be useful regardless of the target population. Their eight guidelines are summarized in Table 8.1. The only addition we would make to their list would be to check the reading level of the written materials. "For the general public, writing at the 6th grade reading level is usually safe. You can check if you're on target by using a readability test such as the SMOG, the Fog-Gunning Index, or the Fry Readability Formula" (USDHHS, 1991, p. 3). You can find such formulas in most reading methods books and on selected computer word-processing programs. Box 8.2 presents the steps in the process of testing readability using the SMOG.

Educational Activities

Educational activities are those usually associated with formal education in courses, seminars, and workshops. This includes educational methods—such as

BOX 8.1 • *Producing Materials for Special Populations*

Although planners should create/select materials that are applicable to each target population, extra attention needs to be given to materials that are prepared for special populations. Consider the following:

A. For culturally diverse populations, remember:
1. Interaction with the target population and "intermediaries" familiar with the culture is especially important.
2. Use of language may vary for different cultural groups (e.g., a word may have different meanings to different groups).
3. Differences in target populations extend beyond language to include diverse values and customs.
4. Different channels of communication may be credible and more capable of reaching certain cultural groups.
5. Don't assume that "conventional wisdom," published research studies or "common knowledge" will hold true for different cultural groups. The degree of assimilation and mainstreaming is ever changing, so current information will be needed to choose the best channels and message strategies.
6. Message appeals should be developed separately for each cultural group, since the perceived needs, values, and beliefs of one culture may differ from others.
7. Print materials should be simply written, reinforced with graphics, and pretested. People perceive graphics and illustrations in different ways, just as their language skills differ.
8. Bilingual materials assure that intermediaries and family members who are most comfortable with English can help the reader understand the content.
9. Print materials should never be simply translated from English; concepts and appeals may differ by culture, just as the words do.
10. Audiovisual materials or interpersonal communication may be more successful for some messages and audiences.

B. For patient populations, remember:
1. Patients and their families facing a disorder or a disease may require different information in different formats at various points in the disease continuum.
2. All patients are not alike, and may have nothing in common except their illness. Therefore, their interests in information and ability to understand the illness may vary.
3. Few patients and family members can handle everything they need to know at once, and may find it particularly difficult to absorb information at the time of diagnosis.
4. Patients' information needs may change as they emotionally adjust to their illness.

Source: Adapted from U.S. Department of Health and Human Services (1989).

lecture, discussion, and group work—as well as audiovisual materials, computerized instruction, laboratory exercises, and written materials (books and periodicals). Figure 8.4 provides a more complete listing of educational activities, and Gilbert and Sawyer (1995) have provided a detailed discussion of these methods.

TABLE 8.1 *Guidelines for Preparing Written Materials*

Guideline	Explanation
1. Needs and target population identification	Identify the topic and the target population (e.g., middle-aged women and mammography).
2. Plan the project	Develop a work plan and budget for your material.
3. Audience research	Segment your target population using such factors as experience, attitude, culture, etc.
4. Material development	
a. Style	Use an active voice with familar terms that highlight key points. If possible, develop a behaviorally oriented interactive message.
b. Organization	Sequence or prioritize the message.
c. Content	Write using words and terms that are understandable to lay people. Use short sentences and paragraphs.
d. Format	Make it appealing to the eye, making sure the reader can identify the main points.
5. Graphics and illustrations	Graphics and illustrations should be positive and easy to understand, and should summarize the message.
6. Pretesting	Make sure the materials work before you use them with the target population. Also, make sure the reading level is appropriate.
7. Printing	Consider paper color, size, and cost.
8. Distribution and training	Develop a distribution system and instructions for use.

Source: Adapted from Meyer and Rainey (1994), pp. 372–374.

Behavior Modification Activities

Behavior modification activities, often used in intrapersonal-level interventions, includes techniques intended to help those in the target population experience a change in behavior. *Behavior modification* is usually thought of as a systematic procedure for changing a specific behavior. The process is based on the stimulus response theory. As applied to health behavior, emphasis is placed on a specific behavior that one might want either to increase (such as exercise or stress management techniques) or to decrease (such as smoking or consumption of fats). Particular attention is then given to changing the events that are antecedent or subsequent to the behavior that is to be modified.

In changing a health behavior, the behavior modification activity often begins by having those in the target population keep records (diaries, logs, or journals) for a specific period of time (24 to 48 hours, one week, or one month) concerning the behavior (such as eating, smoking, or exercise) they want to alter. Using the information recorded, one can plan an activity to modify that behavior.

BOX 8.2 • *The SMOG Readability Formula*

To calculate the SMOG reading grade level, begin with the entire written work that is being assessed, and follow these four steps:

1. Count off ten consecutive sentences near the beginning, in the middle, and near the end of the text.
2. From this sample of thirty sentences, circle all of the words containing three or more syllables (polysyllabic), including repetitions of the same word, and total the number of words circled.
3. Estimate the square root of the total number of polysyllabic words counted. This is done by finding the nearest perfect square, and taking its square root.
4. Finally, add a constant of three to the square root. This number gives the SMOG grade, or the reading grade level that a person must have reached if he or she is to fully understand the text being assessed.

A few additional guidelines will help to clarify these directions:

- A sentence is defined as a string of words punctuated with a period (.), an exclamation point (!), or a question mark (?).
- Hyphenated words are considered as one word.
- Numbers that are written out should also be considered, and if in numeric form in the text, they should be pronouned to determine if they are polysyllabic.
- Proper nouns, if polysyllabic, should be counted, too.
- Abbreviations should be read as unabbreviated to determine if they are polysyllabic.

Not all pamphlets, fact sheets, or other printed materials contain thirty sentences. To test a text that has fewer than thirty sentences:

1. Count all of the polysyllabic words in the text.

2. Count the number of sentences.
3. Find the average number of polysyllabic words per sentence as follows:

$$\text{Average} = \frac{\text{Total \# of polysyllabic words}}{\text{Total \# of sentences}}$$

4. Multiply that average by the number of sentences *short of thirty*.
5. Add that figure to the total number of polysyllabic words.
6. Find the square root and add the constant of three.

Perhaps the quickest way to administer the SMOG grading test is by using the SMOG conversion table. Simply count the number of polysyllabic words in your chain of thirty sentences and look up the appropriate grade level on the chart.

SMOG Conversion Table*

Total Polysyllabic Word Counts	Approximately Grade Level (±1.5 Grades)
0–2	4
3–6	5
7–12	6
13–20	7
21–30	8
31–42	9
43–56	10
57–72	11
73–90	12
91–110	13
111–132	14
133–156	15
157–182	16
183–210	17
211–240	18

*Developed by Harold C. McGraw, Office of Educational Research, Baltimore County Schools, Towson, Maryland.

Source: U.S. Department of Health and Human Services (1989).

FIGURE 8.4 *Commonly Used Educational Activities*

A. Audiovisual materials and equipment
  1. Audiotapes, records, and CDs
  2. Bulletin, chalk, cloth, flannel, magnetic, and peg boards
  3. Charts, pictures, and posters
  4. Films and filmstrips
  5. Instructional television
  6. Opaque projector
  7. Slides and slide projectors
  8. Transparencies and overhead projector
  9. Video disks and tapes
B. Computer based
  1. World Wide Web
  2. Desktop Publishing
  3. Presentation programs
  4. Individualized learning programs
  5. Video conferencing
C. Printed educational materials
  1. Instructor-made handouts and worksheets
  2. Pamphlets
  3. Study guides (commercial and instructor made)
  4. Text and reference books
  5. Workbooks
D. Teaching strategies and techniques for the classroom
  1. Brainstorming
  2. Case studies
  3. Cooperative learning
  4. Debates
  5. Demonstrations and experiments
  6. Discovery or guided discovery
  7. Discussion
  8. Group discussion
  9. Guest speakers
  10. Lecture
  11. Lecture/discussion
  12. Newspaper and magazine articles
  13. Panel discussions
  14. Peer group teaching/coaching
  15. Poems, songs, and stories
  16. Problem solving
  17. Puppets
  18. Questioning
  19. Role playing and plays
  20. Simulation, games, and puzzles
  21. Tutoring
  22. Values clarification activities
E. Teaching strategies and techniques for outside of the classroom
  1. Community resources
  2. Field trips
  3. Health fairs
  4. Health museums
  5. Health education centers

For example, facilitators of smoking cessation programs often will ask participants to keep a record of all the cigarettes they smoke from one class session to the next (see Figure 8.5 for an example of such a record). After keeping the record, participants are asked to analyze it to see what kind of smoking habit they have. They may be asked questions such as these: "What three cigarettes seem to be the most important of the day to you?" "In what three places or activities do you find yourself smoking the most?" "With whom do you find yourself smoking most often?" "Is there a primary reason or mood for your smoking?" "When during the day do you find yourself smoking the most and the least?" Once the participant

FIGURE 8.5 *Twenty-Four-Hour Cigarette Count*

Name _____

Date _____

Number of Cigarettes during the Day	Time of Day	Need Rating*	Place of Activity	With Whom	Mood or Reason
1.	_____	1 2 3	_____	_____	_____
2.	_____	1 2 3	_____	_____	_____
3.	_____	1 2 3	_____	_____	_____
4.	_____	1 2 3	_____	_____	_____
5.	_____	1 2 3	_____	_____	_____
6.	_____	1 2 3	_____	_____	_____
7.	_____	1 2 3	_____	_____	_____
8.	_____	1 2 3	_____	_____	_____
9.	_____	1 2 3	_____	_____	_____
10.	_____	1 2 3	_____	_____	_____
11.	_____	1 2 3	_____	_____	_____
12.	_____	1 2 3	_____	_____	_____
13.	_____	1 2 3	_____	_____	_____
14.	_____	1 2 3	_____	_____	_____
15.	_____	1 2 3	_____	_____	_____
16.	_____	1 2 3	_____	_____	_____
17.	_____	1 2 3	_____	_____	_____
18.	_____	1 2 3	_____	_____	_____
19.	_____	1 2 3	_____	_____	_____
20.	_____	1 2 3	_____	_____	_____
21.	_____	1 2 3	_____	_____	_____
22.	_____	1 2 3	_____	_____	_____
23.	_____	1 2 3	_____	_____	_____
24.	_____	1 2 3	_____	_____	_____
25.	_____	1 2 3	_____	_____	_____
26.	_____	1 2 3	_____	_____	_____
27.	_____	1 2 3	_____	_____	_____
28.	_____	1 2 3	_____	_____	_____
29.	_____	1 2 3	_____	_____	_____
30.	_____	1 2 3	_____	_____	_____

*Need rating: How important is the cigarette to you at this time?
1 = Most important; I would miss it very much.
2 = Average
3 = Lease important; I would not miss it.

has answered these questions, appropriate interventions can be designed to deal with the problem behavior. For example, if a participant says she only smokes when she is by herself, then activities would be planned so that she does not spend a lot of time alone. If another participant seemed to do most of her smoking while drinking coffee, an activity would be developed to provide some type of substitute. If a person seemed to smoke the most while sitting at the table after meals, activities could be planned to get the person away from the dinner table and doing something that would occupy her hands.

Another way of leading into a behavior modification activity is through a health status evaluation, or what is often referred to as a *health screening*. Such screenings could happen at home (e.g., BSE, TSE, hemocult, etc.), at a community health fair (e.g., blood pressure, cholesterol), or in the office of a health care professional (e.g., breast examination). Like record keeping via diaries, logs, or journals, health screenings can "grab the attention" (develop awareness) of those in the target population to begin the behavior modification process.

Environmental Change Activities

Another group of activities that have proved useful in reaching desired outcomes falls into the category of environmental change. Cheadle and colleagues (1992) define environmental intervention activities as the measures that alter or control the legal, social, economic, and physical environment. (*Note:* For the purpose of this presentation, the legal aspects are placed in a section titled Regulatory Activities, and economic aspects are placed in a section titled Incentives and Disincentives.). These activities are characterized by changes in those things "around" individuals that may influence their awareness, knowledge, attitudes, skills, or behavior. Some of these activities provide a "forced choice" situation, as when the selection of foods and beverages in vending machines or cafeterias is changed to include only "healthy" foods. If people want to eat foods from these sources, they are forced to eat certain types of foods. French and colleagues (1997) used a similar idea to the forced choice idea when they lowered the price by 50% on low-fat snacks in vending machines to try to influence food choices. Other activities in this category may provide those in the target population with health messages and environmental cues for certain types of behavior. Examples would be posting of no-smoking signs, eliminating ashtrays, providing lockers and showers, using role modeling by others, playing soft music in a work area, organizing a shuttle service or some other type of transportation system to get seniors to congregate meals or to a health care provider, and providing point-of-purchase education, such as a sign on a vending machine or food labeling on the food lines in the cafeteria.

Regulatory Activities

Regulatory activities include executive orders, laws, ordinances, policies, position statements, regulations, and formal and informal rules. These could be classified as mandated activities or regulated activities because they are activities that are required by an administrator, board, or legislative body to guide individual or collective behavior (Schmid, Pratt, & Howze, 1995). Examples include state laws requiring the use of safety belts and motorcycle helmets or raising the taxes on cigarettes, company policy stating that there will be no smoking in corporate offices and company-owned vehicles, and a board of education adopting a position statement that it will provide only well-balanced meals in its cafeterias. "An example of an executive order is a ban on tobacco advertising on city-owned buses" (Brownson et al., 1995, p. 479).

This type of intervention activity may be controversial. It has been criticized by some because it mandates a particular response from an individual. It takes away individual freedoms and sometimes plays on a person's pride, "pocketbook," and psyche. This type of activity must be sold on the basis of "common good." That is, the justification for this type of societal action is to protect the public's health. Regulatory activities exist for the protection of the community and of individual rights.

> Officials are willing to intercede into the private activities and lives of people in order to protect the larger population. When such intervention occurs it is usually very narrow and very specifically defined. There also tend to be sanctions attached if people do not comply. For example, in the case of inoculations, if a mother and father did not have their child inoculated that child cannot attend school. If parents do not send their child to school they are in violation of the law, and there are criminal and civil penalties that are involved. (Rich & Sugrue, 1989, p. 33)

Some would say that regulatory activities do not allow for the "voluntary actions conducive to health" that are suggested by Green and Kreuter (1999, p. 27) in their definition of health education. But, at the same time, this kind of activity can get people to change their behavior when other strategies have failed. For example, before the passage of safety belt laws, most states were reporting about a 14% use rate by drivers of automobiles and were trying to attack the problem through educational activities using the mass media. Now that safety belt laws are in effect in many states, usage rates in those states are closer to 50%; in some states where there is strict enforcement, usage rates approach 80%. Another example is the work of Sorensen and colleagues (1991), which showed a 21% reduction in the number of employees who smoked in a company that put a nonsmoking policy in effect. Both of these examples show that regulatory activities are necessary to reinforce and support prevention messages.

Since regulatory activities are mandatory, it is particularly important to use good judgment and show respect for others when implementing them. In some instances, program planners will be faced with ethical decisions. If a program will make use of regulatory intervention activities, the planner should remember that, as in any political process, there is likely to be both pro and con feelings toward the "mandatory" action. Thus, when developing and implementing any mandatory action, planners should bear in mind the following points:

1. Have top-level support for the mandated action (Emont & Cummings, 1989; Mikanowicz & Altman, 1995).
2. Have a representative group (committee) from the target population help formulate the "mandatory" action.

3. Consider surveying those in the target population to gain additional information regarding policy change (Mikanowicz & Altman, 1995).
4. Make sure expert advice on the subject of the mandated action is available to the group developing it.
5. Seek a legal opinion if necessary.
6. Examine the work of others and review the issues they faced when implementing "mandatory" actions.
7. Be sure that regulatory activities are based on sound principles and, if possible, good research.
8. Seek input and debate/discussion concerning the mandated action from the target population while it is being formulated.
9. Develop regulatory activities that are written simply and include a rationale, a general policy statement, specific areas affected, and clearly defined complaint, grievance, and enforcement procedures (Mikanowicz & Altman, 1995).
10. Consider phasing in the new regulation a little bit at a time. For example, if a no-smoking policy is going to be implemented, the planner may want to begin by restricting smoking in certain areas before banning it altogether. This not only helps people change gradually but it also expresses concern for them.
11. Provide education and behavior change programs to assist those in the target population with the implementation of the "mandatory" actions (Mikanowicz & Altman, 1995).
12. Ensure that, once formulated, the "mandatory" actions
    a. are actively communicated to those in the target population.
    b. are reviewed on a regular basis for the purposes of evaluating and revising if necessary.
    c. apply to all in the target population and not just to select groups.
    d. are consistently enforced. Be prepared to deal with the complaint and grievance processes (Mikanowicz & Altman, 1995).
    e. are enforced as a shared responsibility of all in the institution.

To help gain a sense of the difficulty of dealing with regulatory activities, let's examine the options available to a group of department heads who are trying to decide whether they should continue to allow the public to smoke in the lobby of the building and employees to smoke in their individual, self-contained offices. Several options are available to this administrative group:

1. Decide to have no explicit policy.
2. Make no changes and continue with the status quo.
3. Eliminate only public smoking in the building.
4. Designate a different area within or outside the building for public smoking.
5. Allow smoking only in individual offices.
6. Designate the entire building as a "smoke-free building."
7. Request that all employees hired in the future be nonsmokers.
8. A combination of items 1–7.

Each of these options poses special concerns for administrative groups. Policies are seldom easy to develop, but looking at others that have already been developed helps in the creation of a new policy. For this reason, a couple examples are provided in the appendices to this book. Appendix C presents the smoking policy of the McSmeltzer Corporation. Appendix D presents the "Model Ordinance Eliminating Smoking in Workplaces and Enclosed Public Places (100% Smokefree)" developed by Americans for Nonsmokers' Rights. (*Note:* Planners interested in developing policies regulating smoking should also review the works of Mikanowicz & Altman [1995] and USDHHS [1985].)

Community Advocacy Activities

Not to be confused with regulatory activities, community advocacy activities are used to influence social change. Community advocacy is a process in which the people of the community become involved in the institutions and decisions that will have an impact on their lives. It has the potential for creating more support, keeping people informed, influencing decisions, activating nonparticipants, improving service, and making people, plans, and programs more responsive (Checkoway, 1989). But community advocacy is not without costs: In most situations it requires time and effort, as well as persistence. Yet it can have a big impact on social change issues involving health. Community advocacy includes community organizing (see Chapter 9), coalition building (see Chapter 9), and education of the community and decision makers (Deeds, 1992). Techniques often used in advocacy activities include: (1) personal visits to educate or lobby the key people; (2) a community rally; (3) telephone call campaigns to the offices of the decision makers; (4) TV or radio appearances to express your views; (5) letter-writing campaigns (see Figure 8.6) to the key people who educate/influence decision makers; (6) letter-writing campaigns to newspaper editors, expressing concern (congratulations or shame-on-you) about the results of a vote by decision makers on a particular issue; and (7) letter-writing campaigns to decision makers, thanking them for support on a key issue.

Auld (1997) offered a set of practical tips for influencing public policy. They are adapted here to apply to influencing public policy at the local as well as the state and federal levels.

1. *Opening doors.* Establish relationships that build trust and rapport with staff, legislative assistants, and, if possible, the elected officials themselves so that you can approach them for their support on an issue of concern. Know on what committees your elected officials sit and how they have voted on the issues.
2. *Identifying the players.* Identify who the stakeholders are on a particular issue and find out why they are.
3. *Making the link.* Find out how the issues you are interested in are linked to the health problems of the population/constituency of the elected officials. For example, if you are interested in chronic diseases, show how they are linked to the elderly in the population/constituency.

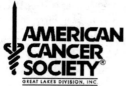

Hope. Progress. Answers.

Senators and Representatives pay attention to their constituents. It is good politics. Responding to constituents is the "bread and butter" of a legislative office. A member knows your approval can be won or lost by his or her response to your concerns.

The most effective means of communication with your legislator, aside from a personal visit, is a personal letter (not a form letter). It should be concise, informed and polite.

Date

Your address

Legislator's address

Dear Senator/Representative:

· Try to stick to one typewritten page. Don't type or write on the back of a page. If writing longhand, take care to write legibly.
· In a short first paragraph, *state your purpose.* Stick with *one* subject or issue. Support your position with the rest of the letter.
· If a bill is the subject, cite it by name and number.
· Be factual and support your position with information about how legislation is likely to affect you and others. Avoid emotional, philosophical arguments.
· Explain how you intend to help the cause. *Ask what else you can do to help change things.* State one more time what you would like your legislator to do.
· Be sure you include your name and address
· Follow up your letter with a phone call.

Sincerely,

Jane Doe

U.S. CONGRESS ADDRESSES

The Honorable ...
U.S. Senate
Washington, DC 20510

The Honorable...
U.S. House of Representatives
Washington, DC 20515

INDIANA LEGISLATURE

The Honorable...
Indiana State House
200 W. Washington St.
Indianapolis, IN 46204

MICHIGAN STATE LEGISLATURE

The Honorable...
Michigan State Senate
P.O. Box 30036
Lansing, MI 48909

The Honorable...
Michigan House of Representatives
P.O. Box 30014
Lansing, MI 48909

FIGURE 8.6 *Tips for Writing Effective Letters*

Source: American Cancer Society, Great Lakes Division, Inc. Used with permission.

4. *Crafting your position.* Make sure your position on the issue(s) is (are) developed on the best available science and data.
5. *Organizing the troops.* Organize others who may be interested in your issue to show broad representation from the population/constituency (see Chapter 9 for organizing techniques).

6. *Visiting policy makers.* Schedule appointments with the elected official or staff to express your views on the issues. Take others with you who can help explain your views. Be on time, be brief, yet be prepared to educate by using practical examples.

7. *Demonstrating the power of press.* Demonstrate your link to the media and how you and your organization can get positive press for the elected official by activating (i.e., letters to the editor, etc.) your link.

8. *Reinforcing your message.* End your visit or follow up the visit with a packet that summarizes your position on the issues. Supporting scientific data should be included. Also, send a thank you letter. As the issue moves through the legislative process, let your elected official know your views on its direction.

9. *Serving as a resource.* Stay in contact with the staff and elected official and offer to be a resource person to help them as needed on the issue.

10. *Responding quickly.* Be prepared to respond quickly when asked to be a resource person or testify to a legislative group. Requests often come at the last minute.

11. *Reaching the finish line.* Follow up on a piece of legislation after it has been passed to help those who have to implement it and to advocate for funding to help the implementation.

A good example of influencing public policy was presented by Heiser and Begay (1997) as they described the campaign to raise the tobacco tax in Massachusetts.

Organizational Culture Activities

Closely aligned with environmental change activities is the category of activities that affect organizational culture. Culture is usually associated with norms and traditions that are generated by and linked to a "community" of people. Organizations, which are made up of people, also can have their own culture. The culture of an organization can be thought of as its personality. The culture expresses what is and what is not considered important to the organization. The nature of the culture depends on the type of organization—corporation, school, or nonprofit group.

Many people think that it takes a long time to establish norms and traditions, and it often does. Still, change can occur very quickly if the decision makers in an organization support it. For example, if organizational decision makers believe exercise is important, they may provide employees with an extra 20 minutes at lunchtime for exercise. Similarly, it is surprising to see how many young executives will use a corporation's exercise facility because the chief executive officer does. Other examples of organizational culture activities might include changing the types of foods found in vending machines; closing the "junk food" machines during lunch periods at school; offering discounts on the health foods found in the company cafeteria; and getting retailers to change the way they have done things in the past, such as moving their tobacco products from in front of a counter to behind a counter, where an employee has to get them for the customer. Because these activities affect groups of people, they are usually used at the organizational or institutional level.

Incentives and Disincentives

The use of **incentives** and **disincentives** to influence health outcomes is a common type of activity. This type of intervention activity is based on many health behavior theories that suggest that it is the anticipation of rewards—and tangible ones at that—that increases the probability of an individual engaging in desired behavior (Lefebvre, 1992). An incentive can increase the perceived value of an activity (Patton et al., 1986), motivate people to get involved, and remind program participants of their commitment to and goals for behavior change (Wilbur, 1983). The key to motivating someone with an incentive is to know what will incite an individual to action. Thus, for this type of activity to work, the planner needs to match the incentives with the needs, wants, or desires of the target population. However, this is not easy, for what is an incentive for one person may be a deterrent for another, and vice versa. It has been suggested that incentives should even be tailored to the socioeconomic characteristics of the participants (Chenoweth, 1987) and, for that matter, the individual characteristics of each person.

For the planners, the task becomes one of matching the needs of the program participant or potential program participant with available incentives. Two approaches have been used to accomplish this. The first is to include questions about incentives as part of any needs assessment conducted in program planning. For example, a workforce needs survey might include a question on incentives, such as "What incentives would entice you to participate in the exercise program?" or "What would it take to get you to participate in this program?" or "What would it take to keep you involved in a health promotion program?" or "Would you continue to participate in an exercise program if you knew you were going to be given a nice tee shirt after logging 100 miles running or walking, or participating for 50 days in an aerobic dance or swimming program?" The responses to these questions should provide some indication of the type of incentives that would be most useful for this target population. The second is the shotgun approach, based on previous experience or the experience reported by others. The shotgun approach offers a variety of incentives to meet the needs of a large percentage of the program's target population. However, the former approach is recommended as being more likely to meet the targeted needs and wants.

Based on the idea that incentives should meet the individual needs of the target population, the number of different types of incentives is almost endless. Feldman (1983) suggests two major categories of incentives or reinforcers. The first group includes incentives that would be considered social reinforcers; the second group includes incentives that are considered material reinforcers, or what may be referred to as economic incentives (see Figure 8.7).

Finally, the following advice is offered to program planners who choose to use incentives:

1. Make sure everyone can receive one, whatever the incentive may be (Kendall, 1984).
2. Make the incentives useful and meaningful (Kendall, 1984).

FIGURE 8.7 *Incentives: Social and Material Reinforcers*

I. Social Reinforcers
   A. Special attention or recognition from instructors, peers, classmates, coworkers, or chief executive officers (Feldman, 1983; Shepard, 1985)
   B. Praise/verbal reinforcement (Feldman, 1983; Shepard, 1985)
   C. Public and other recognition (i.e., name in newsletter, name on bulletin board) (Koffman et al., 1998)
   D. Encouragement (Feldman, 1983; Shepard, 1985)
   E. Friendship (Feldman, 1983; Shepard, 1985)
   F. Inclusion of family members in the program (Feldman, 1983; Shepard, 1985)
   G. Personal letter to those reaching goals (Bensley, 1991)

II. Material Reinforcers
   A. Inexpensive "token" incentives
      1. T-shirts, hats, caps, visors, warm-up jackets, calendars, key chains, flashlights, pens, windshield scraper, wallets, tape measures, vacuum bottles, mugs, home fire extinguishers, smoke detectors, and auto safety kits (Cinelli, Rose-Colley, & Hayes, 1988; Kendall, 1984)
      2. Certificates
      3. Pins, buttons, patches, and decals that can be worn and plaques or markers that can be displayed in the work area
      4. Towels, lockers
      5. Preferred or free parking
   B. Program cost sharing between employer and employee
      1. Cost of registering for a program (Pollock et al., 1982)
      2. Membership at a fitness center/club
      3. Sliding-scale fee based on the ability to pay
      4. Refund of part or all of program fee based on participant's completion of a activity
      5. Money to be used as an incentive (Koffman et al., 1998)

   C. Health Insurance
      1. Sharing between employer and employee of money saved on health insurance from one year to the next (Toufexis, 1985)
      2. Alteration of fringe benefit package to reward good health practices
      3. Employer picking up more of the insurance costs to reward good health practices (Toufexis, 1985)
      4. Provision of a fund for each employee to pay for the person's health care costs during the year, with any unused money from this account given to the employee at the end of the year (Hosokawa, 1984; Toufexis, 1985)
      5. Lower premiums for employees with fewer health risks (i.e., nonsmoker or exerciser) (Hosokawa, 1984)

   D. Monetary
      1. Tokens, Monopoly-style dollars, stamps, coupons, or points that are redeemable at a company store or a retail store, or for catalog shopping for prizes or merchandise (Kendall, 1984; Piniat, 1984; Toufexis, 1985)
      2. Drawings, lotteries, and raffles open to those who have participated or met a goal (Cinelli et al., 1988; Emont & Cummings, 1992; Health Insurance Association of America, 1983; Toufexis, 1985)
      3. Bonus, extra pay, or just plain pay for completion of contract, participation, not smoking on the job, or quitting (DiBlase, 1985; Toufexis, 1985)
      4. Financial rewards for both individuals and groups who have fewer and/or no work accidents during the year (DiBlase, 1985) or better smoking cessation rate (Koffman et al., 1998)

(continued)

FIGURE 8.7 Continued

5. "Well pay" for unused sick days (DiBlase, 1985)
6. Gift certificates, from a small value, such as for a free ice cream cone, to something of greater value, such as a U.S. savings bond (Kendall, 1984)

E. Work Hours
 1. Flex-time (flexible work hours) in order to participate
 2. Released time to participate
 3. Time off (Cinelli et al., 1988)

F. Contracts
 1. Contract (competition) with a buddy
 2. Contract with instructor to reach a specific goal, with a material incentive provided by instructor
 3. Forfeiture of money or time to charity for not fulfilling a contract (Bloomquist, 1981)

4. Contract is entered into with the instructor in which money is withheld (via payroll deduction) while the person is enrolled in the program, so that if goal is met, the money is refunded; if not, it is forfeited (Bensley, 1991; Forster et al., 1985)

III. Miscellaneous
 A. Special medical examinations and screenings for those who participate.
 B. Special events, such as contests or luncheons (Kendall, 1984; Patton et al., 1986)
 C. Providing special "space," such as a table in the lunchroom for those on a special diet (Bensley, 1991)

---

3. Ensure that the ground rules are fair, understandable, and followed by everyone (Kendall, 1984).
4. Make a big deal of awarding the incentive.
5. Use incentives that are consistent with health promotion philosophies. For example, avoid incentives of alcoholic beverages, high fat or high sugar foods, or other mixed-message prizes.

Just as incentives can be used to get people involved in behavior change, **disincentives** can be used to discourage a certain behavior. For example, Penner (1989) reports on the use of a surcharge for health insurance to influence the behavior of those who continue to use tobacco products. Other examples include placing user taxes on a product to deter its use in a target population (e.g., cigarettes and adolescents), levying fines for health-harming behavior (e.g., not wearing safety belts), and not allowing the use of something because of a certain behavior (e.g., not allowing smokers to use the teachers' lounge or company vehicles).

As a final comment on incentives, several authors (French, Jeffery, & Oliphant, 1994; Jeffery et al., 1993; Matson, Lee, & Hopp, 1993; Price et al., 1992) have reported on the effectiveness of using incentives for program participation and behavior change. From these works, it appears that incentives are useful in getting people to participate and change their behavior for a short period of time. Their effectiveness in long-term behavior change is not so clear.

Health Status Evaluation Activities

An activity aimed at making those in the target population more aware of their current health status is often used as part of a multiactivity intervention. These activities have involved the completion of a health risk appraisal (HRA) form (see Chapter 4 for a discussion of HRAs), self-screenings (e.g., breast self-examination or testicular self-examination), clinical screenings (e.g., blood pressure and cholesterol), and professional health check-ups and examinations. The settings for such activities have included health fairs, worksites, personal residences, mobile units (e.g., vans equipped with mammography units), and health care facilities. These activities usually have high credibility with target populations because of their link with health care providers.

Social Activities

The importance of social support for behavior change and its relationship to health have been noted by several researchers (Becker & Green, 1975; Berkman & Syme, 1979; Cohen & Lichtenstein, 1990; Colletti & Brownell, 1982; Horman, 1989; Kviz et al., 1994; Kaplan & Cassel, 1977; Cummings, Becker, & Maile, 1980). Many people find it much easier to change a behavior if those around them provide support or are willing to be partners in the behavior change process. One of the major reasons why worksite health promotion programs have been so well received is because of the built-in social support from coworkers (Behrens, 1983).

Reference has already been made to how social support could work as an incentive. That would be one form of a social activity. Other social interventions could include support groups or buddy support, social activities, and social networks. These intervention activities have been used in both micro and macro interventions with much success.

Support Groups and Buddy System.   The importance of support groups as part of comprehensive interventions has been well established. One need only look to the 12-step programs (such as Alcoholics Anonymous, Overeaters Anonymous, and Gamblers Anonymous) and commercial programs (such as Weight Watchers) to realize the importance of people coming together to share their experiences and support one another's efforts. A support group need not be large; it might be as small as just two people. A buddy system is an example of a two-person group. A buddy system can take one of two different forms. In the first, both individuals are trying to change a behavior. In such a relationship, the two individuals support each other, whether this means helping each other stay on a special diet or meeting each other at 6 A.M. for exercise. In the other form, only one of the two is trying to change a behavior. The one not changing the behavior may have already changed (e.g., has already quit smoking or is exercising regularly) and is acting as a mentor to the one trying to change, or may not be trying to change but provides support at regular intervals or as problems arise.

Special elements that can be added to the support group or buddy system are the use of competition or a contract. Competition can take place between individual group members over such things as who can lose the most weight, who can walk/run the most miles, or who can go the longest without a cigarette. Competition could also be based on teams within the target population (such as two different companies, two schools, or departments within an organization), using similar criteria but now based on group total figures (pounds, miles, or cigarettes). See Chapter 11 for more on competitions.

Contracts could be used by having one member of the target population enter into an agreement with another member or with another person (such as the program facilitator, a friend, or spouse) over a change in some health behavior. The major component of a contract is the contingency. The *contingency* is a statement of what will happen if a contract is met or not met. For example, if a person meets the terms of his contract by losing 10 pounds in five weeks, he can then expect to receive something specified (an intangible, such as praise, or a material object) from the person who agreed to the contract. If the terms are not met, then the person for whom the contract was written must forfeit something specified (perhaps time volunteered to a community service or a material object of his own). See Chapter 11 for more on contracts.

Social Activities.   Social activities can be an an important type of social intervention. Bringing together people who may be confronting similar problems for the purpose of purely social interaction not related to the problem can indirectly help them deal with the problem. Examples of such activities might be single parents having a cookout or a group of senior citizens attending a play. Although these activities do not deal directly with these people's common problems, they do help fill voids in their lives and thus indirectly help with the problem.

Social Networks.   Social networks are another type of social intervention. *Networks* are matrices linked by relationships or "ties." The nature of a tie can be quite varied, consisting of almost anything that creates a special feeling: need, concern, loyalty, frustration, power, affection, or obligation, to name just a few. When people are "networking," they are said to be looking for relationships that would be useful in helping them with their concerns, such as problem solving, program development, resource identification, and others. As part of a health promotion intervention, social networking may take the form of having program participants trade telephone numbers for the purpose of calling each other when they are trying to resist smoking a cigarette or trying to locate a needed resource to solve a problem.

It should also be noted that although most social support and buddy systems take place between individuals, they can also be established at the institutional level. Like individuals, institutions can be paired up to help one another. For example, if two companies are interested in establishing health promotion programs, they could work together on their programs and share information and resources where appropriate. Or, if one company has a well-established program in place, then that company could "mentor" another company in setting up a program.

Technology-Delivered Activities

Traditionally, many health education and health promotion programs have been delivered via face-to-face contact between the provider of the program and the target population. However, with the use of technology, health education and health promotion programs can be delivered in a variety of ways. For example, since the widespread use of personal computers, much has been written about the pros and cons of computer-assisted instruction (Gilbert & Sawyer, 1995). More recently, computers have been used by members of target populations to identify educational materials on the World Wide Web and to communicate with their health care providers via electronic mail.

One piece of technology that many do not think of as "technology" because of its longer history, as compared to personal computers, is the telephone. Over the years, the telephone has been used in a variety of ways by health educators, including "gathering information, disseminating information, providing health education and counseling, promoting health education programs, offering cues to action and social support" (Soet & Basch, 1997, p. 760). Health education delivered by telephone "can be classified into two broad categories: *individual initiated*, where the individual must actively seek contact and assistance from a health information hotline; and *outreach*, where the individual is called by a health educator or counselor" (Soet & Basch, 1997, p. 760). Individual-initiated health information hot lines usually provide information, and sometimes education and counseling, whereas outreach activities range from brief, one-time preappointment reminders to long-term interactive professional health counseling (Soet & Basch, 1997). Telephone-delivered intervention activities have been created for a variety of topics, including but not limited to cancer screening (Davis et al., 1997; Ludman et al., 1999; McDowell, Newell, & Rosser, 1989b), medical appointments (Linkins et al., 1994), hypertension screening (McDowell, Newell, & Rosser, 1989a), smoking cessation (Koffman et al., 1998; Simmons, 1998), and weight loss (Hellerstedt & Jeffery, 1997). Soet and Basch (1997) present a generic process for developing a telephone intervention activity that includes three areas: "designing the intervention protocol, selection and training of the health educator/counselor(s), and developing the documentation and data collection protocol" (p. 763).

Designing Health Promotion Interventions

Once program planners have completed a needs assessment, written program goals and objectives, and considered different types of intervention activities, they are in a position to begin designing an appropriate intervention.

Criteria and Guidelines for Developing a Health Promotion Intervention

There is no one best way of intervening to accomplish a specific program goal that can be generalized to all target populations. Each target population has its own needs and wants that must be addressed. Nevertheless, successful and responsible health promotion programs generally adhere to some common set of guidelines, standards, or criteria around which their interventions are planned (Ad Hoc Work Group, 1987). Such guidelines help standardize and ensure the quality of the program, give credibility to a program, help with program accountability, provide a legal defense if a liability situation might arise, and identify ethical concerns that need to be addressed as a part of planning, implementing, and evaluating programs.

In 1987, the American Public Health Association (APHA), in collaboration with the Center for Health Promotion and Education of the Centers for Disease Control (CDC), developed a set of criteria to serve as guidelines for establishing the feasibility and/or the appropriateness of health education and promotion programs in a variety of settings (industrial, hospital, worksite, voluntary and official agencies) before making a decision to implement them. The criteria were not developed to assure successful programs, but rather to suggest issues that need to be considered in the decision-making process leading to the allocation of resources or the setting of program priorities (Ad Hoc Work Group, 1987, pp. 89–92). The five criteria suggested by the Work Group are:

1. A health promotion program should address one or more risk factors that are carefully defined, measurable, modifiable, and prevalent among the members of a chosen target group, and these factors that constitute a threat to the health status and the quality of life of target group members.
2. A health promotion program should reflect a consideration of the special characteristics, needs, and preferences of its target group(s).
3. Health promotion programs should include interventions that will clearly and effectively reduce a target risk factor and are appropriate for a particular setting.
4. A health promotion program should identify and implement interventions that make optimum use of the available resources.
5. From the outset, a health promotion program should be organized, planned, and implemented in such a way that its operation and effects can be evaluated.

In addition to the criteria set forth by APHA and CDC, other agencies and organizations have suggested criteria and guidelines. The Society of Prospective Medicine has developed the Ethics Guidelines for the Development and Use of Health Assessments (SPMBoD, 1999). Some organizations and professionals have set guidelines, criteria, or **codes of practice** for specific types of health promotion programs. Examples are the criteria set forth by the American College of Sports Medicine (1998) for exercise programs, the guidelines established by the American

TABLE 8.2   *Conceptual Model for Designing an Intervention*

Goal	Objectives	Theory/Model	Level of influence	Intervention activities	Evaluation
	Administrative	Stimulus response theory	Intrapersonal	Communication	Process
	Learning		Interpersonal	Educational	Impact
	Awareness	Social cognitive theory	Institutional/ Organizational	Behavior modification	Outcome
	Knowledge	Theory of planned behavior	Community	Regulatory	
	Attitudes		Public policy	Community advocacy	
	Skills	Theory of freeing			
	Behavioral	Problem-behavior theory		Organizational culture	
	Environmental			Incentives/ Disincentives	
	Program	Health belief model		Health status evaluations	
		Transtheoretical model		Social	
		Cognitive-behavioral model of the Relapse Process		Technology delivered	

College of Obstetricians and Gynecologists for exercise during pregnancy, and the clinical practice guidelines for smoking cessation available from the Agency for Health Care Policy and Research (AHCPR, 1996) as well as those by Bartlett and colleagues (1986). Obviously, these guidelines and criteria are not all that are available. Prudent planners should seek out, through inquiry and networking, other criteria and guidelines that apply to programs they are planning.

A Model for Designing Interventions

What should be included in a health promotion intervention? This question is constantly asked by those who are responsible for planning programs. The criteria and guidelines listed earlier in this chapter and the theories presented in Chapter 7 provide a partial answer to this question, but more guidance is needed to help planners in the development of well-conceived interventions. For this reason, it is important to present a model that would be useful in planning an intervention.

   The conceptual model (see Table 8.2) begins with the review of the goal(s) and objectives of the program you are planning. What outcomes are expected from the program? What theory or model best aligns with the expected outcomes.? What specific constructs are being used and how are they translated to variables? Next, the level of influence must be considered. Different intervention activities will be selected at the same time the level of influence is being considered. For example, if the level of influence selected was at the intrapersonal level, a communication intervention activity would be different than if the level of influence was public policy. And finally, as a program planner, you will need to decide how and when the intervention will be evaluated. The evaluation should be closely linked to the objectives of the program. That is, how and when will you be able to measure the program outcomes? No matter whether program planners use this model or another, they should devote much thought to the health problem or concern, the desired program outcome(s), at what points to intervene, and the most effective intervention activities for the problem.

Summary

Interventions are activities used by program planners to bring about the outcomes identified in the program objectives. These activities are also sometimes referred to as *treatments.* Although many times an intervention is made up of a single activity, it is more common for planners to use a variety of activities to make up an intervention for a program. In this chapter, intervention activities were categorized into the following groups:

1. Communication activities
2. Educational activities or methods
3. Behavior modification activities
4. Environmental change activities
5. Regulatory activities
6. Community advocacy activities
7. Organizational culture activities
8. Economic and other incentives
9. Health status evaluation activities
10. Social intervention activities
11. Technology-delivered activities

Additionally, this chapter identified the need for program planners to be aware of recommended standards/criteria/guidelines when planning program interventions. Some examples were reviewed of general, as well as program-specific, guidelines that have been set forth by both professional organizations and individual professionals. Finally, this chapter presented a model that planners can use in developing health education interventions.

Questions

1. What is an intervention?

2. What are the advantages of using a multi-activity intervention over one that includes a single activity? Are there any disadvantages? If so, what are they?

3. What are the major categories of interventions? Explain each.

4. Why should program planners be concerned with program guidelines that have been developed by professional organizations?

5. What are some of the documents and sponsoring groups that have suggested standards, criteria, or guidelines for program development?

6. Briefly discuss the conceptual model set forth in this chapter for creating an intervention.

Activities

1. Create a multiactivity intervention for a program you are planning.

2. Create a multiactivity intervention for a program that has as its goal "to get third-grade students to wear helmets while riding their bicycles."

3. Create a multiactivity intervention for a program that has as its goal "to eliminate smoking of all employees of Company X."

4. Create a multiactivity intervention for a program that has as its goal "the rehydration of young children in the small village of Y in the Third World country of Q."

5. Design and present on a 8½" × 11" piece of paper a bulletin board that could be used as part of the multiactivity intervention you are planning. Divide the piece of paper that represents the bulletin board into six equal sections and indicate what you will include in each section.

6. Interview a classmate to find out information about his or her health risks. Then, assuming you are a patient educator in a health clinic, create a one-page *tailored* letter to the person, urging him or her to seek an appropriate screening for the health risk(s).

7. Develop a three-fold pamphlet that can be used as an informational piece for a program you are planning.

8. With other students in your class, write a PSA script for a program you are planning. Then rehearse the script and have it videotaped.

9. Write a two-page, double-spaced news release that describes a program you are planning.

10. Write a letter to your state or federal senators or representatives and request their support of a piece of health-related legislation that is currently being considered.

Activities on the Web

1. Visit the advocacy page of the website for either the Americans for Nonsmokers' Rights (**<http://www.no-smoke.org/advo. html>** or the American Heart Association **<http://www.americanheart.org/support/ advocacy/>**. Find out what the organization is advocating for and the process it presents for doing so. Download the information you find, then write a draft of a letter that would support the cause.

2. Using a search engine (i.e., *Excite, GoTo.com, Snap,* or *Lycos*), conduct a search on "readability." Identify a website that contains a readability scale. Using the readability scale presented, check the readability level of two pamphlets that you have obtained from a voluntary health organization (e.g., American Cancer Society, American Lung Association, or American Heart Association). One of the pamphlets should be targeted for children and the other targeted for adults. Take your work to class.

3. Box 8.1 stressed the importance of producing materials that are applicable to the

target population. Visit one or all of the following websites that present information on a variety of cultural groups. After visiting the sites, create a list of at least 10 items you have learned about creating materials for special populations. Provide the appropriate bibliographic citation for each item you list and provide a downloaded copy of the home page for each site you visit:

a. The Cross Cultural Health Care Program <**http://www.xculture.org**>

b. Multi-cultural Educational Services <**http://www.mcedservices.com/**>

c. The Center for Cross-Cultural Health <**http://www.crosshealth.com**>

d. Minority Health Program at University of North Carolina, Chapel Hill <**http://www.minority.unc.edu**>

e. National MultiCultural Institute <**http://www.nmci.org/**>

9

Community Organizing and Community Building

After reading this chapter and answering the questions at the end, you should be able to:

- Define *community, community organizing, community building,* and *coalitions.*
- Outline the processes for organizing and building a community.
- Explain the term *mapping community capacity.*
- Provide an overview of PATCH.

Key Terms

active participants
bottom-up
citizen initiated
coalitions
community
community building
community organizing
executive participants

gatekeepers
grass-roots
locality development
mapping community capacity
occasional participants
ownership
PATCH
potential building blocks

primary building blocks
secondary building blocks
social action
social planning
stakeholders
supporting participants

A significant portion of the work of health educators involves implementing health promotion programs with small communities of people. **Community** means

> a locale or domain that is characterized by the following elements: (1) membership—a sense of identity and belonging; (2) common symbol systems—similar language, rituals, and ceremonies; (3) shared values and norms; (4) mutual

influence—community members have influence and are influenced by each other; (5) shared needs and commitment to meeting them; and (6) shared emotional connection—members share common history, experiences, and mutual support. Communality may be geographically bounded (e.g., a neighborhood) but is not necessary (e.g., an ethnic group). (Israel et al., 1994).

Thus, it is not uncommon for health educators to implement a smoking cessation program in a corporate setting, organize a support group for families affected by a chronic disease, or present a drug education program for school-age children. However, health educators sometimes work with large communities, a task that involves organizing the people in a community to work together to implement a solution to a communitywide problem, concern, or issue. This chapter addresses the fundamental elements of organizing large communities for action.

Community Organizing and Its Assumptions

In recent years, there has been a shift in the focus of the work of health educators and others in the helping professions. Where once the work of health educators focused almost solely on the individual, today the focus is on broadening to the community. *Citizen participation, grass-roots participation, community participation, macro practice, community based, community empowerment,* and *community partnerships* are among the many terms that are being used more frequently by health agencies, outside funders, and policy makers (Minkler, 1997b). There are good reasons for the use of these terms and most revolve around the need for communities to organize.

In the early history of the United States, a sense of community was inherent in everyday life (Green, 1989). It was natural for communities to pool their resources to deal with shared problems. As time has passed, technology has improved greatly, resources have become more centralized, and U.S. society has become more mobile. As a result of these changes, communities have become more dependent on those outside the community and have fewer reasons to interact with neighboring communities.

> From self-sufficient farming communities of colonial America to the single-industry towns of the westward expansion and the industrial revolution to the Silicon Valleys of today's information and service era, communities have become increasingly dependent on other communities and on higher levels of organization and government to facilitate, coordinate, and regulate their interdependence. (Green, 1990, p. 165)

Because of these changes in community social structure and the resources necessary to meet the needs of communities, it now takes specific skills to organize a community to act for the collective good.

"The term *community organization* was coined by American social workers in the late 1880s to describe their efforts to coordinate services for newly arrived immigrants and the poor" (Minkler & Wallerstein, 1997, p. 31). More recently, *community organization* has been used by a variety of professionals, including health educators, and refers to various methods of intervention to deal with social problems. "Community organization is important in health education in part because it reflects one of the field's most fundamental principles, that of starting where the people" (Minkler & Wallerstein, 1997, p. 31). More formally, **community organizing** has been defined as "a process through which communities are helped to identify common problems or goals, mobilize resources, and in other ways develop and implement strategies for reaching their goals they have collectively set" (Minkler & Wallerstein, 1997, p. 30). It is not a science but rather an art of building consensus within the democratic process (Ross, 1967). (See Figure 9.1 for definitions of related terms.)

Although community organization may not be as "natural" as it once was, communities can still organize to analyze and solve problems through collective action. In working toward this end, those who try to organize communities must make several assumptions. Ross (1967, pp. 86–92) has stated these as follows:

1. Communities of people can develop capacity to deal with their own problems.
2. People want to change and can change.
3. People should participate in making, adjusting, or controlling the major changes taking place in their communities.
4. Changes in community living that are self-imposed or self-developed have a meaning and permanence that imposed changes do not have.
5. A "holistic approach" can deal successfully with problems with which a "fragmented approach" cannot cope.

FIGURE 9.1 *Terms Associated with Community Organizing*

Citizen Participation	The bottom-up, grass-roots mobilization of citizens for the purpose of undertaking activities to improve the condition of something in the community.
Community Development	"A process designed to create conditions of economic and social progress for the whole community with its active participation and the fullest possible reliance on the community's initiative" (United Nations, 1955, p. 6).
Community Participation	"A process of involving people in the institutions or decisions that affect their lives" (Checkoway, 1989, p. 18).
Empowered Community	"One in which individuals and organizations apply their skills and resources in collective efforts to meet their respective needs" (Israel et al., 1994).
Grass-Roots Participation	"Bottom-up efforts of people taking collective actions on their own behalf, and they involve the use of a sophisticated blend of confrontation and cooperation in order to achieve their ends" (Perlman, 1978, p. 65).
Macro Practice	The methods of professional change that deal with issues beyond the individual, family, and small group level.

6. Democracy requires cooperative participation and action in the affairs of the community, and that the people must learn the skills which make this possible.
7. Frequently communities of people need help in organizing to deal with their needs, just as many individuals require help in coping with their individual problems.

The Processes of Community Organizing and Community Building

There is no one specific method for organizing a community (Clapp, Packard, & Stanger, 1993). In fact, Rothman and Tropman (1987, pp. 4–5) have stated, "We should speak of community organization methods rather than the community organization method." Over the years, several different community organization methods have been used, including revolutionary techniques (Alinsky, 1971). However, in recent years, three models of community organization have been developed (Rothman & Tropman, 1987). They are locality development, social planning, and social action. **Locality development** is most like community development and seeks community change through broad self-help participation from the local community. "It is heavily process oriented, stressing consensus, and cooperation and aimed at building group identity and a sense of community" (Minkler & Wallerstein, 1997, p. 34). **Social planning** "is heavily task oriented, stressing rational-empirical problem-solving" (Minkler & Wallerstein, 1997, p. 34) and includes various levels of participation, ranging from a little to a lot, and involves outside planners. **Social action** "is both task and process oriented" (Minkler & Wallerstein, 1997, p. 34) and deals with organizing a disadvantaged segment of the population. It aims at making changes in institutions and communities and often seeks a redistribution of resources and power. Although this model is no longer used as often as it once was, it was most useful during the civil rights and gay rights movements.

Each of the above-noted approaches to community organizing varies slightly from the others. However, they all revolve around a common theme: the work and resources of many have a much better chance of solving a problem or meeting a goal than the work and resources of a few.

At the risk of violating Rothman and Tropman's (1987) maxim that there are various ways of organizing a community based on existing resources and problems, and since the purpose of this chapter is to provide an overview of community organizing, a very general or generic approach is presented here (see Figure 9.2). It does not include everything planners need to know about community organizing, but it does present the basic elements. The model relies heavily on social planning but also includes some specific elements from locality development, social action, and community building, a term defined later. For further information about community organizing, refer to any of several references (Archer, Kelly, & Bisch, 1984; Brager, Specht, & Torczyner, 1987; Checkoway, 1989; Minkler, 1997a; Langton, 1978; Rifkin, 1986; Ross, 1967; Rothman & Tropman, 1987; Rubin & Rubin, 1992) that are devoted entirely to the subject. Also, there are several

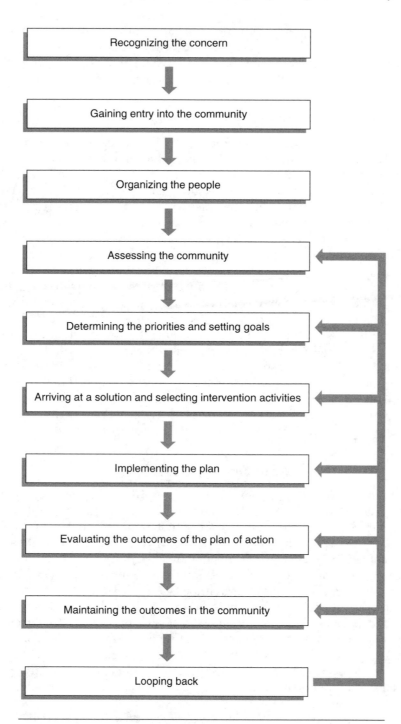

FIGURE 9.2 *Summary of the Steps in Community Organizing and Building*

works that deal specifically with the application of community organization to health promotion activities (Blackburn, 1983; Kumpfer, Turner, & Alvarado, 1991; Maccoby & Solomon, 1981; McAlister et al., 1982; Pentz et al., 1989; Wallenstein, Sanchez-Merki, & Dow, 1997).

Recognizing the Concern

The processes of community organizing and building begin when someone recognizes that a concern or issue exists in the community and that something needs to be done about it. This person (or persons) is referred to as the *organizer.* For the purposes of this discussion, assume that the concern is a health problem, but remember that the community organization process may be used with any type of problem found in a community. Concerns can be as specific as trying to get a certain piece of legislation passed or as general as advocating for a drug-free community.

The recognition of a health concern can occur from inside or outside the community. A citizen or a church leader from within the community may point out the problem, or it may first be identified by someone outside the community, such as an employee of a local or state health department, a state legislator, or someone from a local voluntary health agency. However, the community organizing efforts that have been most successful have been those that are recognized from the inside. The primary reason for this is that those within the community are much more likely to take ownership of the effort. It is difficult for someone from the outside coming in and telling community members that they have problems or issues that need to be dealt with and they need to organize to take care of them. When there is internal recognition of the issue or concern, it is referred to as **grass-roots, citizen-initiated,** or **bottom-up** organizing.

Gaining Entry into the Community

Recognition of a concern does not mean that people should immediately set about correcting it. Instead, they should follow a set of steps to deal with it, gaining proper "entry" into the community is the first step. Braithwaite and colleagues (1989) have stressed the importance of tactfully negotiating entry into a community with the individuals who control, both formally and informally, the "political climate" of the community. These individuals are referred to as **gatekeepers.** The term infers that one must pass through the "gate" in order to get at the people in the community (Wright, 1994). These "power brokers" know their community, how it functions, and how to accomplish tasks within it. Long-time residents are usually able to identify the gatekeepers of their community. They may include people such as business leaders, education leaders, heads of law enforcement agencies, leaders of community activist groups, parent and teacher groups, clergy, politicians, and others. Their support is absolutely essential to the success of any attempt to organize a community.

Organizers must approach the gatekeepers on the gatekeepers' terms and "play" the gatekeepers' "game." However, before making this contact, organizers must first be familiar with the community with which they are working. They must (1) know with whom the power lies, (2) know what type of political interactions take place within the community, (3) understand the culture or cultures that exist in the community, and (4) know whether the concern has been recognized before, and, if so, how was it addressed. In other words, community organizers must have a thorough knowledge of the community and the people living there before they try to enter the informal boundaries of the community (Braithwaite et al., 1989). Having a thorough understanding of the community and tactfully approaching its gatekeepers will help community organizers develop credibility and trust with those in the community, and, as noted earlier, it is not easy to bring a concern to the attention of those in the community. Few people are glad to know they have a problem, and fewer still like others to tell them they have a problem. Move with caution, and do not be too aggressive!

When the top-down approach is being used, organizers might find it advantageous to enter the community through an already established, well-respected organization or institution in the community, such as a church, a service group, or another successful local group. Green (1990) has suggested that the academic health center might be the ideal convener to address health services, health protection, or health promotion issues. "It has the deep roots in the community, it is not typically beholden to an out-of-state master, it can cut deals with local organizations, and it can draw upon resources to leverage commitments and resources from other organizations" (Green, 1990, p. 175). If such an organization/institution can be convinced that the problem exists and needs to be solved, it can help smooth the way to gaining entry and achieving the remaining steps in the process.

Organizing the People

Obtaining the support of the community members to deal with the concern is the next step in the process. It is best to begin with those individuals who are already interested in addressing the concern. This is not the time to try to convert people to the cause or to make sure that all the key players of the community are involved. It is best to begin with a core group of people who want to see change occur. Make sure this group includes people who are most affected by the concern. For example, if you are dealing with a teenage drug problem, include teens in the core group. If you are trying to help low-income individuals who need housing, make sure they are involved. More often than not, this core group will be small and will consist of people who are committed to the resolution of the concern, regardless of the time frame. Brager and colleagues (1987) have referred to this core group as **executive participants.** From among the core group, a leader or coordinator must be identified. If at all possible, the leader should be someone with leadership skills and a good knowledge of the concern. One of the early tasks of the leader will be to help build group cohesion.

Not everyone is cut out to be an organizer or a leader. Researchers have found that good organizers are successful because of a combination of skills and attributes. These skills and attributes fall into three main areas: change vision attributes, technical skills, and interactional or experience skills. *Change vision attributes* are closely aligned with the organizer's view of the world political terms. These people see a need for change and are personally dedicated and committed to seeing the change occur—so much so that they are willing to put other priorities aside to see the project through (Mondros & Wilson, 1994).

Technical skills include two areas: those related to efficacy on issues and those related to organizational health and effectiveness. The former includes being able to analyze issues, opponents, and power structure; develop and implement change strategies; achieve goals; and have outstanding communication and public relation skills. Organizational health and effectiveness skills include building structures for the recruitment and involvement of others, forming and maintaining task groups, and implementing skills of fund-raising and organizational management (Mondros & Wilson, 1994).

The third characteristic of a good organizer is possessing *interactional or experience skills*. These include an ability to respond with empathy, to assess and intervene with individuals and groups, and to be able to identify, develop, educate, and maintain organizational members and leaders (Mondros & Wilson, 1994).

With the core group and leader in place, the next step is to expand the group to build support for dealing with the concern—that is, to broaden the constituency. Brager and colleagues (1987) have noted that other group participants will include active, occasional, and supporting participants. The **active participants** (who may also be executive participants) take part in most group activities and are not afraid to do the work that needs to be done. The **occasional participants** become involved on an irregular basis and usually only when major decisions are made. The **supporting participants** are seldom involved but help swell the ranks and may contribute in nonactive ways or through financial contributions. When expanding the group, look for others who may be interested in helping, and ask current group members for names of people who might be interested. Look for people who may already be dealing with the concern through their present work or who have resources to contribute. This search should include existing social groups, such as voluntary health agencies, agricultural extension services, church groups, hospitals, health care providers, political officeholders, policy makers, police, educators, lay citizens, or special-interest groups. (See Box 9.1 on tips for understanding the diversity in a working group.)

Over the last few decades, in many communities the number of people interested in volunteering their time has decreased. Today, if you ask someone to volunteer, you may hear the reply, "I'm already too busy." There are two primary reasons for this response. First, there are many families in which both husband and wife work outside the home. Between 1970 and 1996, the proportion of married women with preschool-aged children who were in the labor force almost doubled, from 30.3% to 62.7%. Also during this same period of time, the proportion of married women with children of school age who were in the labor force jumped from 49.2% to 76.7%. In 1996, 70% of married couples with children reported that both husband and wife were employed outside the home. Second, there are more single-parent households. Today, they constitute about one-third (32%) of all family households with children, and most (27% vs. 5%) are headed by women (USBC, 1997). (See Box 9.2 for tips on working with volunteers).

BOX 9.1 • *Understanding Diversity*

Members of a group come from many different backgrounds. Some members may be much older or much younger than other members; some may represent different cultural, racial, or ethnic groups; some may represent different educational levels and abilities. Extra awareness and flexibility are required for the facilitator and other group members to remain sensitive to different backgrounds. Below we suggest a few ways to improve your awareness of differences. In general, new information is acquired so that different perspectives can be understood and appreciated.

- Become aware of differences in the group by asking questions and getting involved in small-group discussions.
- Seek involvement and input and listen to persons of different backgrounds without bias, and avoid being defensive.

- Learn the beliefs and feelings of specific groups about particular issues.
- Read about current and emerging issues that concern different groups, and read literature that is popular among different groups.
- Learn about the language, humor, gestures, norms, expectations, and values of different groups.
- Attend events that appeal to members of specific groups.
- Become attuned to cultural cliches, stereotypes, and distortions you may encounter in the media.
- Use examples to which persons of different cultures and backgrounds can relate.
- Learn the facts before you make statements or form opinions about different groups.

Source: Centers for Disease Control and Prevention (no date), p. A2–15.

These expanded community groups are sometimes referred to as *coalitions*. A **coalition** can be defined as a temporary union of two or more individuals and/or organizations to achieve a common purpose (often, to compensate for deficits in power, resources and expertise). The underlying concept behind coalitions is collaboration, for several individuals, groups, or organizations where their collective resources have a better chance of solving the problem than any single entity. "Building and maintaining effective coalitions have increasingly been recognized as vital components of much effective community organizing and community building" (Minkler, 1997b, p. 15). For those wanting more information about coalition development, Goldstein (1997) has presented a self-assessment instrument for gauging the developmental stage of coalitions.

Figure 9.3 provides a modified list of guidelines (Lindsay & Edwards, 1988) for keeping a coalition dynamic, viable, and effective.

Assessing the Community

Earlier in this chapter reference was made to the Rothman and Tropman's (1987) typology of community organization: locality development, social planning, and

BOX 9.2 • *Tips on Working with Volunteers*

Volunteers work for self-satisfaction, personal growth, fun, and other intangible rewards. Each volunteer should be treated as a colleague and recognized as an official part of the team. However, offer volunteers more flexibility than you can to employees, and adjust your expectations accordingly. For example, because volunteers cannot contribute as much time as paid, full-time workers do, they cannot complete tasks as quickly. When scheduling activities, be realistic about how long a busy PATCH participant will need to complete it.

Get to know each volunteer personally so that you can learn about special abilities and limitations and match responsibilities to skills. Vary responsibilities as desired by volunteers.

Be sure to assign specific and clearly defined tasks and to explain procedures and expectations. Develop a work plan or job description for the volunteer to help ensure that roles and responsibilities are understood. Provide training and give credit for work done. Give lots of feedback, encouragement, and signs of appreciation. Be willing to change the placement of volunteers, if that seems appropriate, or even dismiss a volunteer if necessary.

Keep in mind the following key points of working with volunteers. They want to be

- appreciated for the work that they do.
- busy with worthwhile and varied tasks.
- provided with clear communication about tasks and expectations.
- developed through training.

Source: Centers for Disease Control and Prevention (no date), p. A2–17.

social action. Each of these community organizing strategies operates "from the assumption that problems in society can be addressed by the community becoming better or differently 'organized,' with each strategy perceiving the problems and how or whom to organize in order to address them somewhat differently" (Walter, 1997, p. 69). In contrast to these strategies is community building. **Community building** "is an orientation to community that is strength based rather than need based and stresses the identification, nurturing, and celebration of community assets" (Minkler, 1997b, pp. 5–6). Thus, one of the major differences between community organization and community building is the type of assessment that is used to determine where to focus the community's efforts. In the community organization approach, the assessment is focused on needs of the community, whereas in community building, the assessment focuses on assets and capabilities of the community. A clearer picture of the community will be revealed and stronger base will be developed for change if the assessment includes the identification of both needs and assets, and involves those who live in the community. Hancock and Minkler (1997, p. 140) provide this illustration:

> For example, a narrowly defined needs assessment designed and conducted by outside experts as a means of justifying and providing raw data for organizing

FIGURE 9.3 *Guidelines for Effective Coalitions*

1. Be sensitive to turf issues.
2. Make sure the coalition is genuine.
3. Clarify the exact purpose of the coalition.
4. Limit the number of agencies involved in the coalition.
5. Allow enough time for decisions to be made.
6. Communicate with other coalitions from other geographic areas dealing with the same problem.
7. Make sure the visibility and recognition of the agencies involved in the coalition are increased as a result of their participation.
8. Secure a financial commitment from agencies involved in the coalition.
9. Have infrequent but worthwhile meetings.
10. Make sure someone is accountable for the work of the coalition.
11. Be sure to distribute the workload of the coalition among participating agencies.

Source: G. B. Lindsay and G. Edwards, "Creating Effective Health Coalitions," reprinted with permission from *Health Education, 19*(4), (1988): 35–36. *Health Education* is now titled *Journal of Health Education* and is a publication of the American Alliance for Health, Physical Education, Recreation and Dance, 1900 Association Drive, Reston, Virginia 22091.

around a predetermined community health need may be effective in achieving its objectives. But by failing to meaningfully involve community members in determining the goals of the assessment process, by focusing solely on needs rather identifying and building on community strengths, and by failing to make empowerment of people a central goal of the assessment process, such an approach would fail to meet several critical criteria of community organizing and community building practice.

Thus, a community assessment conducted by the community and for the community will produce needs data that will identify the deficiencies (Hancock & Minkler, 1997). But the assessment will also uncover the capacities and assets of a community. It is from these capacities and assets that communities are built (McKnight & Kretzmann, 1997).

The steps to complete the needs identification of an assessment have already been discussed in this book (see Chapter 4). But what has not yet been discussed is the process of assessing the capacities and assets. McKnight and Kretzmann (1997) provide a technique for completing this portion of assessment called **mapping community capacity.** They have categorized assets into three different groups based on their availability to the community and refer to them as *building blocks.* **Primary building blocks** are the most accessible assets. They are located in the neighborhood and are largely under the control of those who live in the neighborhood. Primary building blocks can be organized into the assets of individuals and those of organizations or associations (see Figure 9.4 for examples of each). The next most accessible building blocks are **secondary building blocks,** which are assets located in the neighborhood but largely controlled by people outside (see Figure 9.4). The least accessible assets are referred to as **potential building blocks.** They are located resources originating outside the neighborhood and controlled by people outside (see Figure 9.4). Knowing both the needs and the assets of the community, organizers can work to identify the true concerns of the community and the capacity to deal with them.

Determining Priorities and Setting Goals

Once the community has been assessed, the community group is ready to develop its goals. The goal-setting process includes two phases. The first phase consists of identifying the priorities of the group—what the group wants to accomplish. The priorities should be determined through consensus rather than through an individual or small group decision (See Box 9.3 for tips on how to reach consensus). The second phase consists of using the priority list to write the goals. To help ensure that the ideals of community organization take hold, the **stakeholders** (those in the community who have something to gain or lose from the community organizing and building efforts) must be the ones to establish priorities and set goals. This may sound simple, but in fact it may be the most difficult part of the process. Getting the stakeholders to agree on priorities takes a skilled group facilitator, because there is sure to be more than one point of view.

When working with coalitions and task forces, one is likely to find that determining priorities and setting goals causes turf struggles. Even though individuals or representatives of their organizations have come together to solve a problem, many people will still be concerned with finding specific solutions to the problems faced by their organization. For example, in the case of drug abuse in the community, consensus may indicate that the majority of people believe the concerns lie in the educational system, but people who work in the treatment centers may believe that they lie in the treatment of drug abuse. The facilitator will need special skills to keep these treatment center people involved after the priority-setting process does not identify their concern as a problem the group will attack. One means of dealing with this is to have subgoals, objectives that can be worked on by special interest subcommittees. Such an arrangement will allow the subcommittee to have a feeling of **ownership** in the process.

Arriving at a Solution and Selecting Intervention Activities

To achieve the goals that it has set, the group will need to identify alternative solutions and—again, through consensus—choose a course of action. Most concerns can be dealt with in any of several ways, however, each alternative has advantages and disadvantages. The group should examine the alternatives in terms of probable outcomes, acceptability to the community, probable long- and short-term effects on the

FIGURE 9.4 *Building Blocks (Assets) of Communities*

Primary Building Blocks

Individual assets
- Skills, talents, and experience of residents
- Individual businesses
- Home-based enterprises
- Personal income
- Gifts of labeled (disabled) people

Organizational assets
- Associations of businesses (i.e., Chamber of Commerce)
- Citizens' associations (i.e., neighborhood watch)
- Cultural organization (i.e., Old West End Festival, British Club)
- Communications organizations (i.e., newspapers, TV, radio)
- Religious organizations

Secondary Building Blocks

Private and nonprofit institutions
- Higher education institutions
- Hospitals and clinics
- Social service groups (i.e., United Way)

Public institutions and services
- Public schools
- Police sheriff and fire departments
- Libraries
- Parks and other recreational facilities

Physical resources
- Vacant land
- Commercial and industrial structures
- Housing
- Energy and waste resources

Potential Building Blocks

Welfare expenditures

Public capital information expenditures

Public information

Source: Adapted from McKnight and Kretzmann (1997), pp. 157–172.

BOX 9.3 • *Reaching Consensus*

Groups sometimes find it hard to reach a consensus, or general agreement. Remind participants of the following guidelines to group decision making.

- Avoid the "one best way" attitude; the best way is that which reflects the best collective judgment of the group.
- Avoid "either, or" thinking; often the best solution combines several approaches.
- A majority vote is not always the best solution. When participants give and take, several viewpoints can be combined.

- Healthy conflict, which can help participants reach a consensus, should not be smoothed over or ended prematurely.
- Problems are best solved when participants try both to communicate and to listen.

If a group has trouble reaching consensus, consider using some special techniques such as brainstorming, the nominal group process, and conflict resolution.

Source: Centers for Disease Control and Prevention (no date), p. A2–12.

community, and the cost of resources to solve the problem (Archer & Fleshman, 1985). Most of the interventions discussed in Chapter 8 are means by which the group deal with the concerns.

Much of the work to identify the appropriate solution(s) can be accomplished through subcommittees. Subcommittees can complete specific tasks that will contribute to the larger plan of action. Their work should yield specific strategies that are culturally sensitive and appropriate for the community. The plan of action is usually written in a proposal format and will be given final approval at a meeting of the full committee or coalition. It is important to take care in putting together this proposal; as many as possible of the ideas of the various subcommittees should be included. This will help to ensure approval of the entire plan. In the end, the real test of the course of action selected is whether it can provide whatever it is the people are seeking (Brager et al., 1987).

Final Steps in the Community Organizing and Building Processes

The final four steps in a community organizing and building processes include implementing the plan, evaluating the outcomes of the plan of action, maintaining the outcomes in the community, and, if necessary, "looping" back to the appropriate point in the process to modify the steps and restructure the work plan. Once the work of the group has been completed (that is, either the problem has been solved or community empowerment achieved), the group can either disband or reorganize to deal with other issues.

Planned Approach to Community Health (PATCH)

So far, this chapter has presented a general description of the processes of organizing and building a community. However, there are some models for the community organization process that have been developed to guide community organizers. One model that has received considerable use and attention in the area of health promotion is the Planned Approach to Community Health, better known by its acronym, **PATCH** (Kreuter et al., 1985). The concept of PATCH emerged in 1983 as the response of the Centers for Disease Control and Prevention (CDC) to the shift in the federal policy regarding the distribution of money to states via categorical (block) grants (Kreuter, 1992). PATCH was designed using the PRECEDE model and was created "to strengthen state and local health departments' capacities to plan, implement, and evaluate community-based health promotion activities targeted toward priority health problems" (Kreuter, 1992, p. 135). Since its development, PATCH has proved to be a useful process with a good "track record for facilitating collaborative, community-based programs" (Speers, 1992, p. 132). The use of PATCH also led to the inspiration for PROCEED (Green & Kreuter, 1992). (See the *Journal of Health Education,* April 1992, for accounts of some of the success stories.) The essential elements of PATCH include community organization with local support, participation, and leadership; community members using local health data to determine the health problems, prioritize the health problems, and set goals and objectives; carrying out interventions; and evaluating the results (Speers, 1992). PATCH is a team approach in which the people of the community make the decisions (via a consensus process) and do the work, with technical assistance from the state and local health departments and the Centers for Disease Control and Prevention. These team members not only facilitate the necessary work but also provide financial support for the project.

The three boxes presented in this chapter have come from the "PATCH Guide for the Local Coordinator" (USDHHS, CDC, no date). For more information on PATCH, contact your local health department, state health department, or the Centers for Disease Control and Prevention.

Summary

Community organization refers to various methods of intervention whereby individuals, groups, and organizations engage in planned collective action to deal with social concerns. The literature on community organizing and building is not distinct; it is often intertwined with such terms as *citizen participation, community empowerment, community participation, grass-roots participation, macro practice, and community development.* The process of community organization has been used for many years in the area of social work, but its history in the area of health promotion is much more recent. Within this chapter generic processes for community organizing and building were presented, which should be an adequate introduction to the process. Finally, a brief overview of the PATCH model was presented.

Questions

1. What is meant by the term *community?*

2. How does community organization relate to community empowerment?

3. Community organization originated out of what discipline?

4. What is the underlying concept of community organization?

5. What are some of the assumptions under which planners work when organizing a community?

6. What are the basic steps in the community organizing and building processes?

7. What is meant by the term *gatekeepers?*

8. What is the difference between the assessments for community organizing and community building?

9. What is meant by *mapping community capacity?*

10. What are the differences among primary, secondary, and potential building blocks (assets)?

11. What does the acronym PATCH stand for? What are the major components of this process?

Activities

1. Assume that a core group of individuals have come together to deal with the concern of a high rate of teenage pregnancy in the community. Identify (by job title/function) others who you think should be invited to be part of the larger group. In addition, provide a one-sentence rationale for inviting each. Assume that this community is large enough to have most social service organizations.

2. Provide a list of at least 10 different community agencies that should be invited to make up an antismoking coalition in your home town. Provide a one-sentence rationale for including each.

3. Assume that you want to make entry into a community, with which you are not familiar, in order to help to organize and build the community. Describe such a community, and then write a two-page paper to tell what steps you would take to gain entrance into the community.

4. If you wanted to find out more about your community's resources regarding exercise programs, with whom would you network? Provide a list of at least five contacts, and provide a one-sentence rationale for why you selected each.

5. Ask your professor if he or she is aware of any community organizing or building efforts in a local community. If such exists, make an appointment along with three of your classmates to interview the organizers. Ask the organizers to respond to the following questions:
   a. What is the concern being tackled?
   b. Who identified the initial concern?
   c. Who makes up the core group? How large is it?
   d. Did the group complete an assessment?
   e. What type of intervention is being used?
   f. What type of community organizing or building model was used?

Activities on the Web

1. Using a search engine (i.e., *Excite, GoTo.com, Snap,* or *Lycos*), enter "community organiz-ing" or "community building." Identify at least two websites that contain information

about how a group of people have organized to deal with a concern. Visit each of the websites, download the home page, and provide a written response to the following questions:

a. What is the URL for the sight?

b. What is the name of the organizing group?

c. What is the concern/problem that the organizing group is dealing with?

d. How is the group going about working on the problem?

e. In reviewing the information at the website, what do you see that is consistent with the general community organizing approach presented in this chapter? What is different?

2. This chapter presented a general approach to community organizing and community building. Many of the steps in the process seem straightforward but can be difficult to implement. The website for the Community Tool Box (<**http://ctb.lsi.ukans.edu/>**) offers a number of different ideas community organizers can use when they run into problems. Find the section titled Community Troubleshooting Guide. Identify a problem associated with community organizing or community building that interests you. Read all that the site has to offer about the problem and how to deal with it. Then write a two-page paper identifying the problem and a summary of how organizers can deal with the problem.

3. Box 9.1 presented information on understanding the importance of diversity. The more program planners know about their target population, and the diversity within it, the better. Visit the web site of Diversity Rx (<**http://www.diversityrx.org>**) to learn more about diversity. While reviewing the site, download a copy of the home page for Diversity Rx and attach a written response to the following questions:

a. What is Diversity Rx?

b. How are the following words defined: *culture, cultural competency, community interpreter service pool,* and *triadic interview?*

c. Why are language and culture important?

d. What are some strategies for overcoming linguistic and cultural barriers locate?

10

Identification and Allocation of Resources

After reading this chapter and answering the questions at the end, you should be able to:

- Define *resources.*
- List the common resources used in most health promotion programs.
- Identify the tasks to be carried out by program personnel.
- Explain the difference between *internal* and *external* resources.
- Define *culturally sensitive* and *culturally competent.*
- Explain what is meant by *canned* health promotion programs.
- Identify questions to ask vendors when they are selling their programs.
- List and explain common means of financing health promotion programs.
- Define *budget.*
- Identify and explain the major components of a grant proposal.

Key Terms

canned program	hard money	request for proposals (RFP)
culturally competent	in-house materials	resources
culturally sensitive	in-kind support	seed dollars
curriculum	internal resources	sliding-scale fee
external resources	ownership	soft money
flex time	peer education	speaker's bureau
grant money	profit margin	vendors
grantsmanship	proposal	

For a program to reach the identified goals and objectives, it must be supported with the appropriate resources. **Resources** include all the people and things needed to carry out the desired program. The quantity or amount of resources needed to plan, implement, and evaluate a program depends on the scope and nature of the program. Most resources carry a "price tag," which planners must take into account. Thus, planners face the task of securing the financial resources necessary to carry out a program. However, several different resources are provided by organizations, mostly voluntary or governmental health organizations, that are free or inexpensive. This chapter identifies, describes, and suggests sources for obtaining the resources commonly needed in planning, implementing, and evaluating health promotion programs.

Personnel

The key resource of any program is the individuals needed to carry out the program. Instead of trying to identify all the individuals necessary to ensure the program's success (because many times the same person is responsible for several different program components), planners should focus on the tasks that need to be completed by the program personnel. These tasks include planning; identifying resources; advertising; marketing; conducting the program, including having the necessary interpreters for those who speak a different language than the one in which the program is offered and accommodating those with disabilities; evaluating the program; making arrangements for space and program materials; handling clerical work; and keeping records (for program sign-up, collection of fees, attendance, and budgeting).

In some cases, the program participants themselves constitute a program resource. In the case of a worksite health promotion program, planners will need to find out whether the employees will participate on company time, on their own time before or after work hours, on a combination of company time and employee time, or on their own anytime during the work day as long as they put in their regular number of work hours. (This last option is known as **flex time**.) The current trend in worksite health promotion programs is to ask the employees to participate at least partially on their own time. The reasoning behind this trend is that this investment by the participant helps to promote a sense of program **ownership** ("I have put something into this program, and therefore I am going to support it") and thus build loyalty among participants.

When identifying the personnel needed to conduct a program, planners have three basic options. One, referred to as **internal resources,** uses individuals from within the planning agency/organization or people from within the target population to supply the needed labor. For example, if a local health department was planning a health promotion program in a community, the employees of the health department might handle the planning, implementation, and evaluation of the program. If that same health department was planning a health promotion program for the faculty and staff of a school district, there would likely be many school employees (school nurse, health educator, physical education instructor, family and consumer science teacher) who have the expertise (knowledge and skills) to carry out much of the program. If the department was planning a worksite program, there would probably be quite a few employees who would be qualified to conduct at least a portion of the program (for example, an employee who is certified to teach first aid or cardiopulmonary resuscitation).

Another internal resource that health promotion planners are using successfully in a variety of settings, especially in schools (from kindergarten to college), is **peer education.** The process is simple: Individuals who have specific knowledge, skills, or understanding of a concept help to educate their peers. For example, college students may work with other college students to help educate them about the dangers of drinking and driving. The major advantages of peer education are its low cost and the credibility of the instructor. Children, for example, are greatly influenced by their peers.

A second source of personnel for a program is to bring in individuals from outside the planning agency/organization or the target population to conduct part or all of the program. Such individuals are considered **external resources.** There are now many companies that offer or sell programs, services, or consulting to groups wanting health promotion programs. These companies are referred to as **vendors.** Some vendors are for-profit groups—such as hospitals, consulting agencies, health promotion companies, or related businesses—whereas others are nonprofit organizations—such as voluntary health agencies, YMCAs, YWCAs, governmental health agencies, universities/colleges, extension services, or professional organizations. Because of the recent growth of interest in health promotion programs, the quality of vendors can vary greatly. Planners should screen vendors carefully before using their services. Harris, McKenzie, and Zuti (1986) provide a checklist for choosing an appropriate vendor (see Appendix E).

An often untapped source of personnel for health promotion programs is experts available through **speaker's bureaus.** Most local offices of voluntary health agencies, hospitals, and other health-related organizations maintain speaker's bureaus. The services of these experts are usually available at little or no cost to groups. With some inquiry and a little networking, it is not difficult for planners to identify organizations that have individuals available to speak on a variety of health-related topics, or health care organizations willing to send their medical experts into the community to share their knowledge. The speaker's bureau is a win-win concept for both the group offering the service and the one receiving it. Groups that take advantage of a speaker's bureau gain access to expert information, but those delivering the information gain in terms of public relations and recognition.

There are advantages and disadvantages connected with using either internal or external personnel to conduct health promotion programs. Table 10.1 lists the pros and cons of each.

One special concern for personnel, regardless of whether they are internal or external, is that they are both culturally sensitive and culturally competent. **Culturally sensitive** means having a basic understanding and appreciation of the importance of sociocultural factors (Kim, McLeod, & Shantzis, 1992). Cultural

TABLE 10.1 *Advantages and Disadvantages of Using Internal and External Personnel*

	Advantages	*Disadvantages*
Internal Program Personnel	1. Reduced costs 2. Internal arrangements can be made to free needed personnel from their work schedules. 3. More control over those involved.	1. Limited by the interest of those on staff. 2. May have to train personnel or be limited by the expertise of those on staff. 3. Can spend more time developing the program than implementing it, thus reaching fewer people.
External Program Personnel	1. Known expertise. 2. The responsibility for conducting the program becomes the work of another. 3. Can request product (program) guarantees. 4. External personnel sometimes more respected than internal personnel just because they are from the outside.	1. Often more costly than using internal resources. 2. Subject to the limitations of any given vendor. 3. Sometimes less control over the program.

competence goes beyond just being culturally sensitive. **Culturally competent** is defined as the "process for effectively working within the cultural context of an individual or community from a diverse cultural or ethnic background" (Campinha-Bacote, 1994, pp. 1–2). Thus, when working with multicultural populations, planners should use indigenous health workers and/or those that are well trained and are bilingual and bicultural.

The third option for obtaining personnel to carry out a program is a combination of internal and external resources. This option is the one most commonly used because it allows the program planners to make use of the advantages of the first two options and avoid many of the disadvantages.

Curricula and Other Instructional Resources

When it comes to selecting the **curriculum** and other instructional materials that will be used to present the content of the program, planners can proceed in three ways: (1) by developing their own materials (in house) or having someone else develop custom materials for them; (2) by purchasing or obtaining "canned" programs from outside vendors; or (3) by using a combination of in-house and canned materials. Each choice has both advantages and disadvantages.

Developing **in-house materials** or having someone else develop custom materials has the major advantage of allowing the developers to create materials that match very closely the needs of the target population. The more "unique" the target population is, the more important this approach may be—especially if the target population possesses cultural differences. Materials must be relevant and culturally appropriate to the target population (Kline & Huff, 1999). However, a serious drawback is the time, money, and effort necessary to develop an original curriculum and other instructional materials. The exact amount of time necessary would obviously depend on the scope of the program and the expertise of those doing the work. No matter who does the work, however, the commitment of time and resources is sure to be considerable. In putting together an in-house program, planners should be aware of several different sources from which they can obtain free or inexpensive materials to supplement the ones they develop. For example, most voluntary and official health agencies have up-to-date pamphlets on a variety of subjects that they are willing and eager to give away in quantity. Also, most communities have a public library with a film/video section that includes some health films/videos. If the public library does not carry health films/videos, almost all local and state health departments offer such a service. Planners who are unsure about what sources of information are available in their community can begin by checking the Yellow Pages of the local telephone directory. Appendix F provides a partial listing of organizations that provide information for planners.

Purchasing or obtaining canned programs from vendors has become very popular in recent years because of the time and money needed to create programs. A **canned program** is one that has been developed by an outside group and includes the basic components and materials necessary to implement a program. Because some vendors are for-profit groups whereas others are nonprofit organizations, the cost of these programs can range from nothing at all to thousands of dollars.

Most canned programs have five major components:

1. A participant's manual (printed material that is easy to follow and read and is handy for participants)
2. An instructor's manual (a much more comprehensive document than the participant's manual, which includes the program content, background information, and lesson and unit plans with ideas for presenting the material)
3. Audiovisual materials that help present the program content (usually including films, video and audiotapes, overhead transparencies, charts, or posters)
4. Training for the instructors (a concentrated experience that prepares individuals to become instructors)
5. Marketing (the "wrapping" that makes the program attractive to both the participants and the program planners who will purchase it to market to the participants)

The advantages and disadvantages of these canned programs are just the opposite of those for materials developed in house. No time is spent on development; however, the program may not fit the needs or the demographics of the target population. For example, using the same canned smoking cessation program with middle-aged adults who realize the long-term hazards of cigarettes and with teenagers who are required to attend a smoking cessation program for disciplinary reasons may not be advisable. Most adults who enter smoking cessation programs are there because they do not want to smoke. Obviously, this is not the case with teenagers who have been caught smoking. The approaches taken with these two programs would have to be very different if both are to be successful. Another example of when use of a canned curriculum program would not be advisable is use of a program that was designed for upper-middle-class suburban adults in a program for low-income inner-city populations. The lifestyles of the two groups are just too different for the same curriculum to be appropriate in both situations. Because of the possible mismatch between the needs and peculiarities (i.e., age, culture, ethnicity, norms, race, sex, socioeconomic status) of a particular target population, planners are urged to move with caution when deciding on the use of a canned program. Make sure there is a good fit.

Many of the agencies and organizations listed in Appendix F offer canned programs for program planners. Canned programs often come attractively packaged and seemingly complete, but this does not mean that they are well conceived and effective programs. Before adopting canned programs for use, planners should consider the following questions:

1. Is the program based on sound theory and tested models? As noted in an earlier chapter, all programs should be based on sound theory and tested models.
2. Does the program include a long-term behavior modification component? There are no "quick fixes" with regard to health behavior change. If behavior modification is used, it should be based on sound health behavior practice over an appropriate time frame.
3. Is the program educational? Not only should the program be based on sound psychological and sociological theory but it should also be based on valid educational theory.
4. Is the program motivational? Health behavior change is not easy to accomplish, and so all programs need to include activities that motivate people to get and stay involved.
5. Is the program enjoyable? Planned programs should be enjoyable. Some people like hard work, but it is difficult to sustain hard work for a long time without some enjoyment.
6. Can the program be modified to meet the specific needs and peculiarities of the target population? As mentioned earlier, not all populations have the same needs, beliefs, traditions, and ways of approaching a problem.

Space

Another major resource needed for most health promotion programs is sufficient space—a place where the program can be held. Depending on the type of program and the intended audience, space may or may not be readily available. For example, an employer may make space available for a worksite program, or a school system may furnish space for a school program. If space is a problem, planners may locate inexpensive space in local schools, colleges, and universities, and in "community service rooms" (rooms that are available free of charge to community groups as a community service) of local businesses. In addition, planners may find educational institutions and local businesses that are willing to cosponsor programs and thus contribute the space necessary to conduct the program. It may also be possible to obtain space by trading for it. For instance, a planner might trade expertise, such as serving as consultant for a program, in return for the use of suitable space. Or it might be possible to trade one space for another, such as trading the use of classrooms for time in the local YMCA/YWCA pool.

Equipment and Supplies

Some programs may require a great deal of equipment and supplies. For example, first aid and safety programs need items such as CPR mannequins, splints, blankets, bandages, dressings, and video equipment. Other programs, such as a stress management program, may need only paper and pencils. Whatever the kinds and amounts of equipment and supplies required, planners must give advance thought to their needs so as to:

1. Determine the necessary equipment and supplies to facilitate the program.
2. Identify the sources where the equipment and supplies can be obtained.
3. Find a way to pay for the needed equipment and supplies.

Financial Resources

To hire the individuals needed to plan, implement, and evaluate a health promotion program and to pay for the other resources required, planners must obtain appropriate financial support. Most programs are limited by the financial support available. In fact, few programs are financed at such a level that planners would say they have all the money they need. Because of this, the planners are often faced with making decisions about how to allocate the funds that are available. Some typical financial questions that planners generally must address are the following:

1. Is it better to run an adequately financed program for a few people or to run a poorly financed program for more people?
2. If funds are limited, where is the first place we should cut?
3. Should we start a program knowing that we will be short of funds, or should we wait until we have appropriate funding before we begin?
4. Is it better to have fewer instructors or to make do with fewer supplies?

Programs can be financed in several different ways. Some sources of financial support are very traditional, whereas others may be limited only by the creativity and imagination of those involved. Following are several established ways of financing programs.

Participant Fee

This method of financing a program requires the participants to pay for the cost of the program. Depending on whether the program is offered on a profit-making basis, this fee may be equal to expenses or may include a profit margin. Participant fees not only are a means by which programs can be financed but they also help motivate participants to stay involved in a program. If people pay to participate in a program, then they may be more likely to continue to participate because they have made an investment—that is, a commitment. This concept has also been referred to as *ownership*. Many participants who pay a fee feel like they are part "owners" of the program. However, it should be noted that not everyone shares in the ownership concept. There are some participants who still would prefer a free or almost free program that has been paid for by others. An example of the ownership and cost issue is the participant fees associated with smoking cessation programs. If planners were looking for vendors of smoking cessation programs, they would find that the costs of such programs range from zero (i.e., American Cancer Society's FreshStart program) to modest (i.e., American Lung Association's Freedom from Smoking program) to expensive (i.e., those offered by private health promotion companies).

Deciding to finance a program through a participant fee may sound easy, but planners need to give serious thought to how much they will charge and who will be charged. Often, those most in need of a health promotion program are the least able to pay. Planners do not want to create a barrier to program participation by charging a fee or a setting the fee too high. If a fee is necessary, then planners should consider creating a fee structure on "ability to pay." One form of this is a **sliding-scale fee**—that is, the less one's income, the lower the participant fee.

Third-Party Support

Most individuals are familiar with insurance companies acting as third-party payers to cover the costs of health care. Although this is not a common means of paying for health promotion programs, it is sometimes used. Third party means that someone other than participants (the first party) or program planners (the second party) is paying for the program. Third-party payers that may cover the cost of health promotion programs are:

1. Employers that pick up the cost for employees, as is often the case in work-site health promotion programs
2. Agencies other than the groups sponsoring the program—for example, when local service or civic groups "adopt" a pet program
3. A professional association or union that financially supports a program

The money used by third-party payers can be generated from a special fund-raising event, from sale of concessions, or with money saved from reduced health care costs, absenteeism, or the remodeling of employee benefit plans.

Cost Sharing

A third means of financing a program is a combination of participant fee and third-party support. It is not unusual to have an employer pay 50% to 80% of a program's costs and let the employee pay the remaining 50% to 20%. Such an arrangement has the advantages of both ownership and a fringe benefit.

Organizational Sponsorship

Many times, the sponsoring organization (health department, hospital, or voluntary agency) bears the cost of the program as a part of its programming or operating budget. For example, the American Cancer Society offers its smoking cessation program free of charge. The program is paid for with the society's program-planning funds.

Grants and Gifts

Another means of financing health promotion programs is through gifts and grants from other agencies, foundations, groups, and individuals. This source of money is often referred to as **grant money**, external money, or **soft money**. The term *soft money* refers to the fact that grants and gifts are usually given for a specific period of time and at some point will be taken away. This is in contrast to **hard money**, which is an ongoing source of funds that is part of the operating budget of an organization from year to year.

Grant money is becoming more important to program planners because of limited resources dedicated to health promotion programming. It thus becomes necessary for program planners to develop adequate **grantsmanship** skills. These skills include (1) discovering where the grant money is located, (2) finding out how to get (apply for) the money, and (3) writing a proposal requesting the money.

Locating Grant Money.   There are four basic types of grant makers: foundations, corporations, voluntary agencies, and government. These grant makers are found at three different levels: local, state, and national. They are not the only grant makers, however. Planners may also find a variety of local organizations (such as service groups like the Lion's Club or the Jaycees, or a community group like the United Way) that may be willing to support specific local causes through a grant. Philanthropic foundations are not-for-profit organizations that award grants to serve the public interest. There are a number of large national foundations (e.g., Robert Wood Johnson Foundation, Rockefeller Foundation, W. K. Kellogg Foundation), but planners may also find state and local foundations too.

Not all corporations have giving programs, but many do as a part of a community service or public relations program. Planners will need to contact the corporations to "ask who is in charge of charitable giving, what subjects they consider for grants, and how the company giving program operates" (Guyer, 1999, p. 1). Library or Internet research will possibly help answer these questions.

Voluntary health agencies also have grant programs. Though most grants from voluntary organizations at the national level are specified for research efforts, planners may find the local or state offices of these organizations are willing to provide **seed dollars** (start-up dollars) or **in-kind support** (such as providing free materials or other resources) for local programs.

Government is the largest grant maker. Government, at all three levels—local, state, and federal—make grants for many purposes. With the other three grant makers (foundations, corporations, and voluntary agencies), planners can ask them to fund any project. However, with the government, only grants that are in one of the subjects specified by the government have a chance of being funded (Guyer, 1999).

When looking for grant makers, planners need to look for a pattern in giving by asking key questions: Has this funder made grants in the past for subject areas like mine? In my geographic area? In the amount I need? For the things I need funded? (Guyer, 1999). The answers to these questions will indicate whether it is a good idea to contact the funder. After doing the initial research, planners should call or write funding sources to ask questions and to obtain any guidelines, grant request forms or applications, and printed material about their grant making. This contact will also help establish a relationship with the funder. Planners not only can obtain needed information but they can also introduce their organization to the funder. This can be done by sending publications about the planners' organization, making personal contacts, and staying in touch (Guyer, 1999).

Planners can identify possible funding sources in a couple of different ways. The first is by networking with others who have been successful in obtaining grant funding in the past. Since seeking grant funding is a competitive process, planners may have to network with others who are not seeking funding from the same grant maker. A second means of identifying funding sources is through library "research." A variety of books on grants may be found in college and university libraries as well as many larger public libraries. For example, there are directories of grant makers for foundations and corporations, and there is usually a directory that lists grant funders that are specific to a state. Most of these books are indexed by subject area.

> In looking for a government grant, examine the *Catalog of Federal Domestic Assistance*, which lists the federal grant programs. For each program the *Catalog* shows who is eligible, what the program is about, and an information contact to whom to write for application information. The *Federal Register*, a daily publication, lists the newest grant opportunities. For state and local government grants, there is no one book to use that is comprehensive. You need to call elected officials or appropriate government departments to inquire about what is available. Be persistent in calling around until you find the person who is in charge of grant making. (Guyer, 1999, p. 2)

A third way of identifying funding sources is through the Internet. There are several advantages to using the Internet for seeking grant makers: convenience, time saving, and being able to reach several grant makers at the same time. Planners do not have to leave their office to conduct a search, thus much "leg work" of finding out if grant maker is a "good fit" with the planner's organization can be found almost instantaneously. In addition, some websites permit an applicant to complete one form for grant consideration at several different funders (Breen, 1999).

The fourth way of identifying grant makers, is the least difficult. Planners should be alert for **requests for proposals,** known as **RFPs.** Many times some funding agency would like to have a project conducted for it, so the group will issue an RFP. If you feel qualified to do the work, you can submit a proposal.

Submitting Grant Proposals.   As noted in the previous section, most funding agencies have specific guidelines outlining who is qualified to submit a proposal (perhaps only nonprofit groups can apply, or only practitioners who hold certain certifications) and the format for making an application. Those seeking money can request or apply for the money by writing a proposal. A **proposal** can be thought of as a written document that represents a request for money. A good proposal is one that is well written and explains how the needs of the funding agency can be met by the group wishing to receive the money. To increase your chances of writing a good proposal, call the funding agency first and speak with the grant officer to find out specifically what he or she is looking for and the format desired.

Because there is a great deal of competition for grant money, it is more than likely that proposals will be read by a busy, impatient, skeptical person who has no reason to give any one proposal special consideration and who is faced with many more requests than he or she can grant, or even read thoroughly. Such a reader wants to find out quickly and easily the answers to these questions:

1. What do you want to do, how much will it cost, and how much time will it take?
2. How does the proposed project relate to the sponsor's interests?
3. What will be gained if this project is carried out?
4. What has already been done in the area of the project?
5. How do you plan to do it?
6. How will the results be evaluated?
7. Why should you, rather than someone else, conduct this project?

As noted, funding agencies request proposals in a variety of different forms. However, there are several components that are contained in most proposals no matter what the funding agency. Figure 10.1 presents these components.

A Combination of Sources

It should be obvious that program planners should not be limited to any single source for financing a health promotion program. In fact, it is more than likely that most programs will be funded via a variety of sources—that is, any combination of the sources listed previously.

FIGURE 10.1 *The Components of a Grant Proposal*

---

1. **Title (or cover) page.** When writing the title, be concise and explicit; avoid words that add nothing.
2. **Abstract or executive summary.** May be the most important part of the proposal. Should be written last and be about 200 words long.
3. **Table of contents.** May or may not be needed, depending on the length of the proposal. It is a convenience for the reader.
4. **Introduction.** Should begin with a capsule statement, be comprehensible to the informed layperson, and include the statement of the problem, significance of the program, and purpose of the program.
5. **Background.** Should include the proposer's previous related work and the related literature.
6. **Description of proposed program.** Should include objectives, description of intervention, evaluation plan, and time frame.
7. **Description of relevant institutional/agency resources.**
8. **List of references.** Should include references cited in the proposal.
9. **Personnel section.** Should include the résumés of those who are to work with the program.
10. **Budget.** Should include budget needs for personnel (salaries and wages), equipment, materials and supplies, travel, services, other needed items, and indirect costs.

Preparing a Budget

Simply put, a budget is a plan that is presented in financial terms using quantitative units such as dollars, pounds, hours, and work force hours (Shim & Siegel, 1994). A budget represents the decision makers' intentions and expectations by allocating funds to achieve desired outcomes (program goals and objectives) (Finkler, 1992; Shim & Siegel, 1994). In financial terms, the budget compares the expected income to the expected expenses in order to estimate the financial results of the program (Finkler, 1992).

A budget can be prepared for any length of time. When programs are planned, budgets are usually created for the entire length of the program. However, when a program is projected to last longer than a year, the overall program budget is typically broken down into 12-month periods.

The purpose of a program has a lot to say about the type of budget created. From a financial standpoint, programs can make money (a profit), lose money, or break even. If a program must make money, the income will have to be greater than the expenses, and the intended profit **(profit margin)** will need to be included in the budgeting process. No matter what the desired bottom line is in a budget, the budget should be put together in sufficient detail that all income and expenses are accounted for. Figure 10.2 presents a sample budget sheet that lists some line items that are typically included in a health promotion program budget.

FIGURE 10.2   *Sample Budget Sheet*

Income	**Amount**
Contribution from sponsors	_____
Gifts	_____
Grants	_____
Participant fee	_____
Sale of curriculum materials	_____
	Total income _____
Expenses	
Curriculum materials	_____
Equipment	_____
Marketing	_____
Print advertising	_____
Other media	_____
Personnel	_____
For planning	_____
Program facilitators	_____
Clerical	_____
Evaluator(s)	_____
Participants	_____
Postage	_____
Space	_____
Supplies	_____
Travel	_____
	Total expenses _____
	Balance _____

Summary

This chapter identified and discussed the most often used resources for health promotion programs: personnel, curriculum and other instructional materials, space, equipment and supplies, and funding. In addition, typical questions were covered regarding how to secure and allocate resources and how to obtain funding.

Questions

1. What are the major categories of resources that planners need to consider when planning a health promotion program?

2. List and explain the different means by which health promotion programs can be funded.

3. Define the terms *ownership, flex time, vendor,* and *canned programs.*

4. What are the advantages and disadvantages of using internal resources? External resources?

5. How might program planners obtain free or inexpensive space for a program?

6. What are some key questions that planners should ask vendors when they try to sell their product?

7. What is meant by the term *profit margin?*

Activities

1. Identify and describe the resources you anticipate needing to carry out a program you are planning. Be sure to answer the following questions that apply to your program:
   a. What personnel will be needed to carry out the program? List the individuals and the duties to be carried out.
   b. What curriculum or educational materials will you use in your program? Why did you select it?
   c. What kind of space allocation will your program require? How will you obtain the space? How much will it cost?
   d. What equipment and supplies do you anticipate using? How will you obtain them?
   e. How do you anticipate paying for the program? Why did you select this method?

2. Visit the local office of a voluntary agency and find out what type of resources it makes available to individuals planning health promotion programs. Ask for a sample of the materials. Also, ask if the agency offers any canned programs. If it does, find out as much as you can about the programs and ask for any available descriptive literature.

3. Collect information on a single type of canned health promotion program (for example, smoking cessation or stress management) from vendors. Then compare the strengths and weaknesses of the programs.

4. Through the process of networking and using the local telephone book, find where in your community there is free or inexpensive space available for health promotion programs.

5. Call three different voluntary agencies and one hospital in your community and find out if they have a speaker's bureau. If they do, find out how to use the bureaus and what topics the speakers can address.

6. Prepare a mock grant proposal for a program you are planning. Make sure it includes all the components noted in Figure 10.1.

7. Outline the major sources of income and expenses that would be associated with the program you are planning by preparing a budget sheet.

Activities on the Web

1. Visit the websites of five of the organizations/agencies presented in Appendix F. Search each site for canned health promotion programs. Download the information from each site and examine the information for each program. Does each program

contain the primary elements of a canned program that were mentioned in this chapter? Make a list of what you see to be the pros and cons of each program. Then compare the information you found; what program do you like best? Why?

2. Again, using the websites presented in Appendix F, locate a canned program that could be used for a program you are planning. Download the information so that it can be incorporated into your written plan.

3. There are a number of websites that can be helpful when writing a grant proposal. Visit at least three of the following sites, download the home page of each, and then create a list (titled What Every Grant Proposal Writer Should Know) of items you found at the sites that you did not know before.
   a. The Community Toolbox **<http://ctb.lsi.ukans.edu/>**
   b. GrantsNet   **<http://www.os.dhhs.gov/progorg/grantsnet>**
   c. The Grantsmanship Center **<http://www.tgci.com>**
   d. The Foundation Center **<http://www.fdncenter.org>**
   e. Philanthropy News Network **<http://www.pj.org>**
   f. National Network of Grantmakers **<http://www.nng.org>**
   g. Foundations On-line **<http://www.foundations.org>**

4. Visit the website of the American Heart Association that contains the canned program Heart at Work **<http://www.americanheart.org/haw/>**. Read the material about the program, then write a two-page report that answers the following questions. Attach a copy of the downloaded web page to your paper.
   a. Describe the program.
   b. What do you see as the benefits of an online health promotion program?
   c. What do you have to do to use this program?
   d. Do you think this would be a program that would be useful for health educators who are employed in worksite health promotion?
   e. What do you like and dislike about the program?

5. The Indiana University Library has a page **<http://www.indiana.edu/~librcsd/eval/checklist.html>** on its website that provides a checklist for evaluating websites. Download the checklist, then visit the site of one of the agencies listed in Appendix F and critique it. Print out a copy of the home page of the agency you visit and attached it to your critique.

11

Marketing

Getting and Keeping People Involved in a Program

After reading this chapter and answering the questions at the end, you should be able to:

- Define *market, marketing, social marketing,* and *target marketing.*
- Explain the diffusion theory.
- Explain how the diffusion theory can be used in marketing a health promotion program.
- Identify the functions involved in the marketing process as outlined by Syre and Wilson (1990).
- Explain the relationship between a needs assessment and a marketing program.
- Explain the four Ps of marketing.
- Define *marketing mix.*
- Name techniques for motivating program participants to continue in a program.

Key Terms

audience segmentation	internal advertising	price
contingencies	laggards	product
diffusion theory	late majority	promotion
early adopters	market	social marketing
early majority	marketing	social support
external advertising	marketing mix	tangible
incentives	market segmentation	target marketing
innovators	placement	
intangible	position the product	

After putting a great deal of work and energy into planning a health promotion program, planners naturally hope that the target population will want to participate in it. They also hope that, once involved in the program, the participants will want to continue with the program for its duration. Hoping is not enough, however. Planners must not just hope these things will occur, but work to make sure they occur. They need to have skills in marketing and psychology in order to get the target population involved and keep them involved. Only when the participants continue the behavior learned in a health promotion program over a long period of time can the health goals of both the individual and the program be met.

Market and Marketing

For the purposes of program planning, the people in the target population make up the market. Kotler and Clarke (1987, p. 108) define **market** as "the set of all people who have an actual or potential interest in a product or service." A key to getting and keeping these people involved in a health promotion program is to be able to market the program effectively. The process of **marketing** operates on the underlying concept of the exchange theory.

> Marketing is the planned attempt to influence the characteristics of voluntary exchange transactions—exchanges of costs and benefits by buyers and sellers or providers and consumers. Marketing is considerably different from selling in that selling concentrates on the needs of the producer (to sell more products), whereas marketing, which may have the same ultimate objective, concentrates necessarily on the needs of the buyer or the public. (Pickett & Hanlon, 1990, p. 231)

"Strip away all the fancy language, and marketing comes down to offering benefits that an identified group of potential customers will pay a price for and be satisfied with" (Novelli, 1988, p. 7).

Applying the definition of marketing to health promotion suggests that program planners would like to exchange costs and benefits with those in the target population. That is to say, program planners would like to exchange the benefits of participation in health promotion programs (the objectives or outcomes of the programs they planned), such as "a longer healthier life, looking and feeling better, and having fewer but healthier children" (Novelli, 1988, p. 6) for the costs of the program, which come from the participants. The cost to the participant may be financial, but often with health promotion programs, the costs are something other than financial. "Consumers may pay a price in terms of the time it takes to learn new information or practice new behaviours [sic]; they expend cognitive and physical efforts; they risk alienating family members and friends when adopting new ideas and practices; and they may be perceived by the community-at-large as being 'different'" (Lefebvre, 1992, p. 157).

For this exchange to take place, program planners must have an understanding of marketing principles. Unfortunately, many health promotion planners have had to learn the hard way—by planning a program and then not have anyone sign up to participate in it. The principles of marketing are not difficult to learn, but their application can be challenging. Applying marketing principles to health promotion programs is not as easy as applying them to the latest model of a car or a new line of clothing. Health promotion programs are social programs; as such, they do not have material objects to market, but instead must market awareness, knowledge, skills, and behavior. The marketing of health promotion programs falls into a special type of marketing called *social marketing.*

The term *social marketing* was introduced by Kolter and Zaltman (1971) to explain the techniques and concepts used to market social issues and causes instead of products and services. More specifically, Lefebvre and Flora (1988, p. 300) define **social marketing** this way: "Social marketing concepts and methods borrow heavily from traditional marketing literature. However, social marketing is distinguished by its emphasis on so-called 'non-tangible' products—ideas, attitudes, lifestyle changes—as opposed to the more tangible products and services that are the focus of marketing in business, health-care, and nonprofit service sectors." They continue, "For example, how does one buy a 'healthier life'? The challenge is to begin to make these 'intangibles' tangible in a way that appeals to the target audience" (Lefebvre & Flora, 1988, p. 306). Thus, in social marketing, the exchange may come down to exchanging an intangible for another intangible, such as the effort to accept a new idea and discard an old custom, or adopt a new behavior and giving up a habit (Lefebvre, 1992). Table 11.1 compares the marketing of a **tangible** (product) and an **intangible** (a program that will improve the quality of life).

Marketing and the Diffusion Theory

One analytical tool that has been most useful in understanding the importance of marketing principles is the **diffusion theory** (Rogers, 1962). The theory provides an explanation for the diffusion of innovations (something new) in populations; stated another way, it provides an explanation for the pattern of adoption of the innovations. If one thinks of a health promotion program as an innovation, the theory describes a pattern the target population will follow in adopting the program. The pattern of adoption can be represented by the normal bell-shaped curve (Rogers, 1983) (see Figure 11.1). Therefore, those individuals who fall in the portion of the curve to the left of minus 2 standard deviations from the mean (this would be

TABLE 11.1 *Marketing a Tangible versus an Intangible*

Concern	Tangible	Intangible
Success	Increase sales 3–5%	Great enough to be cost effective
Changes	One-time sales	Lasting a lifetime
Target population	Most likely to respond	Least likely to respond

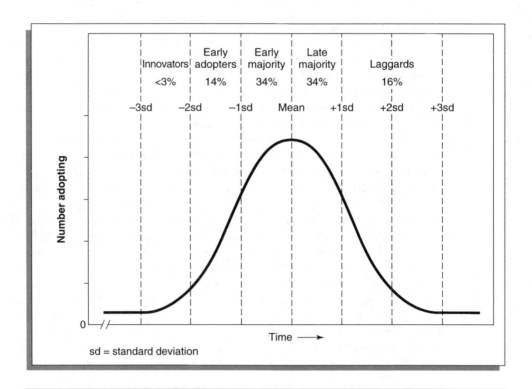

FIGURE 11.1   *Bell-Shaped Curve and Adopter Categories*

Source: Adapted from Rogers (1983), p. 247.

between 2% and 3% of the target population) would probably become involved in the program just because they had heard about it and wanted to be first. These people are called **innovators.** They are venturesome, independent, risky, and daring. They want to be the first to do things, and they may not be respected by others in the social system.

The second group of people to become involved are those represented on the curve between minus 2 and minus 1 standard deviations. This group would include about 14% of the target population; they are called **early adopters.** These people are very interested in the innovation, but they are not the first to sign up. They wait until the innovators are already involved to make sure the innovation is useful. Early adopters are respected by others in the social system and looked at as opinion leaders.

The next two groups are the **early majority** and the **late majority.** They fall between minus 1 standard deviation and the mean and between the mean and plus 1 standard deviation on the curve, respectively. Each of these groups comprises about 34% of the target population. Those in the early majority may be interested in the health promotion program, but they will need external motivation to become involved. Those in the early majority will deliberate for some time before making a decision. It will take more work to get the late majority involved, for they are skeptical and will not adopt an innovation until most people in the social system have done so. Planners may be able to get them involved through a peer or mentoring program, or through constant exposure about the innovation.

The last group, the **laggards** (16%), are represented by the part of the curve greater than plus 1 standard deviation. They are not very interested in innovation and would be the last to become involved in new health promotion programs, if at all. Some would say that this group will not become involved in health promotion programs at all. They are very traditional and are suspicious of innovations. Laggards tend to have limited communication networks, so they really do not know much about new things.

Figure 11.2 presents an *s*-shaped curve showing the cumulative prevalence of adopters at successive points in time. At first, only a few people adopt (innovators). However, over time, the curve begins to climb as additional individuals decide to adopt the innovation (early adopters, early majority, and late majority). The curve then levels off as adoption of the innovation ceases, leaving a few who have not adopted (laggards) (Goldman, 1998; Rogers 1994).

The real plus of using the diffusion theory when trying to market a health promotion program is that "the distinguishing characteristics of the people who fall into each category of adopters from 'innovators' to 'early adopters' to middle majority categories to 'late adopters' [laggards] tend to be consistent across a wide range of innovations" (Green, 1989). Therefore, different marketing techniques can be

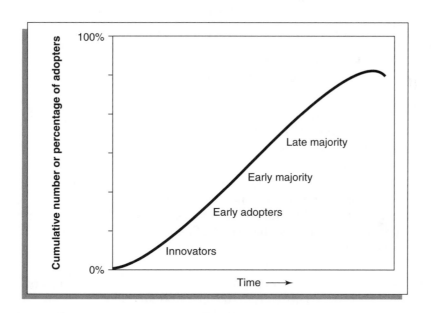

FIGURE 11.2 *S-Shaped Curve and Cumulative Adoption*

Source: Adapted from Rogers (1983), p. 95.

used depending on the type of people the program planners are trying to attract to a program. For example, smoking cessation programs have been around for many years. In the last 30 years, the percentage of adult smokers in the United States has dropped from just over 50% to less than 25%. Thus, taking into account that there will always be some new smokers, one could safely assume that the majority of smokers in the United States today are probably not innovators, early adopters, or early majority, at least with regard to smoking cessation programs. Instead, they are likely to be those who would be much more difficult to reach—late majority and laggards. Therefore, according to the diffusion theory, the marketing techniques that were used to get people to stop smoking right after former U.S. Surgeon General Terry's report in 1964 probably would be less effective if used today.

Figure 11.3 lists some generalizations drawn from the work of various researchers on innovations and reported in Rogers (1983). These generalizations could have an application to the innovation of health promotion programs.

The application of the diffusion theory to health promotion programs is quite common now. To learn more about the concept and its application to health promotion programs, review some other references to see how they have applied the concept in a variety of health promotion and health education settings (Anderson & Portnoy, 1989; Basch, 1984; Basch & Sliepcevich, 1983; Dishman, 1988; Goldman, 1994, 1998; Greer, 1977; Kolbe & Iverson, 1981; Monahan & Scheirer, 1988; Orlaldi, 1986; Parcel at al., 1989; Steckler et al., 1992; USDHHS, 1987; Wolfe, Slack, & Rose-Hearn, 1993).

One of the more interesting uses of the diffusion theory has been its use to "conceptualize the transference of health promotion programs from one locale to another" (Steckler et al., 1992). Steckler and colleagues (1992) developed a series of six questionnaires to measure the extent to which health promotion programs are successfully disseminated. Program planners should refer to this work if they are interested in trying to measure diffusion.

The Marketing Process and Health Promotion Programs

If everyone in a given population were an innovator or early adopter, there would be no need for marketing plans. Since that is not the case, there is a need for program planners to understand the marketing process and be able to apply its principles.

Syre and Wilson (1990) have identified five distinct functions of the marketing process as they relate to the health care field:

1. Using marketing research to determine the needs and desires of the present and prospective clients from the target population.
2. Developing a product that satisfies the needs and desires of the clients.
3. Developing informative and persuasive communication flows between those offering the program and the clients.

FIGURE 11.3 *Generalizations about Selected Variables and Innovation*

Socioeconomic Characteristics

1. Earlier adopters have more years of education than later adopters have.
2. Earlier adopters are more likely to be literate than are later adopters.
3. Earlier adopters have higher social status than do later adopters.
4. Earlier adopters have a greater degree of upward social mobility than do later adopters.
5. Earlier adopters are more likely to have a commercial (rather than a subsistence) economic orientation than are later adopters.

Personality Variables

1. Earlier adopters have a greater ability to deal with abstractions than do later adopters.
2. Earlier adopters have a more favorable attitude toward change than later adopters have.
3. Earlier adopters are more able to cope with uncertainty and risk than are later adopters.
4. Earlier adopters have a more favorable attitude toward education than do later adopters.
5. Earlier adopters have a more favorable attitude toward science than do later adopters.
6. Earlier adopters have higher levels of achievement motivation than do later adopters.
7. Earlier adopters have higher aspirations (for education, occupations, and so on) than later adopters have.

Communication Behavior

1. Earlier adopters have more social participation than do later adopters.
2. Earlier adopters are more highly interconnected in the social system than are later adopters.
3. Earlier adopters are more cosmopolitan than later adopters are.
4. Earlier adopters have more change agent contact than do later adopters.
5. Earlier adopters have greater exposure to mass media communication channels than do later adopters.
6. Earlier adopters have greater exposure to interpersonal communication channels than later adopters have.
7. Earlier adopters have a higher degree of opinion leadership than later adopters have.
8. Earlier adopters are more likely to belong to highly interconnected systems than are later adopters.

Source: Adapted from Rogers (1983), pp. 251–259.

4. Ensuring that the product is provided in the appropriate form, at the right time and place, and at the best price.
5. Keeping the clients satisfied and loyal after the exchange has taken place.

Next, each of these functions will be discussed.

Using Marketing Research to Determine Needs and Desires

This particular function involves conducting a marketing needs assessment. Since the needs assessment process was discussed in detail in Chapter 4, the discussion will not be repeated here. However, the focus of marketing research is a bit different than that of a traditional needs assessment for a program. The types of data that planners try to uncover in marketing research are "audience segment needs and characteristics, market analyses to determine positioning strategies, pretesting of concepts and messages, and pilot tests of message/product/service acceptability and effectiveness" (Lefebvre, 1992, p. 160). Some market research can be conducted as part of a regular needs assessment, such as collecting information that would help segment the market (see the next section for a discussion of market segmentation) or finding out how best to position a program for a specific market. But other components, such as pretesting and pilot tests, will need to be conducted while the program is being developed. When this is the case, it is referred to as *formative research*.

If planners want to gather marketing research data as part of primary data collection for a program needs assessment, they may want to consider questions such as:

1. What type of health promotion programs would you participate in if they were offered in the community?
2. Where would you like the program offered?
3. On what days of the week would you like the program offered?
4. At what time of the day would you like the program offered?
5. How much would you be willing to pay to attend the program?
6. What might be the best way to notify you of future programs?
7. Do you think other members of your family would like to attend these programs? If yes, which members?

Developing a Product That Satisfies the Needs and Desires of Clients

The steps involved in developing a high-quality, marketable product (health promotion program) were discussed in earlier chapters. One key to developing a marketable product is knowing as much as possible about the target population. The more they know about a population, the better program planners can describe the population. By describing the population, planners are then able to divide the population based on certain characteristics, a process called **audience segmentation** or **market segmentation.** Figure 11.4 shows the concept of market segmentation, identifying black teenagers for a dietary excess intervention. "Audience segmentation has two major goals: (1) define homogeneous subgroups for message and product design purposes, and (2) identify segments that will target distribution and communication channel strategies" (Lefebvre & Flora, 1988, p. 303). Segmentation permits planners to develop programs that will meet the specific needs and desires of the target population, thus greatly increasing the chances for an exchange between the two parties. For example, there are certain employee segments that are more likely than others to read health newsletters distributed by their company (Davis, 1990; Golaszewski et al., 1989; Miller & Golaszewski, 1992). Segmentation is especially useful when trying to reach "high-risk" and "hard-to-reach" groups. This type of marketing is referred to as **target marketing** and allows program planners to strongly **position the product** (health promotion program) in the community by focusing on the sociodemographic, psychological, and behavioral characteristics of a specific group of people.

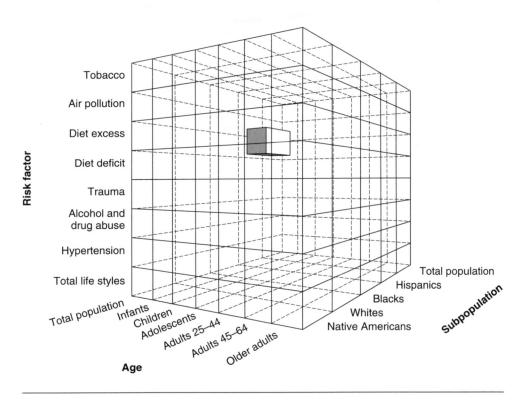

FIGURE 11.4 *Example of Market Segmentation, Identifying Black Teenagers for a Dietary Excess Intervention*

Source: U.S. Dept. of Health and Human Services (1986a), p. 41.

Planners can carry out the segmentation of groups of people before surveying them (a priori) by examining demographic variables—such as age, gender, income, marital status, occupation, religion, ethnicity, and socioeconomic status—or on the basis of a relevant model or theory. Or planners can conduct segmentation after surveying (a posteriori) the target population and collecting data, such as psychographics (attitudes, values, and lifestyle), risk factors, health history, or personal health behaviors. For example, the National Cancer Institute (NCI) used attitudes and lifestyle to identify different segments of the target population for communications about cancer. They found that one group, which they called the naive optimists, were generally optimistic, self-involved, and complacent about their health. They did not make any effort to stay healthy or seek health information and did not worry about their health. This group of people was young with high incomes and made up about 12% of the population (Freimuth & Mettger, 1990). Segmentation is thus most helpful in developing a market plan for this group of people.

Kotler and Clarke (1987, p. 236) indicate that "there is no one, or right, way to segment a market." Demographic segmentation has been the most common means of segmentation in commercial marketing (Hertoz et al., 1993). However, it may not be the most efficient for social marketing. Program planners will need to experiment with the various variables to determine what works best for them. Figure 11.5 includes many of the major segmenting variables identified by several different authors (Hertoz et al., 1993; Kotler & Clarke, 1987; Romer & Kim, 1995; Williams & Flora, 1995).

It should also be noted that segmentation need not be limited to just individuals. In situations when planners are trying to influence the target population at the organizational/institutional, community, or public policy levels, the segmentation process can be of social systems.

> Social systems are easily divided into sector "segments"—educational, industry, government, health, etc. These sectors can be further segmented by location (e.g., urban vs. rural health departments), membership size of composite units (e.g., larger school districts vs. smaller ones), type of business (e.g., service industries vs. manufacturing vs. agricultural), current practices (e.g., businesses with active health promotion programmes [sic] for employees), organizational factors (e.g., innovativeness, leadership style, employee participation, community involvement), characteristics associated with organizational innovativeness (e.g., centralization, complexity, formalization, interconnectedness, organizational slack, size: Rogers, 1983), and many other variables. (Lefebvre, 1992, p. 159)

Developing Informative and Persuasive Communication Flows

The third function of marketing is developing informative and persuasive communication flows; that is, what avenues will planners use to get the "message" out about their product, and how can they phrase the "message" in such a way that will make the product (the health promotion program) appealing to the target population? Several authors (Kline & Huff, 1999; Lefebvre & Flora, 1988, Rice &

FIGURE 11.5 *Segmentation and Variables*

1. Geographic segmentation
   a. Nations
   b. States
   c. Regions
   d. Service areas
   e. Counties
   f. Cities, towns, villages
   g. Neighborhoods
2. Demographic segmentation
   a. Age
   b. Stage of life cycle
   c. Disease or diagnostic category
      • Health history
      • Risk factors
   d. Gender
   e. Health insurance
   f. Income
   g. Education
   h. Religion
   i. Race/ethnicity
3. Psychographic segmentation
   a. Social class
      • Upper upper (less than 1% of population)
      • Lower upper (2%)
      • Upper middle (12%)
      • Lower middle (30%)
      • Upper lower (35%)
      • Lower lower (20%)
   b. Lifestyle
   c. Attitudes
   d. Values
   e. Personality
      • Self-image
      • Self-concept
4. Behavioristic segmentation
   a. Purchase occasion
   b. Benefits sought
   c. User status
   d. Usage rate
   e. Loyalty status
   f. Stages of buyer readiness
   g. Health behavior
5. Multivariable segmentation (i.e., males age 42 living in Indiana)
6. Constructs of behavior theories and models

Atkin, 1989) have made suggestions on items that planners should consider when developing the communication message and flow:

1. What are the media habits of the target population?
2. What medium (electronic or print, visual or auditory, combination of several) should be used?
3. What are the costs of each medium versus the worth?
4. Can the medium's capability build on or multiply the effects of another medium?
5. Will the message reach a significant portion of the target population?
6. Can the message be sent through several different channels?
7. Is the message culturally appropriate?
8. Through how many intermediaries must the message travel to reach the target population?
9. How frequently should the message be delivered?
10. Can a medium be overused to the point that it will "turn off" the target population to the message?

Ensuring That the Product Is Provided in an Appropriate Manner

The fourth marketing function outlined by Syre and Wilson (1990) can best be explained by McCarthy's (1978) four Ps: product, price, placement, and promotion. The particular blend of these four marketing variables that planners use to achieve their objective(s) in the target market is referred to as the **marketing mix** (Kotler & Andreasen, 1991; Kotler & Clarke, 1987; Wilson & Olds, 1991).

Product.   **Product** refers to the actual program you are planning: The program is your product. A goal for all planners is to develop the best product possible with the resources available. In Chapter 8, it was indicated that a health promotion program can be comprised of a variety of intervention activities and thus take many different forms. Lefebvre (1992) came up with a classification system of putting the health promotion product into three categories. The first is *messages,* or the *communication of information.* These are the most common social marketing programs. "The dissemination of 'information products' comprises the major thrust of public information, or health communication, campaigns. The creation of messages that are both scientifically sound in content and possess the creative ability to capture attention and reliably communicate the content to the desired audience are necessary features of social marketing programmes [sic]" (p. 163). An example of such a program, would be a media blitz aimed at the U.S. population about the dangers of HIV/AIDS.

The second category of health promotion products is *tangible products.* "These products might range from condoms in family planning projects to school curricula for AIDS education to self-help materials for smoking cessation in various formats (print, electronic video)" (Lefebvre, 1992, p. 164). The third type of health promotion product is *service delivery,* which can include screening, counseling, education programs, self-help and support groups, telephone hotlines, health care, and social welfare assistance to name a few.

As noted in Chapter 2, the CDCynergy planning model uses a similar classification as Lefebvre (1992) for describing a product. However, in CDCynergy (1999a) the categories are labeled *communication, engineering, policy,* and *health services.*

Price.   "Prices can be thought of in a variety of ways; in addition to economic reasons, there are social, behavioral, psychological, temporal, structural, geographic, and physical reasons for exchanging or not exchanging" (Lefebvre & Flora, 1988, p. 307). In other words, price is the sum of costs the consumer must accept to engage in the exchange process (Neiger, 1998). From an economic standpoint, **price** refers to charging the appropriate amount for the product (program) being provided. As was mentioned in Chapter 10, there are many ways to finance a program. If you are "selling" participation in the program, then the price must match the participants' ability and willingness to pay. When considering the amount to be charged for a product (program), planners should determine:

1. Who are the clients?
2. What is their ability to pay?

3. Are copayers involved?
4. Is the program covered under an insurance program?
5. What is the mission of the planner's agency?
6. What are competitors charging?
7. What is the demand for the program?

The price of a program and who pays for it help determine how a program should be marketed. Whether the program is intended to make a profit will have a great impact on the price. Does the program have to make money? Break even? Or can it lose money? It is a real art not to overprice or underprice the program. Demand and location (placement) will also influence price. If a program is in high demand, obviously the price can be higher than if it is not. For example, a stress-management program in a large metropolitan area may be able to command a higher price than one located in a small rural area.

Not only do the demand and the location influence the amount one might charge for a program, but so can the psychological mindset of those in the target population. There are some individuals who would not participate in a free or inexpensive program because "how could such a program be any good?" Some people believe they have to put out a lot of money to get anything of worth. Also, sometimes when programs are offered free of charge, people may be less likely to attend regularly because they have not "invested" financially in the program. On the other hand, there are some people who, if given the choice of a free program versus one with a cost, will always take the free program, even if they are financially able to pay. Being able to segment the target population with regard to these economic issues can help in setting the right price. Figure 11.6 provides several examples of "price," other than economic, that the target population may face when participating in a health promotion program.

Placement.   The third marketing variable is **placement,** which can be thought of as distribution. Where is the best place to offer the program? How large is the service area? How many distribution points should there be? A good example of the importance of placement is worksite health promotion programs. The advantages of providing health promotion programs in this setting include the following:

1. Access to a large portion of the adult population
2. An effective internal communication channel to employees
3. Stable social support
4. Opportunity to create environments that support healthy behaviors
5. Convenient access for employees (O'Donnell, 1992; O'Donnell & Ainsworth, 1984; Sciacca et al., 1993; Sloan, Gruman, & Allegrante, 1987)

In placing a program, it is also important to avoid areas where people do not normally go or places where they would not feel comfortable or safe.

Two other good examples concerning program placement can be found in the literature. Scandrett (1994) presents a case for the church as a place to deliver

FIGURE 11.6   *Other Prices of Participation in a Health Program*

Behavioral

What can I do to replace my old behavior/habit? What will I do when confronted with a high-risk (potential relapse) situation?

Geography

Is the place where the program offered convenient? Is it safe?

Physical

Will I physically hurt when I make the change? Will it be painful?

Psychological

What if I am not successful with the change? Will the change be worth all I have to go through to achieve it?

Social

Will my peers pressure me not to change my behavior? Will there be social support for my change? How will my friends react to my change? Will my spouse/mate support me?

Structural

Will I be able to make the change in the environment in which I work? Recreate? Eat?

Temporal

Is the timing right for this change? Would it be better to wait until _____ to make change?

Source: Adapted from Lefebvre (1992), pp. 153–181 and Bensley (1989), pp. 86–89.

programs in the African American community, and Sutherland and colleagues (1994) suggest the beauty shop as a place to deliver health information.

The timing of a program is closely associated with its placement. When is the program best offered? If a worksite program was offered in the evenings, so that the workers had to return to the worksite after dinner, that probably would not be much different from driving across town from work to attend a program. Offering a program right after a shift or on a lunch hour would be much more appealing to most workers. Obviously, planners should be concerned about placing their program in a desirable locale (where they are wanted and needed) at the best possible time.

Promotion.   The fourth marketing variable is **promotion.** "Promotion consists of the integrated use of advertising, public relations, promotion, media advocacy, personal selling and entertainment vehicles. The focus is on creating and sustaining demand for the product" (Weinreich, 1999, p. 1). This means taking the necessary steps to make people aware that you have a product (program) in which they would be interested. Such communication should be both informative and persuasive. The choice of a title for a program is an important element in its promotion, since the title can make a difference in whether someone from the target population will be interested in a program. Creating a title is part of the marketing process used to develop informative and persuasive communication flows between the providers of a program and those in the target population. More likely than not, a program title will be the first contact that someone in the target population will have with the product (health promotion program). A title to a program is analogous to the headline of a newspaper article. When most people read a newspaper, they do not read every article; rather, they skim the headlines of the articles and then read those articles that appeal to them. It is the headlines that grab their attention. The same concept applies in advertising a product. "A good headline ought to compel members of the target audience to read the rest of the message" (Granat, 1994, p. 58), or, in the case of a health promotion program, create enough interest that those in the target audience want to find out more about the program. Which of these program titles do you think would attract more attention: "Alcohol and You" or "Not Knowing Your Company's Drug Policy Can Cost You Your Job"?

In addition to creative titles, acronyms are useful in bringing attention to a program. For example, Foldcraft, a company in Minnesota, uses the acronym H.E.A.L.T.H. as the name of its health program. It stands for "Hey everyone always learns the hardway." Program titles and acronyms seem to be limited only by the planners' creativity. Table 11.2 shows additional examples of program titles and acronyms.

Promotion can be thought of as advertising the program. As with product development, planners should consider the segmentation of the target population when promoting the program. For example, advertising for a program to reach high-risk new mothers would be very different from that for one intended for all new mothers. Depending on the type of program planned and the setting for the program, the techniques of advertising the program will vary. If the program is being promoted through **internal advertising**—that is within an organization, say for the employees of a business or for the faculty and staff of a school—promotion might include such elements as posters, bulletin boards, brochures, displays, table tents, newsletters, envelope stuffers, and announcements made through groups that represent the target population, such as unions or professional organizations. If the program is being promoted through **external advertising**—that is, not within an organization but in a community at large—some of the same techniques can be used. Posters, bulletin boards, brochures, and displays are also useful when trying to attract members of a larger community. Other useful techniques for external advertising might include the following:

1. Advertising through the mass media (newspapers; television, including the use of message boards that run across the bottom of a television screen on cable stations; and radio)
2. Direct contact with specific groups that might be at high risk and in need of the programs (contacting recent heart attack patients about a program on the need to eat in a "heart healthy" way)
3. Contact with specific professionals who would be in a position to make referrals to your program

TABLE 11.2   *Example Program Names and Acronyms*

Title (topic)	Acronym (if appropriate)	Organization/Company
A Plan for Life (general health)		IBM
Freedom from Smoking (smoking)		American Lung Association
FreshStart (smoking)		American Cancer Society
Heart at Work (cardiovascular health)		American Heart Association
Hey everyone always learns the hardway	H.E.A.L.T.H.	Foldcraft (Minnesota)
Live for Life (general health)		Johnson & Johnson
Live Well—Be Well (general health)		Quaker Oats
Time Out for Life (general health)		Colonial Life and Accident Insurance Company
Total Life Concept (general health)	TLC	AT&T
United Way at Work (general health)		United Way
Lifestyle Improvements for Everyone (general health)	LIFE	Physicians' Health Plan (Ft. Wayne, IN)
Life after Work Program (general health)		Physicians' Health Plan (Ft. Wayne, IN)
Start Smart (prenatal care)		Key Care Health Resources (Indianapolis, IN)
StayWell (general health)		Control Data
Up with Life (general health)		Dow Chemical
Work Well (general health)		Washtenaw County (MI) government

Of these techniques, the first, advertising through the mass media, requires a special set of skills in order to be used effectively. High on the list of these skills is the ability to interact with media representatives (newspaper reporters and television or radio journalists, and advertising staff). Before a program is ready to be marketed, planners should meet with the advertising staff, the health editor and/or writers, and the health/consumer reporters. These people can provide insight into the type of advertising to be used. They know what attracts their readers, listeners, and watchers to an advertisement. They can also provide additional insight into how to prepare news releases and stage newsworthy activities that can lead to stories and articles in the media. Such stories can be thought of as free advertising, since the space or time is not paid for.

Other techniques that can be useful in promoting a program either internally or externally are as follows:

1. Providing incentives for people to become involved, such as free tee-shirts, extra vacation time, a free introductory offer, free health appraisal, flex time, or money
2. Gaining the endorsement of key people in an organization (those who are admired, a supervisor or the boss) or a famous person or someone well known in the community
3. Distributing mailbox or door-to-door stuffers
4. Making a personal contact with an individual, such as a friend or a superior or boss who is already involved
5. Setting up a mentoring program where someone already in the program works with a beginner
6. A special kickoff, countdown, ribbon-cutting, or health party to get a program started

Keeping Clients Satisfied and Loyal

Keeping clients satisfied and loyal involves two key concepts. The first is that satisfied and loyal clients can add much to future marketing efforts by providing word-of-mouth advertising. They can provide a lot of favorable advertising, free of charge. Second, and more important, is the value of keeping those in the target population involved in the health-enhancing behavior that they began as a result of being involved in the health promotion program. Becoming involved in a program is important, but maintaining a health-enhancing behavior is a more important objective. There is strong evidence that people are not very likely to maintain health behavior change over a long period of time. The problem of recidivism to past behaviors, such as substance abuse, has been known for quite a while (Hunt, Barnett, & Branch, 1971). More recently, however, researchers have warned health education and health promotion program planners of recidivism and dropout problems associated with exercise (Dishman, Sallis, & Orenstein, 1985; Horne, 1975), weight loss (Stunkard & Braunwell, 1980), and smoking cessation (Leventhal & Cleary, 1980; Marlatt & Gordon, 1980). (A detailed discussion of relapse can be found in Chapter 7.)

Why do people behave the way they do? Why do some people begin and continue with health promotion programs, whereas others make a strong start but drop out, and still others never begin? Research has shown that the reasons are many and varied. Participation in health promotion programs may be influenced by a variety of factors—including demographic, behavioral, and psychosocial variables—and program structure. "Lack of time, failure to recognize significance of participation, inconvenience to the participant, failure to achieve personal goals, and lack of enjoyment of participation are some of the reasons why individuals drop out of wellness [health promotion] programs" (Bensley, 1991, p. 89). Proper motivation is one way of preventing dropouts.

Motivation.   A key element for initial involvement and continued participation in a health promotion program seems to be motivation, which has been described as a concept that is both simple and complex. "The concept of motivation…is simple because the behavior of individuals is goal-directed and either externally or internally induced. It is complex because the mechanism which induces behavior consists of the individual's needs, wants, and desires and these are shaped, affected, and satisfied in many different ways" (Rakich, Longest, & O'Donovan, 1977, p. 262). Feldman (1983) suggests a variety of ways in which participants may be motivated to adopt a new health behavior. These means are seldom independent of each other, but from a planning standpoint, they are usually viewed separately. The key to motivation is matching the means of motivating with those things that seem to reinforce the individual program participants. What motivates one individual may not be the least bit motivating to another individual, and vice versa.

Two approaches are commonly used. The first is to include questions about motivation as part of any needs assessment conducted in program planning. For example, if the planners are surveying a target population regarding their needs, they could include questions on reinforcers, such as "What incentives would entice you to participate in the exercise program?" or "What would it take to get you to participate in this program?" or "What would it take to keep you involved in a program?" The responses to these questions should provide some direction concerning the type of reinforcers that would be most useful for the target audience. The second is the "shotgun" approach based on a planner's previous experience or the experience reported by others. Using the shotgun approach, a program planner would offer a variety of reinforcers to meet the needs of a large percentage of the program's target population. The former approach is recommended in most cases, but sometimes motivation is not considered when a needs assessment is completed. In such a case, the latter approach is used. The remaining portions of this chapter provide ideas for motivating program participants.

Using Contracts to Motivate.   A *contract* is an agreement between two or more parties that outlines the future behavior of those parties. Contracts are a common part of everyday living. People enter into contracts when they sign a lease for an apartment or a residence hall agreement, take out an insurance policy, borrow money, or buy something over a period of time. The same concept can be applied to getting and keeping people motivated in health promotion programs. Each program participant would enter into a contract with another person (the program facilitator, a significant other, or a fellow participant) and then work toward an objective or agreement specified in the contract. The contract would also specify contingencies— that is, what happens as a result of the contract's either being met or not being met.

For an exercise program, this system might work as follows. The program participant and program facilitator would draw up a contract based on the participant's present status in the program (e.g., exercising for 20 minutes once a week) and on what would be a reasonable goal for the near future (e.g., eight weeks). Thus, the contract might state that the participant will exercise for 20 minutes twice a week for the first week, 20 minutes three times a week for the second week, and so forth, building up gradually to the final goal of exercising for 50 minutes three or four times a week at the end of eight weeks. The outcome should focus on a behavior that can be maintained at the end of the contract period. For a weight loss program, the goal might be written as eliminating snacking in the evening, increasing fruits and vegetables in the diet to five servings per day, and walking for 20 minutes three times a week. These are behaviors that can reasonably be maintained after the weight loss.

The parties to the contract then decide on what the contingencies will be. Thus, the participant might offer to make a contribution to some local charity or state that she will continue in the program for another eight weeks if she does not meet the contract goal. The facilitator might promise the participant a program tee-shirt if she fulfills the contract during the specified eight-week period. Other ideas for contingencies might include granting a kickback on fees for completing a certain percentage of the classes, or earning points towards products or services. No matter what the contingencies are, it seems to help if the contract is completed in writing. A sample contract is presented in Appendix G.

Using Social Support to Motivate.   It has long been recognized that whatever the behavior may be, it is almost always easier to do if people have the support of those around them. Long-standing examples of the concept of **social support** in the area of health education and health promotion are programs such as Weight Watchers and Alcoholics Anonymous. They are based on the support of others who are experiencing the same behavior change. One of the key reasons why worksite health promotion programs are so effective is that the working environment lends itself to social support. Being around other individuals who are engaging in the same behavior change provides a good support system.

Another means of helping program participants develop the necessary support system might be to pair them with other participants in a "buddy" arrangement. People find it harder to let others down than to disappoint themselves. Another technique that is being used increasingly is to incorporate the help of family members or significant others to provide the needed motivation. It is easier for someone to quit smoking if all members in the household try quitting at the same time, than to "go it alone" while others in the household continue to smoke.

Using Media to Motivate.   Another technique for keeping people motivated to continue in a health promotion program is to recognize them publicly through some medium available to those in the program. Examples of such media include organization newsletters or newspapers, community newspapers, local television and radio stations, bulletin boards at the location where the program is being offered or public bulletin boards elsewhere, and letters sent to the significant others of the participants (family members, job superiors, etc.) noting the participants' progress in the program.

It is important for program planners to exercise caution when recognizing people through the different types of media. Not everyone likes to see their name publicized. Before you publicly acknowledge individual participants, make sure they do not mind if you do so.

Using Incentives to Motivate.   In Chapter 8, **incentives** were discussed as an intervention strategy, but they are also useful in keeping people involved in programs (Jason et al., 1990). Dunbar, Marshall, and Howell (1979) state that reinforcement may be any consequence that would increase the probability of a behavior's being repeated. Wilson (1990, p. 33) defines incentive as "some reward for achieving a level of performance or goal." It has been reported (Frederiksen, 1984) that incentives seem to be most effective if they are provided in small quantities, are frequent in nature, are tailored to those in the target population, address behaviors over which the individual has control, and do not conflict with any organizational policies. Many ideas for different types of incentives were presented in Chapter 8, but one only needs to study the incentives used by those in consumer marketing to create other incentive ideas for social marketing.

Competition as a Means of Motivating.   Wilson (1990, p. 33) reports that competitions have been a useful means of "introducing and promoting health promotion programs and achieving significant initial participation rates." A *competition* can be described as a contest between two teams (groups) or individuals in which the object is to try to outperform the other competitor. In a health promotion context, this could mean competing to lose the most pounds, smoke the fewest cigarettes, walk the most miles, swim the most laps, or plan the most nutritious meals. Competitions are a good method of introducing a health promotion program, but they are probably not useful as an ongoing recruitment tool (Wilson, 1990).

Final Comment on Marketing

Planners who intend to use a canned program should be sure to ask the vendor if there is a marketing plan that goes along with the program. The good programs will usually include some useful marketing strategies, if not an entire plan. A word of caution about the marketing materials: Like the canned programs themselves, they are usually aimed at a general target population, not one that has been segmented. Therefore, they may have to be adapted to meet local needs.

Summary

An important aspect of any health promotion program is being able to attract participants initially and to keep them involved once they have begun the program. An understanding of the diffusion theory is helpful in determining strategies for marketing a program. The actual marketing mix for a program should take into account the four Ps of marketing: product, price, placement, and promotion. Special attention should be given to segmenting the target population. Once people are enrolled in a program, they need to be motivated to remain involved. Strategies of contracts, social support, media recognition, incentives, and competition can be most helpful in motivating people to continue their participation in a program.

Questions

1. Define the following terms: *market, marketing, social marketing,* and *target marketing.*

2. What is the relationship between marketing and needs assessment?

3. How does the diffusion theory relate to marketing a program?

4. What are the five different groups of people described in the diffusion theory? When would each group most likely join a health promotion program?

5. What is the difference between marketing a tangible product and an intangible product?

6. What are the four Ps of marketing? Explain each one.

7. What is meant by *marketing mix?*

8. What are the three types of health promotion products described by Lefebvre (1992)? The four types described by CDCynergy (1999a)?

9. What are five techniques for motivating people to stay involved in a health promotion program?

Activities

1. Respond to the following statements/questions with regard to a program you are planning:
   a. Describe your product.
   b. Describe your segmented population.
   c. How much will you charge for the program? Explain the rationale on which you based your decision. What other "prices" do you see for this program?
   d. Where will you place your program (location, days, and time)? Why are you placing it this way?
   e. How will you promote your program? How, when, and where will you advertise?

2. Create a one-page advertisement that could be used as a table tent, a newspaper ad, or a flyer for your program. This advertisement should include both text and graphics.

3. Give an example of how you could use each of the four methods described in the chapter for motivating program participants to stay in a program.

Activities on the Web

1. Visit the website for any voluntary health organization. If you do not know the address for a site, use a search engine (i.e., *Excite, GoTo.com, Snap,* or *Lycos*) to find one. Once at the site, identify a health promotion program offered by the organization. Then analyze the marketing of the program by seeing how the organization used the 4Ps. After reviewing the material, write four paragraphs (one for each P) describing how the organization presented each of the Ps.

2. This chapter provided the basic concepts of the social marketing process. Because of the many different areas of planning, implementing, and evaluating covered in this textbook, not everything there is to know about social marketing could be presented. Visit one or more of the following websites and look for additional information about social marketing. From the websites, create a list of 10 more things that your learned about social marketing that you did not know before visiting the site(s). Make your written description of the 10 items detailed enough that you can discuss them in class.

   a. The Social Marketing Network **<http://www.hc-sc.gc.ca/hppb/socialmarketing/>**

   b. Population Services International **<http://www.psiwash.org/>**

   c. Weinreich Communications **<http://www. social-marketing.com/>**

12

Implementation
Strategies and Associated Concerns

After reading this chapter and answering the questions at the end, you should be able to:

- Define *implementation.*
- Identify several different strategies for implementing health promotion programs.
- List the concerns that need to be addressed before implementation can take place.

Key Terms

acts
beneficence
commission
implementation

informed consent
liability
logistics
nonmaleficence

omission
phased in
pilot testing
prudent

Once a program has been planned and marketed, it must then be implemented. Ross and Mico (1980, p. 225) state that **implementation** "consists of initiating the activity, providing assistance to it and to its participants, problem-solving issues that may arise, and reporting on progress." To accomplish all of this, program planners must select the most appropriate implementation strategy and see that any special concerns associated with implementation are handled properly.

Strategies for Implementation

Planners decide on the best way to implement the program they have planned based on the resources available and the setting for which the program is intended.

Two models for implementing a program are presented here. The first combines some of our ideas with those of Parkinson and Associates (1982). The second model was developed by Borg and Gall (1989) for research and development projects. Both models are flexible and can be modified to meet the circumstances of different programs.

First Implementation Model

Parkinson and Associates (1982) suggest three major ways of implementing a program: by using a piloting process; by phasing it in, in small segments; and by initiating the total program all at once. These three strategies are best explained by using an inverted triangle, as shown in Figure 12.1. The triangle represents the number of people from the target population who would be involved in the program based on the implementation strategy chosen. The wider portion of the triangle at the top would indicate offering the program to a larger number of people than is represented by the point of the triangle at the bottom.

These three different implementation strategies exist in a hierarchy. All programs should go through all three of the strategies, starting with piloting, then phasing in, and finally implementing the total program. However, keep in mind that limited time and resources may not always allow planners to work through all three strategies.

Pilot Testing.   **Pilot testing** (or piloting or field testing) the program is a crucial step. Even though planners work hard to bring a program to the point of implementation, it is important to try to identify any problems with the program that

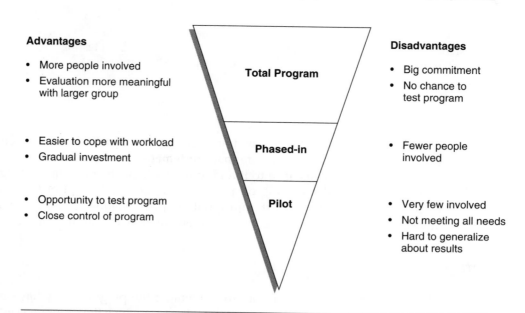

FIGURE 12.1 *Implementation Strategies*

might exist. Pilot testing allows planners to work out any bugs before the program is offered to a larger segment of the target population, and also to validate the work that has been completed up to this point. For the most meaningful results, a newly developed program should be piloted in a similar setting and with people like those who are eventually to use the program. Use of any other group may fail to identify problems or concerns that would be specific to the target population. As an example of the piloting process, take the case of a hospital developing a worksite health promotion program. It would be best if the program was piloted on a worksite group before it was marketed to worksites in the community. The hospital could look for a company that might want to serve as a pilot group, or it might use its own employees.

As part of piloting the program, planners should check on the following:

1. The intervention activities work as planned.
2. Adequate program logistics have been worked out.
3. The program participants are asked to evaluate the program.

It is important to have the program participants critique such aspects of the program as content, approaches used, instructor's effectiveness, space, accommodations, and other resources used. Such feedback will give planners insight into how to revise the program. If many changes are made in the program as a result of piloting, planners may want to pilot it again before moving ahead. This evaluation process during the piloting phase is part of formative evaluation and will be discussed further in Chapter 13.

Phasing In.   Once a program has been piloted and revised, the program should be **phased in** rather than implemented in its entirety. This is especially true when there is a very large target population. Phasing in allows the planners to have more control over the program and helps to protect planners and facilitators from getting in over their heads. There are several ways in which to phase in a program:

1. By different program offerings
2. By a limit on the number of participants
3. By choice of location
4. By participant ability

Say a comprehensive health promotion program was being planned for Blue Earth County, Minnesota. To phase in the program by different offerings, planners might offer stress-management classes the first six months. During the next six-month period, they could again offer stress management but also add smoking cessation programs. This process would continue until all offerings are included.

If the program was to be phased in by limiting the number of participants, planners might limit the first month's enrollment to 25 participants, expand it to 35 the second month, to 45 the third month, and so on, until all who wanted to participate were included. To phase in the program by location, it might initially be offered only to those living in the southwest portion of the county. The second year, it might expand to include those in the southeast, and continue in the same manner until all were included. A program planned for a college town might be offered first on campus, then off campus to the general public. A program phased in by participant ability might start with a beginning group of exercisers, then add an intermediate group, and finally include an advanced group.

Total Implementation.   Implementing the total program all at once would be a mistake. Rather, planners should work toward total implementation through the piloting and phasing-in processes. The only exceptions to this might be "one-shot" programs, such as programs designed around a single lecture, and possibly screening programs, but even then piloting would probably help.

Second Implementation Model (Borg and Gall)

The second model for implementation provides program planners with another way of approaching implementation. Borg and Gall (1989) have presented a 10-step research and development cycle, of which the last 7 steps can be used as an implementation model for health promotion programs. Figure 12.2 lists the major steps in the model.

The implementation portion of the model begins with the fourth step in the process—the preliminary field test. This step is performed "to obtain an initial qualitative evaluation" (Borg & Gall, 1989, p. 790). The preliminary test would include implementation of the program as it has been developed to date, followed by the collection of feedback from both those who receive the program (target population) and those who facilitate it. These individuals would be asked questions such as, "What do you like about the program? What do you dislike? If given a chance to do so, what would you change about the program?" Only a very small number from the target population would participate in this test. The fifth step deals with the revision of the program based on information gained from the preliminary testing. All aspects of the program would be reviewed and revised as appropriate. The revised program would then be tested again with a slightly larger group from the target population. This second testing of the program makes up the sixth step and is called the *main field test*. The purpose of the main field test is to determine whether the program under development meets the program objectives set forth in the earlier stages of planning. If it was found that the program did not meet the objectives, it would be revised accordingly and the main field test would be repeated. In practice, if the program did not meet the objectives during this second main field test, it would more than likely be abandoned. However, if it met the objectives, minor adjustments would be made (step 7), and the program would be readied for the eighth step—operational field testing (Borg & Gall, 1989). The operational field test should very much resemble the final implementation. One could think of this step as the final "dress rehearsal."

The purpose of the first eight steps is to determine whether the program is fully ready for implementation without the presence of the program planner. In order to be fully ready for use, the program must be completely and thoroughly

FIGURE 12.2 *Major Steps of Borg and Gall's Research and Development Cycle Applied to Creating a Health Promotion Program*

1. *Research and information collecting:* Includes needs assessment, review of the literature, small-scale research studies, and preparation of report on the state of the art.

2. *Planning:* Includes defining skills to be learned, stating and sequencing the objectives, identifying learning activities, and small-scale feasibility testing.

3. *Development of preliminary form of program:* Includes preparation of instructional materials, procedures, and evaluation instruments.

4. *Preliminary field testing:* Program given to just a few individuals from the target population. Interview, observational, and questionnaire data collected and analyzed.

5. *Main program revision:* Based on results of preliminary field test.

6. *Main field testing:* Program given to approximately twice as many as in preliminary field test. Pre- and postprogram quantitative data on participants collected; results examined with respect to program objectives and compared to control/comparison group, when possible.

7. *Operational program revision:* Based on results of the main field test.

8. *Operational field testing:* Program given to approximately twice as many as in main field test. Interview, observational, and questionnaire data collected and analyzed.

9. *Final program revision:* Based on results of the operational field test.

10. *Dissemination and implementation:* Program shared with others and implemented where appropriate.

Source: Adapted from Borg and Gall (1989), pp. 784–785.

tested in every respect. In step 9, the final program is revised based on the operational test. The tenth step would include dissemination and final implementation. This includes distributing the program to those who are to use it and helping them to use it properly (Borg & Gall, 1989).

Remember, Borg and Gall's model was originally presented as a research and development cycle, not as an implementation model; however, the last seven steps of the cycle make up a well-conceived and thorough implementation model. Some might say this model is too thorough because it requires so much testing before implementation and does not take into account the frequent lack of time and money for program development; however, planners may modify the model as needed to meet specific needs and available resources.

First Day of Implementation

No matter what implementation model or strategy the planners choose, there will be a "first day" for the program. The first day of the program is just an extension of the fourth P of marketing, promotion (see Chapter 11). The focus of promotion is on creating and sustaining demand for the product (Weinreich, 1999). The creation of the demand for the product leads to the initiation of the program. The first day of the program might include some special event, such as a ribbon cutting, appearance by a celebrity, or some other event that starts off the program on a positive note. Celebrities need not be individuals with national or international recognition, but may be individuals such as the chief executive officer (CEO) of the company, a supervisor, a visible or well-known person (Anspaugh, Hunter, & Savage, 1996) in the community (i.e., the mayor or a coach), or a common person who has been affected by the health problem. Consideration should be given to obtaining news coverage (print and/or broadcast) for the first day to further publicize the program.

Dealing with Problems

With the program up and running, the task of the planners is to deal with problems that might arise and to do so in a constructive manner (Ross & Mico, 1980). Even if a program has been piloted, problems can still arise. The problems that could be encountered can range from petty concerns to matters of life and death. Problems might involve **logistics** (room size, meeting time, or room temperature), participant dissatisfaction, or a personal or medical emergency. Whatever the problem, it should be worked out as much as possible to the satisfaction of all concerned. If there is a question of whether to accommodate a program participant or the program personnel, 99% of the time the participants should be satisfied. They are the lifeblood of all programs. As a part of this implementation step, it might be a good idea to conduct a one-month evaluation asking questions similar to the ones asked in the piloting evaluation.

Reporting and Documenting

Planners need to give attention to reporting or documenting the ongoing progress of the program to interested others (Ross & Mico, 1980). Planners should keep others informed about the progress of the program for several different reasons, including (1) accountability, (2) public relations, (3) motivation of present participants, and (4) recruitment of new participants. The exact nature of the reporting or documenting will vary, but it is important for planners to keep all stakeholders informed.

Implementation Timetable

To provide some guidance in implementing a program, it is helpful to compile a tentative timetable for implementation. It might even be useful to include the entire planning process. Figure 12.3 presents an example of a planning and implementation timetable using a Gantt chart.

Tasks Year 1	Months											
	J	F	M	A	M	J	J	A	S	O	N	D
Develop program rationale	✔	✔										
Conduct needs assessment			✔									
Develop goals and objectives				✔								
Create intervention					✔							
Conduct formative evaluation						✔						
Assemble necessary resources						✔						
Market program						✔	✔					
Pilot test program								✔				
Refine program									✔			
Phase in intervention #1										✔		
Phase in intervention #2											✔	
Phase in intervention #3												✔

Tasks Year 2	Months											
	J	F	M	A	M	J	J	A	S	O	N	D
Phase in intervention #4	✔											
Total implementation		✔	✔	✔	✔	✔	✔	✔	✔	✔	✔	✔
Collect and analyze data for evaluation			✔									
Prepare evaluation report				✔								
Distribute report					✔							
Continue with follow-up for long-term evaluation						✔	✔	✔	✔	✔	✔	✔

FIGURE 12.3 *Sample Planning and Implementation Timetable*

Concerns Associated with Implementation

There are many matters of detail to be considered before the implementation actually takes place. The exact order in which they are considered is not as important as just making sure that they have been taken care of. Therefore, we list and describe these items in no specific order.

Legal Concerns

Liability is on the mind of many professionals today because of the concern over lawsuits. With this in mind, all personnel connected with the planned health promotion program, no matter how small the risk of injury to the participants (physical or mental), should make sure that they are adequately covered by liability insurance. In addition, program personnel should have an understanding of informed consent, negligence, and approval of appropriate professional groups. (See Chapter 8 for information about guidelines from professional groups.)

Informed Consent.   Individuals should not be allowed to participate in any health promotion program without giving their **informed consent.** As a part of the process of obtaining informed consent from participants, program facilitators should:

1. Explain the nature and purpose(s) of the program.
2. Inform program participants of any inherent risks or dangers associated with participation and any possible discomfort they may experience.
3. Explain the expected benefits of participation.
4. Inform participants of alternative programs (procedures) that will accomplish the same thing.
5. Indicate to the participants that they are free to discontinue participation at any time.

In addition, planners must ask if the participants "have any questions, answer any such questions, and make it clear they should ask any questions they may have at any time during the program. Informed consent forms should be signed by participants before they enter the program" (Patton et al., 1986, p. 236).

Program planners must be aware that informed consent forms (sometimes called *waiver of liability* or *release of liability*) do not protect them from being sued. There is no such thing as a waiver of liability. If you are negligent, you can be found liable. However, informed consent forms do make participants aware of special concerns. Further, because people must sign the forms, they may not consider legal action even if they have a case, feeling that they were duly warned. Appendix H provides a sample consent form.

Negligence.   Negligence is failing to act in a **prudent** (reasonable) manner. If there is a question whether someone should or should not do something, it is generally best to err on the side of safety. Negligence can arise from two types of **acts:**

omission and **commission.** An act of *omission* is not doing something when you should, such as failing to warn program participants of the inherent danger in participation. An act of *commission* is doing something you should not be doing, such as leading an aerobic dance program when you are not trained to do so.

Reducing the Risk of Liability.   The real key to avoiding liability is to reduce your risk by planning ahead. Patton and colleagues (1986, p. 236) offer the following tips for reducing legal problems in exercise programs; however, similar advice would apply to all types of health promotion programs:

1. Be aware of legal liabilities.
2. Select certified instructors [in the activity and emergency care procedures] to lead classes and supervise exercise equipment [and for that matter all types of equipment].
3. Use good judgment in setting up programs and provide written guidelines for medical emergency procedures.
4. Inform participants about the risks and danger of exercise [or other activities] and require written informed consent.
5. Require that participants obtain medical clearance before entering an exercise program [or other strenuous programs].
6. Instruct staff not to "practice medicine," but instead to limit their advice to their own area of expertise.
7. Provide a safe environment by following building codes and regular maintenance schedule for equipment.
8. Purchase adequate liability insurance for all staff.

With regard to item 8 in the preceding list, Breckon (1997, p. 88) recommends that "a million dollar per claim liability policy for all employees" be obtained. Planners should check on the availability of liability insurance through (1) their employer, (2) their homeowner's or renter's policy, or (3) special coverage from a professional organization.

Medical Concerns

Does the program put the participants at any special medical risk so that they would need medical clearance (for example, cardiovascular exercise programs)? If so, the necessary steps need to be taken so that the participants can provide proof of clearance. Appendix I presents an example of a medical clearance form.

Program Safety

Necessary steps must be taken to ensure the health and safety of those participating in the program and all staff members. Providing a safe environment includes finding a safe program location (e.g., low-crime area), ensuring that classrooms and laboratories are free of hazards, providing qualified facilitators, supplying first-aid equipment, and developing an emergency care plan. Figure 12.4 provides

FIGURE 12.4   *Checklist of Items to Consider when Developing an Emergency Care Plan*

_____   1. Duties of program staff in an emergency situation are defined.

_____   2. Program staff are trained (CPR and first aid) to handle emergencies.

_____   3. Program participants are instructed what to do in an emergency situation (e.g., medical, natural disaster).

_____   4. Participants with high-risk health problems are known to program staff.

_____   5. Emergency care supplies and equipment are available.

_____   6. Program staff has access to a telephone.

_____   7. Standing orders are available for common emergency problems.

_____   8. There is a plan for notifying those needed in an emergency situation.

_____   9. Responsibility for transportation of ill/injured is defined.

_____   10. Accident report form procedures are defined.

_____   11. Universal precautions are outlined and followed.

_____   12. Responsibility for financial charges incurred in the emergency care process are defined.

_____   13. The emergency care plan has been approved by the appropriate personnel.

_____   14. The emergency care plan is reviewed and updated on a regular basis.

a checklist of items that should be considered when creating an appropriate emergency care plan.

Program Registration and Fee Collection

If the program you are planning requires people to sign up and/or pay fees, you will need to establish registration procedures. Program registration and fee collection may take place before the program (preregistration), by mail, in person, via an indirect method like payroll deduction, or at the first session. Planners should also give thought to the type of payment that will be accepted (cash, credit card, or check).

Procedures for Recordkeeping

Almost every program requires that some records be kept. Items such as information collected at registration, medical information, data on participant progress, and evaluations must be accounted for. In addition, planners must decide whether participant files will be kept in a traditional way, with paper and pencil, or using a computer software program. It is not unusual today to find participants in health promotion programs keeping online records of attendance and daily activities.

Program Logistics

Before implementation, program planners need to make sure that arrangements are made for a number of small but *important* program details. These are often referred to as program **logistics,** defined as the procurement, maintenance, and transportation of materials, facilities, and personnel (Woolf, 1979). Reserving space where the program is to be held, making sure audiovisual equipment is available when requested, ordering the correct number of participant education packets, and arranging for interpreters when working with a multicultural population are examples of program logistics that are important to the success of the program.

Moral and Ethical Concerns

There are times when certain behavior is legal but not moral or ethical. Program planning and evaluation provide the health educator with almost daily opportunities to make decisions that affect other people. Some of these decisions are easy to make; others raise the question of what is the right or wrong decision. In other words, because of the nature of health promotion, program planners are confronted with many moral and ethical decisions.

Who is to judge what is right and wrong? Most often, these decisions are compared to a standard of practice that has been defined by other professionals in the same field. For health promotion planners, the standard of practice is outlined in the Code of Ethics for the Health Education Profession developed by the Coalition of National Health Education Organization, USA (CNHEO) (see Appendix J). However, even a code of ethics cannot spell out all the rights and wrongs of the many decisions that must be made. The interpretation of the code still creates some gray areas. Although the purpose of this section is not to say what is right or wrong, health promotion planners should be alerted to some of the more common ethical issues that they will face.

The first is respect. Even though one may not agree with the values, behavior, and goals of others, it is important to respect them. The program planner's role is not to judge but to facilitate. Fennell and Beyrer (1989) have written a thought-provoking article on some ethical issues concerning AIDS and the health educator.

Autonomy is another issue with which program planners must deal. Should letting people voluntarily adopt health behavior be the guiding principle? Or is there a place for manipulation and coercion in health promotion? Figure 12.5 presents a hierarchy of autonomy.

A third issue concerns informed consent. Although this was discussed earlier with regard to legal concerns, it is often also an ethical concern. Program planners

FIGURE 12.5 *Hierarchy of Autonomy*

1. *Facilitation:* Assist in achieving objectives set by a target group. Examples: putting safety belts in cars or teaching people the skills necessary to perform CPR.
2. *Persuasion:* Argue and reason. Examples: tell people about the importance of wearing safety belts or taking blood pressure medicine.
3. *Manipulation:* Modify the environment around a person or the psychic disposition of the person. Example: automatic safety belts.
4. *Coercion:* Threat of deprivation. Example: safety belt or motorcycle helmet laws and fine.

are faced with questions such as these: Even though the benefits outnumber the risks, do we scare people away by telling them the risks? Is it okay to withhold information if it could affect the results of an evaluation?

Program planners also have to consider the concept of **nonmaleficence**—not causing harm or not doing evil. For example, is it permissible to use an aversive behavior technique to get someone to stop smoking? Which is worse, smoking cigarettes or receiving some physical punishment for doing so?

The concept of **beneficence**—that is, bringing about or doing good—can also be related to ethical issues. Can there be any question whether it is right to do good? If the good comes at the expense of another, then it raises ethical concerns.

Justice and fairness are also involved in ethical issues. For example, the question of fairness might arise in pricing a program. The program needs to show a profit, but the clients cannot afford the price that would be necessary to achieve a profit. (Legal concerns can enter into this area, too.) Issues of sexism, racism, and other cultural biases also involve concepts of justice and fairness.

Finally, the concepts of confidentiality and privacy are involved in ethical issues. Should a program planner be barred from releasing information about a person without his or her consent, even though it will benefit that person? Consider a high school sophomore who approaches the health teacher with confidential information that she is pregnant. Should the health teacher tell anyone else, such as the girl's parents?

The opportunities for dealing with ethical issues are many, and program planners need to be prepared to handle them.

Procedural Manual and/or Participant's Manual

Depending on the complexity of a program, there may be a need to develop manuals or to purchase them from a vendor. Manuals may outline procedures for program facilitators; some refer to these as *training manuals*. Manuals may also provide the participants with detailed information. Developing either type of manual in-house would be a major task; therefore, adequate resources and time need to be given to developing manuals.

Training for Facilitators

If a program that is being planned needs a specially qualified person (certified or licensed) to facilitate it, every effort should be made to secure such a person. This may mean having to hire a vendor to provide such a service. If funds to hire one are not available, others will need to be trained appropriately. This may mean running your own training program or sending people to other training classes to become qualified facilitators.

Summary

A great deal of work goes into developing a program before it is ready for implementation. The process used to implement a program may have much to say about its success. This chapter presents two models for program implementation. The first, a modification of the Parkinson and Associates (1982) model, includes three commonly used strategies: piloting, phasing in, and total implementation. The second, Borg and Gall's (1989) research and development cycle, can be modified to provide a thorough implementation strategy. Also presented in this chapter are matters that need to be considered and planned for prior to implementation.

Questions

1. What is meant by the term *implementation?*

2. What are three strategies from the modified model of Parkinson and Associates (1982) for implementing health promotion?

3. Why are the final seven steps of Borg and Gall's (1989) research and development cycle considered a thorough implementation model?

4. Name the fourth P of marketing and explain how it leads into implementation.

5. What are the legal concerns planners need to be aware of when implementing a program?

6. What is logistics and why is it important to program planners?

7. What is the difference between an act of omission and an act of commission?

8. What role does autonomy play in the ethical decisions a program planner must make?

Activities

1. Explain how you would implement a program you are planning, using a pilot study, phasing in, and total implementation. Also explain what you plan to do to "kick off" the program.

2. Explain how you would implement a program you are planning, using the final seven steps of the Borg and Gall (1989) research and development cycle.

3. Develop an informed consent form that outlines the risks inherent in a program you

are planning. Make sure the form includes a place for signatures of the participant and a witness and the date.

4. In a one-page paper, identify what you see as the biggest ethical concern of health promotion programming, and explain your choice.

5. Write a one-paragraph statement outlining the ethical stand your organization will take with regard to program implementation.

Activities on the Web

1. Use a search engine (i.e., *Excite, GoTo.com, Snap,* or *Lycos*) to locate websites that deal with "informed conformed." Visit several of the sites with the purpose of gathering information that you could use to create a informed consent form for the program you are planning. After visiting several

sites, create a draft of a form. Also, print out a copy of the home pages for each of the sites you use and attach them to your form.

2. Use a search engine (i.e., *Excite, GoTo.com, Snap,* or *Lycos*) to locate websites that include program registration forms. Type in

the words *program registration.* Many different sites will come up for a variety of programs. Visit several of the sites with the purpose of gathering information that you could use to create a registration form for the program you are planning. After visiting several sites, create a draft of a form. Also, print out a copy of the home pages for each of the sites you use and attach them to your form.

13

Evaluation

An Overview

After reading this chapter and answering the questions at the end, you should be able to:

- Compare and contrast the various types of evaluation.
- Identify some of the problems that may hinder an effective evaluation.
- List reasons why evaluation should be included in all programs.
- Explain the difference between internal and external evaluation.
- Describe several considerations in planning and conducting an evaluation.

Key Terms

baseline data	formative evaluation	outcome evaluation
evaluation	impact evaluation	stakeholders
evaluation consultant	informal evaluation	summative evaluation
external evaluation	internal evaluation	
formal evaluation	process evaluation	

Whether they realize it or not, program planners are constantly evaluating their health promotion efforts by asking questions such as: Did the program have an impact? How many people stopped smoking? Were the participants satisfied with the program? Should we change anything about the way the program was offered? What would happen if we just changed the time we offer the program? Should we expect a greater turnout than what we got tonight? Although all these questions are linked to evaluation, some will be of greater importance than others.

The evaluation process that program planners engage in can be classified into two categories of evaluation. The one most commonly used by health educators is **informal evaluation,** which has been characterized as "impromptu unsystematic procedures" (Williams & Suen, 1998, p. 308). Such evaluation processes are used when making small changes in programs, such as changing the time of the program, adding an additional class session, consulting colleagues about a program concern, or making program changes based on participant feedback. Though these evaluation processes are adequate in making minor changes in programs, when the stakes of program evaluation are high (i.e., conducting programs that have significant impact on the stakeholders), evaluation procedures need to become formal, explicit, and justifiable (CDC, 1999c). When these more major decisions are made, there is a need to use formal evaluation processes. **Formal evaluation** processes are characterized by "systematic well-planned procedures" (Williams & Suen, 1998, p. 308). They are processes that are designed to control a variety of extraneous variables that could produce evaluation outcomes that are not correct. Table 13.1 presents several different characteristics associated with formal and informal evaluation processes. Since informal evaluation has fewer restrictions on it than formal evaluation, and since informal evaluation skills are often learned on the job, the focus of the evaluation processes presented in this book are on formal evaluation.

Evaluation is critical for all health promotion programs. It is the only way to separate successful programs from those that are not; it is a driving force for planning new effective health promotion programs, improving existing programs, and demonstrating the results of resource investments (CDC, 1999c). For example, evaluation can help a program planner determine whether participants were satisfied with a weight loss program, whether a smoking cessation workshop actually changed smoking behavior, or whether an exercise program should continue

TABLE 13.1 *Characteristics of Formal and Informal Evaluation*

Characteristic	Formal	Informal
a. Degree of freedom	Planned activities	Spontaneous activities
b. Flexibility	Prescribed procedures or protocols	Flexible procedures or protocols
c. Information	Precision of information	Depth of information
d. Objectivity	Objective scores of measurement	Subjective impressions
e. Utility	Maximal comparability	Maximal informativeness
f. Bias	Potential narrowed scope	Subjective bias
g. Setting	Controlled settings	Natural settings
h. Inference	Strong inferences	Broad inferences

Source: Williams and Suen (1998). Permission granted by PNG Publications, publisher of *American Journal of Health Behavior.*

or not. Without adequate evaluation, accurate information is not gained, and decisions are based on speculation.

In order to generate useful and meaningful data about programs, the evaluation must be designed early in the process of program planning. As mentioned in Chapter 6, evaluation begins when the program goals and objectives are being developed. Evaluation will not only help determine whether program goals and objectives are met but it will also answer questions about the program as it is being implemented. If the evaluation is not designed until the program has ended, the information cannot be used to improve the program as it progresses. For example, low enrollment in a stress-management workshop might reflect an inadequate setting, inconvenient hours, or lack of publicity. All of these problems could be reduced or eliminated if evaluation was conducted in the planning stage.

The process of designing an evaluation should be a collaborative effort of program **stakeholders** (those individuals who have a vested interest in the program). Evaluation results must be relevant to the stakeholders in order to be used most effectively. For example, program planners, administrators, program facilitators, and the representatives from the funding source all have specific questions they would like answered regarding the program's development and outcome. Program planners may want to know if the program met the needs of the target population; program administrators may want to know if the program is making any money; program facilitators may want to know if participants changed their behavior as a result of the program; and representatives from the funding source may be interested in knowing if the program was cost effective. These questions can all be answered if the evaluation is properly planned and implemented.

Although evaluation is a necessary component of health promotion programs, program planners need to understand that evaluation can be a political process. If evaluation is seen as a way to judge a program or determine its worth, it can be threatening. Judgment often "carries the possibilities of criticism, rejection, dismissal, and discontinuation" (Green & Lewis, 1986, p. 16). Thus, program planners may feel that negative results from an evaluation may reduce program funding and eliminate staff, parts of a program, or an entire program.

McDermott and Sarvela (1999) describe additional situations in which evaluations may be political. Results may be intentionally skewed by reporting only successes and not weaknesses to decision makers in order to prevent the elimination of a program. Even when results are reported fairly, political ramifications may occur—reviewing an unpopular but highly visible program, complying with governmental regulations, or complying with the evaluator's desire to publish the results. McDermott and Sarvela (1999) also indicate that an evaluation can be a political "hot potato." For example, if objective results lead to the recommendation that a drug abuse program serving poor, pregnant minority women be eliminated, what are the implications for the agency with regard to morale, racial harmony, and trust in governmental agencies?

Since evaluations may also have ethical considerations for the individuals involved, most colleges, universities, and school systems have boards to review the evaluation design. These groups are sometimes referred to as *institutional review* boards (IRBs) or *human subject review committees.* The purpose of these boards is to safeguard the rights, privacy, health, and well-being of the participants.

Basic Terminology

A variety of definitions of the term **evaluation** have been written; most include the concept of determining the value or worth of the object of interest (the health promotion program) against a standard of acceptability (Green & Lewis, 1986; Weiss, 1998). Table 13.2 lists commonly used standards of acceptability for evaluating health promotion programs.

When determining the value of a program, planners can use several types of evaluation. The type of evaluation reflects whether the results are needed to improve a program before or during implementation, to assess the effectiveness of a program, or to determine whether the program met the goals and objectives.

Evaluations generally use one of two sets of evaluation terms. Some authors use the terms *process, impact,* and *outcome* to identify types of evaluation used to determine the value of a program. Other authors use the terms *formative* and *summative* to describe the evaluation that occurs during the program and after the program, respectively.

- **Process evaluation:** "Any combination of measurements obtained during the implementation of program activities to control, assure, or improve the quality of performance or delivery. Together with preprogram studies, makes up formative evaluation" (Green & Lewis, 1986, p. 364). Getting reac-

TABLE 13.2   *Standards of Acceptability*

Standard of Acceptability	Examples
Mandate (policies, statutes, laws) of regulating agencies	Percent of children immunized for school; percent of target population wearing safety belts
Target population health status	Rates of morbidity and mortality compared to state and national norms
Values expressed in the local community	Type of school curriculum expected
Standards advocated by professional organizations	Passing scores, certification, or registration examinations
Norms established via research	Treadmill tests or percent body fat
Norms established by evaluation of previous programs	Smoking cessation rates
Comparison or control groups	Used in experimental or quasi-experimental studies

tions from program participants about the times programs are offered or about program speakers are examples. Such measurements could be collected with a short questionnaire or focus group.

- **Impact evaluation:** Focuses on "the immediate observable effects of a program, leading to the intended outcomes of a program; intermediate outcomes" (Green & Lewis, 1986, p. 363). Measures of awareness, knowledge, attitudes, skills, and behaviors yield impact evaluation data.
- **Outcome evaluation:** Focuses on "an ultimate goal or product of a program or treatment, generally measured in the health field by morbidity or mortality statistics in a population, vital measures, symptoms, signs, or physiological indicators on individuals" (Green & Lewis, 1986, p. 364).
- **Formative evaluation:** "Any combination of measurements obtained and judgments made before or during the implementation of materials, methods, activities or programs to control, assure or improve the quality of performance or delivery" (Green & Lewis, 1986, p. 362). Examples include, but are not limited to, a needs assessment, pretesting a target population, or pilot testing a program.
- **Summative evaluation:** "Any combination of measurements and judgments that permit conclusions to be drawn about impact, outcome, or benefits of a program or method" (Green & Lewis, 1986, p. 366).

Even though the sets of terms are used to describe evaluation activities, there is some overlap among the terms. Process evaluation occurs during the program and is a form of formative evaluation. Impact and outcome evaluation occur at the completion of the program and are considered forms of summative evaluation. Both sets of evaluation (process, impact, and outcome; formative and summative) take into account the need to conduct evaluation before and/or during the program, and at the end of the program. All types of evaluation should be in place before or during program implementation.

Purpose for Evaluation

Basically, programs are evaluated to gain information and make decisions. The types of evaluation are distinguished by how the information is going to be used. The information may be used by program planners during the implementation of a program to make improvements in services (process evaluation). It may be used to see if certain immediate outcomes—such as knowledge, attitude, skills, and behavior change—have occurred (impact evaluation). It may also be used at the end of a program to determine whether long-term goals and objectives have been met (outcome evaluation). Capwell, Butterfoss, and Francisco (2000) identify six general reasons why stakeholders may want programs evaluated:

1. *To determine achievement of objectives related to improved health status:* Probably the most common reason for program evaluation is to determine if objectives

of the program have been met. Evaluation for this reason may also be used to determine which of several programs was most effective in reaching a given objective.

2. *To improve program implementation:* Program planners should always be interested in improving a program. Through program evaluation, weak elements can be identified, removed, and replaced (Green & Lewis, 1986).

3. *To provide accountability to funders, community, and other stakeholders:* Many stakeholders are interested in the value of a program to a community, or if the program is worth its cost. Thus, an evaluation may provide decision makers with the information to determine if the program funding should continue, discontinue, or expand.

4. *To increase community support for initiatives:* The results of an evaluation can increase the community awareness of a program. Positive evaluation information channeled through the media can help sell a program, which in turn may lead to additional funding.

5. *To contribute to the scientific base for community public health interventions:* Program evaluation can provide findings that can lead to new hypotheses about human behavior and community change, which in turn may lead to new and better programs.

6. *To inform policy decisions:* Program evaluation data can be used to impact policy within the community. For example, a number of communities have passed local ordinances based on the results of evaluative studies on secondhand smoke.

The Process for Evaluation

The process of evaluating a program or activity begins with the initial program planning. Those involved in developing new programs need to be aware of the importance of a well-defined evaluation plan. The following list provides guidelines for planning and conducting an evaluation:

Planning
- Review the program goals and objectives.
- Meet with the stakeholders to determine what general questions should be answered.
- Determine whether the necessary resources are available to conduct the evaluation; budget for additional costs.
- Hire an evaluator, if needed.
- Develop the evaluation design.
- Decide which evaluation instrument(s) will be used and, if needed, who will develop the instrument.
- Determine whether the evaluation questions reflect the goals and objectives of the program.

- Determine whether the questions of various groups are considered, such as the program administrators, facilitators, planners, participants, and funding source.
- Determine when the evaluation will be conducted; develop a time line.

Data Collection
- Decide how the information will be collected: survey, records and documents, telephone interview, personal interview, observation.
- Determine who will collect the data.
- Plan and administer a pilot test.
- Review the results of the pilot test to refine the data collection instrument or the collection procedures.
- Determine who will be included in the evaluation—for example, all program participants, or a random sample of participants.
- Conduct the data collection.

Data Analysis
- Determine how the data will be analyzed.
- Determine who will analyze the data.
- Conduct the analysis, and allow for several interpretations of the data.

Reporting
- Determine who will receive the results.
- Choose who will report the findings.
- Determine how (in what form) the results will be disseminated.
- Discuss how the findings of the process or formative evaluation will affect the program.
- Decide when the results of the impact, outcome, or summative evaluation will be made available.
- Disseminate the findings.

Application
- Determine how the results can be implemented.

Practical Problems in Evaluation

Certain problems may exist that may impede an effective evaluation. Solomon (1987, pp. 366–368) identifies seven types of problems that can hinder an effective evaluation. The eighth practical problem is noted by Glasgow, Vogt, and Boles (1999).

1. The planner failed to build evaluation into program planning.
2. Adequate procedures cost time and resources.

3. Changes sometimes come slowly.
4. Some changes do not last.
5. It is often difficult to distinguish between cause and effect.
6. Conflict can arise between professional standards and do-it-yourself attitudes.
7. Sometimes people's motives get in the way.
8. It is difficult to properly evaluate multilevel interventions.

Examples of these problems in health promotion programs include not collecting initial information from participants because evaluation plans were not in place, failing to budget for the cost of the evaluation (e.g., printing questionnaires, additional staff, postage), or conducting the evaluation before a change can occur (e.g., changes in cholesterol level) or too long after program completion (e.g., long-term effects of a weight loss program). Those without evaluation expertise may conduct an evaluation without a sound design, such as not using random sampling to select participants. Program managers, who have a motivation to make their programs look cost effective, may minimize costs and exaggerate program benefits.

Awareness of these problems and development of strategies to deal with them may improve the accuracy of program evaluation. This chapter discusses many approaches that can help minimize these problems, such as including evaluation in the early stages of program planning, determining who will conduct the evaluation, carefully considering the evaluation design, increasing objectivity, and developing a plan to use the evaluation results. Glasgow, Vogt, and Boles (1999) have created the RE-AIM (an acronym for *reach, efficacy, adoption, implementation,* and *maintenance*) evaluation model to deal with evaluating multilevel interventions. Although this is a useful evaluation framework, limitation of space prevents us from presenting it here.

Evaluation in the Program-Planning Stages

As discussed in Chapter 6, the evaluation design must reflect the goals and objectives of the program. The results of the evaluation will determine whether the goals and objectives were met. To be most effective, the evaluation must be planned in the early stages of program development and must be in place before the program begins. Results from evaluations conducted early in the program-planning process can assist in improving the program. Having a plan in place to conduct an evaluation before the end of a program will make collecting information regarding program outcomes much easier and more accurate.

Discussion on how evaluation plans can be included in program planning will focus on examples of formative and summative evaluations. The formative evaluation should provide feedback to the program administrator, with program monitoring beginning in the early stages. Collecting information and communicating it to the administrator quickly allows for the program to be modified and improved.

Data reflecting the initial status or interests of the participants **(baseline data)** or data from a needs assessment can be used for comparison to the early data collected from program participants. Additional information from the formative evaluation may indicate that the necessary staff have been hired, the program sites are available, brochures have been printed, participants are satisfied with the times the programs are offered, and classes are offered with the needs of the prospective participants in mind.

Early data regarding the program should be analyzed quickly to make any necessary adjustments to the program. This type of evaluation can improve both new and existing programs. Information from the formative evaluation can be useful in answering questions, such as whether the programs are provided at convenient locations for the community members, whether the necessary materials arrived on time, and whether people are attending the workshops at all the various times they are offered.

By developing the summative evaluation plan at the beginning of the program, planners can ensure that the results will be less biased. Early development of the summative evaluation plan ensures that the questions answered reflect the original objectives and goals of the program. This type of evaluation can provide answers to many questions, such as whether the group approach or the individual approach was more effective in reducing tobacco use among the participants in a smoking cessation program, whether the participants in a weight loss program lost weight and kept the weight off, and how many people in the target population increased their knowledge, changed their attitudes, or reduced their risks.

Who Will Conduct the Evaluation?

At the beginning of the program, planners must determine who will conduct the evaluation. The program evaluator must be as objective as possible and should have nothing to gain from the results of the evaluation. The evaluator may be someone associated with the program or someone from outside.

If someone trained in evaluation who is personally involved with the program conducts the evaluation, it is called an **internal evaluation.** An internal evaluator would have the advantage of being closer to the program staff and activities, making it easier to collect the relevant information. Conducting an internal evaluation is also less expensive than hiring additional personnel to conduct the evaluation. The major drawback, however, is the possibility of evaluator bias or conflict of interest. Someone closely involved with the program has an investment in the outcome of the evaluation and may not be completely objective. After all, a positive evaluation of the program may result in future funding that would secure the positions of the staff members.

An **external evaluation** is one conducted by someone who is not connected with the program. Often an external evaluator is referred to as an **evaluation consultant.** This type of evaluator is somewhat isolated, lacking the knowledge and experience of the program that the internal evaluator possesses. Evaluation of this nature is also more expensive, since an additional person must be hired to carry out the work. However, external evaluation can provide a more objective outlook and a fresh perspective, and it helps ensure an unbiased outcome evaluation. Thompson and McClintock (1998) have developed a list of characteristics (see Figure 13.1) that program planners should look for when selecting an external evaluator.

Whether an internal or external evaluator conducts the program evaluation, the main goal is to choose someone with credibility and objectivity. The evaluator must have a clear role in the evaluation design, accurately reporting the results regardless of the findings.

Evaluation Results

The question of who will receive the evaluation results is also an important consideration. The evaluation can be conducted from several vantage points, depending on whether the results will be presented to the program administrator, the funding source, the organization, or the public. These stakeholders may all have different sets of questions they would like answered. The evaluation results must be disseminated to groups interested in the program. Different aspects of the eval-

---

FIGURE 13.1   *Characteristics of a Suitable Consultant*

- Is not directly involved in the development or running of the program being evaluated
- Is impartial about evaluation results (i.e., has nothing to gain by skewing the results in one direction or another)
- Will not give in to any pressure by senior staff or program staff to produce particular findings
- Will give the staff the full findings (i.e., will not gloss over or fail to report certain findings for any reason)
- Has experience in the type of evaluation needed
- Communicates well with key personnel
- Considers programmatic realities (e.g., a small budget) when designing an evaluation
- Delivers reports and protocols on time
- Relates to the program
- Sees beyond the evaluation to other programmatic activities
- Explains both the benefits and risks of evaluation
- Educates program personnel about conducting evaluation, thus allowing future evaluations to be done in house
- Explains material clearly and patiently
- Respects all levels of personnel

Source: Thompson and McClintock (1998), p. 13.

uation can be stressed, depending on the group's particular needs and interests. A program administrator may be interested in which approach was more successful, the funding source may want to know if all objectives were reached, and a community member may want to know if participants felt the program was beneficial.

The planning process of the evaluation should include a determination of how the results will be used. It is especially important in process and formative evaluation to implement the findings rapidly to improve the program. However, an action plan is needed in summative, impact, and outcome evaluation to ensure that the results are not filed away, but are used in the provision of future health promotion programs.

Summary

Evaluation can be thought of as a way to make sound decisions regarding the worth or effectiveness of health promotion programs, to compare different types of programs, to eliminate weak program components, to meet requirements of funding sources, or to provide information about programs. The evaluation process takes place before, during, and after program implementation. If the evaluation is well designed and conducted, the findings can be extremely beneficial to the program stakeholders.

Questions

1. Give an example of a question that could be answered in a process evaluation, impact evaluation, and outcome evaluation.

2. What are some of the general reasons for evaluating a program?

3. Why can an evaluation be viewed as political?

4. What types of problems can block an effective evaluation?

5. What different types of information could an evaluation provide for the various stakeholders (program planners, the funding source, the administrators, and the participants)?

6. Why is it important to begin the evaluation process in the program-planning stages?

7. Explain how feedback from an evaluation can be used in program planning.

8. What are the components of the process of evaluation?

9. In what type of situation would an internal evaluation be more appropriate than an external evaluation?

10. What are the desirable characteristics of an external evaluator (evaluation consultant)?

Activities

1. Describe how process, impact, and outcome evaluation could be used in a stress-management program for college students.

Describe how formative and summative evaluation could be used.

2. Write a rationale to a funding source for hiring an external evaluator (evaluation consultant).

3. Review the evaluation component from a health promotion program in your community and/or discuss an evaluation plan with a program planner or evaluator. Look for the planning process used, the rationale for the data collection method, and how the findings were reported.

4. Assume you are responsible for selecting an evaluator for a health promotion program you are planning. Would you select an internal or an external evaluator? Explain your rationale. If you select an external evaluator (evaluation consultant), where do you think you could find such a person?

Activities on the Web

1. Visit the website for the American Evaluation Association <http://www.eval.org/>. Provide a written answer to the following questions:
   a. What is the mission of this organization?
   b. What types of publications are available from this organization?
   c. Do you see this organization being of assistance to health educators? Why or why not?
   Print out a copy of the home page for this organization and attach it to your answers.

2. The CDC Evaluation Working Group has compiled a list of additional resources for program evaluation. The list can be obtained through the Working Group's website <http://www.cdc.gov/eval/index.htm>. Visit the site and find one resource for each of the following:

   a. Evaluation and ethics
   b. Evaluation-related organization
   c. Step-by-step evaluation manual
   d. An evaluation journal or online publication
   e. Standards for program evaluation
   Print out a copy of the home page for this organization and attach it to your answers.

3. The National Network for Family Resiliency has compiled a list of Electronic Resources for Evaluators. The list has been posted at <http://www.nnfr.org/parented/links.html>. Visit the site and find five other websites that should be helpful in program evaluation. Write a few sentences about each of the sites you selected, indicating why you think each would be helpful. Print out a copy of the home page for each of the five sites.

14

Evaluation Approaches, Framework, and Designs

After reading this chapter and answering the questions at the end, you should be able to:

- Describe the various evaluation approaches outlined.
- Identify the six steps and four standards of the framework for program evaluation.
- List some considerations in selecting an evaluation design.
- Compare and contrast quantitative and qualitative methods of evaluation.
- List the various qualitative methods that can be used in program evaluation.
- Differentiate among experimental, control, and comparison groups.
- Compare and contrast the major types of evaluation design.
- Identify the threats to internal and external validity and explain how evaluation design can increase control.

Key Terms

behavioral objectives
   approach
blind
comparison group
control group
cost-benefit analysis
cost-effectiveness analysis
cost-identification analysis
cost-utility analysis
decision-making approach
deductive

double blind
evaluation design
evaluation framework
experimental design
experimental group
external validity
generalizability
goal attainment
goal based
goal-free approach
inductive

internal validity
measurement
nonexperimental design
posttest
pretest
qualitative method
quantitative method
quasi-experimental design
systems analysis approach
triple blind

This chapter presents several approaches to program evaluation, a framework for program evaluation, and a variety of evaluation designs. Washington (1987) indicates that each approach to evaluation represents a certain way of thinking, which in turn defines the evaluation questions that should be asked. For example, the evaluation questions may focus on the goals and objectives of the program, the effects of the intervention, the cost-benefit ratio of the program, and the behavior of the participants. The **evaluation framework** can be thought of as the "skeleton" of a plan that can be used to conduct an evaluation. It puts in order the steps to be followed.

An **evaluation design** is used to organize the evaluation and to provide for planned, systematic data collection, analysis, and reporting. A well-planned evaluation design helps ensure that the conclusions drawn about the program will be as accurate as possible. The design is developed during the early stages of program planning and has program goals and objectives as its focus. Program planners must give consideration to the audience and/or stakeholders who will read the results of the evaluation; the design must produce information that will answer their evaluation questions.

Evaluation Approaches

In setting up the program evaluation, evaluators have a variety of approaches from which to select; a single approach need not be selected. In fact, Popham (1988) suggests an eclectic approach. He believes that approaches can rarely be used in their pure form, so that choosing parts or categories may be more beneficial to the evaluator.

House (1980) has done a nice job of categorizing the different evaluation approaches. A brief description of each is presented here:

- *Systems analysis* uses output measures, such as test scores, to determine if the program has demonstrated the desired change. It also determines whether funds have been efficiently used, as in cost analyses.
- *Behavioral objectives*, or goal-based evaluation, uses the program goals and collects evidence to determine whether the goals have been reached.
- *Decision making* focuses on the decision to be made and presents evidence about the effectiveness of the program to the decision maker (manager or administrator).
- *Goal-free evaluation* does not base the evaluation on program goals; instead, the evaluator searches for all outcomes, often finding unintended side effects.
- *Art criticism* uses the judgment of an expert in the area to increase awareness and appreciation of the program in order to lead to improved standards and better performance.
- *Professional (accreditation) review* uses professionals to judge the work of other professionals; the source of standards and criteria is the professionals conducting the review.

- *Quasi-legal evaluation* uses a panel to hear evidence considering the arguments for and against the program; a quasi-legal procedure is used for both evaluating and policy making.
- *Case study* uses techniques such as interviews and observations to examine how people view the program.

Because some of these evaluation approaches are used more than others by health educators, it is important to provide a more detailed discussion of those that are more often used.

Systems Analysis Approach

A **systems analysis approach** of evaluation is based on efficiency—determining which are the most effective programs. It focuses on the organization, determining whether appropriate resources are devoted to goal activities (and to nongoal activities, such as staff training or maintenance of the system). This approach is centrally concerned with the measurement of general goals, but it does not focus on the achievement of a specific goal. This is due to the recognition that organizations function at different levels with various goals at each level.

Economic evaluations are typical strategies used in the systems analysis approach. Control over rising health care costs has forced many administrators and planners to be concerned about the cost of health promotion programs. Using cost analyses, decisions can be made regarding which programs are most effective within a certain budget. In order to be able to perform cost analyses, evaluators need to be able to measure both the costs and the outcomes associated with a program.

Some costs may be quite easy to determine, such as those for staff, books, and medical equipment. Other costs are more difficult to determine, such as those associated with years of productive life lost due to accidental death, loss of productivity due to absenteeism, and cost of pain and suffering.

Outcomes can be determined by a number of factors, including health care costs saved due to health promotion programs, years of life saved, number of smokers who quit, reduced absenteeism, and number of pounds lost.

Several different types of cost analysis can be used (McDermott & Sarvela, 1999). **Cost-identification analysis** is used to compare different interventions available for a program, often to determine which intervention would be the least expensive. With this type of analysis, planners identify the different items (i.e., personnel, facilities, curriculum, etc.) associated with a given intervention, determine a cost for each item, total the costs for that intervention, and then compare the total costs associated with each of several interventions. For example, if a health department was interested in providing a tobacco control program for a school district, it could conduct a cost-identification analysis on three different interventions: (1) teacher led, (2) peer education, and (3) voluntary agency provided. Costs for each of these interventions—such as staff time, staff benefits, curriculum materials, and volunteer training—would be identified, compared, and analyzed.

Cost-benefit analysis looks at how resources can best be used. It will yield the dollar benefit received from the dollars invested in the program. **Cost-effectiveness analysis** is used to quantify the effects of a program in monetary terms. It is more appropriate for health promotion programs than cost-benefit analysis, because a dollar value does not have to be placed on the outcomes of the program. Instead, a cost-effectiveness analysis will indicate how much it costs to produce a certain effect. For example, based on the cost of a program, the effect of years of life saved, number of smokers who stop smoking, or morbidity or mortality rates can be determined. A thorough explanation of both cost-benefit and cost-effectiveness analysis is presented in Appendix K in an article written by McKenzie (1986).

As noted in Appendix K, cost-benefit and cost-effectiveness analyses are not easy to carry out. You are referred to two sources (CDC, 1999; Goetzel et al., 1998) presented in Chapter 3 that should be useful in understanding more fully the complexities of these cost analyses.

A fourth type of cost analysis that is used with health promotion programs is **cost-utility analysis.** This approach is different from the others in that the values of the outcomes of a program are determined by their subjective value to the stakeholders rather than their monetary cost. For example, an administrator may select a more expensive intervention for a program just because of the good public relations (i.e., the subjective value in the administrator's eye) for the organization. Or an administrator may survey those in the target population to determine what outcomes they value from a program. Then, based on these data, the administrator selects the appropriate intervention.

Two advantages of the systems analysis approach are that the findings are objective and that the findings can convince decision makers that a program is effective in improving health status. A disadvantage, however, is that this is only one part of the data to be considered when making program decisions: information from program participants is not included. The fate of a program should not be based on a cost analysis alone.

Behavioral Objectives, Goal-Attainment Approach, and Goal-Based Approach

One of the most commonly used types of evaluation models is the **behavioral objectives approach,** which focuses on the stated goals of the program. Approaches using this type of goal-directed focus are also known as **goal attainment** and **goal based.** Data are collected to determine whether the predetermined goals have been met. Success or failure is measured by the relationship between the outcome of the program and the stated goals. This type of approach is based on behavior, and the dependent variable is defined in terms of behaviors the program participant should be able to demonstrate at the end of the intervention.

In the behavioral objective approach, the program goals serve as the standards for evaluation. This type of evaluation was first used in education, to assess student behaviors. Competency testing is an example of goal-attainment evaluation, determining whether a student is able to pass an exam or advance to the next grade. Goal attainment was later used in other fields, and more emphasis was placed on how objectives are to be measured. This approach is also found in business, where organizations use "management by objectives" to determine how well they are meeting their objectives.

Washington (1987, pp. 373–374) identifies five steps in measuring goal attainment:

1. Specification of the goal to be measured
2. Specification of the sequential set of performances that, if observed, would indicate that the goal has been achieved
3. Identification of the performances that are critical to the achievement of the goal
4. Description of the "indicator behavior" of each performance episode
5. Collective testing to find whether each "indicator behavior" is associated with each other

Within the general goal statement is the outcome behavior of the individual. The goal should be operationally defined—that is, it should consist of measurable objectives—and those objectives most critical in achieving the goal should be identified. An indicator of a performance episode refers to a measurable, observable behavior, based on normative criteria. Measurement should be standardized in order to compare outcomes from one behavior to another. (See Chapter 6 for a discussion of writing goals and objectives.)

A strength of the behavioral objective approach is its objectivity. The values of the evaluator do not interfere with the outcome of the evaluation. Another strength is that the goal is predetermined: The evaluation is based on whether the goal was met, not on whether it was appropriate. The goal can be expressed as measurable objectives, making it easier to determine whether the goal was met.

A possible limitation of this approach is how the goal is set, since the outcome of the evaluation is determined by the specification of the goal. The goal reflects the values or interests of the funding source, program staff, or consumers. Who sets the goal is an important factor, and consideration must be given to whose interests the goal represents.

Another limitation of this approach is that only those items included in the objectives are evaluated. There may be other very positive outcomes of a program, but they will not be identified or evaluated because they were not included in the objectives. An example would be to include only behavior change in the objectives of a program; any other positive changes, such as in attitudes or knowledge, would be overlooked in the evaluation.

Decision-Making Approach

According to Stufflebeam and colleagues (1971), the developer of the **decision-making approach,** there are three steps to the evaluation process: delineating (focusing of information), obtaining (collecting, organizing, and analyzing information), and providing (synthesizing information so it will be useful). The decision maker, usually a manager or administrator, wants and needs information to help answer relevant questions regarding a program.

The four types of evaluation in this approach include context, input, process, and product (CIPP), with each providing information to the decision maker. Context evaluation describes the conditions in the environment, identifies unmet needs and unused opportunities, and determines why these occur. The purpose of input evaluation is to determine how to use resources to meet program goals. Process evaluation provides feedback to those responsible for program implementation. The purpose of product evaluation is to measure and interpret attainments during and after the program (Stufflebeam et al., 1971). It is the decision maker, not the evaluator, who uses this information to determine the worth of the program.

The main advantage to this type of approach is the increased likelihood that the information will actually be used by the decision makers. The information most relevant to them will be obtained by this type of evaluation. The advantage for the evaluator is that the evaluation is focused, with criteria already determined. A limitation of the decision-making approach is that the amount of input from administrators may reduce the objectivity of the evaluation.

Goal-Free Approach

The **goal-free approach** of evaluation was developed in response to the limitations of the goal-attainment model. Scriven (1973), who developed the goal-free approach, believed that evaluation should not be based on goals in order to enable the evaluator to remain unbiased. The evaluator must search for all outcomes, including unintended positive or negative side effects. Thus, the evaluator does not base the evaluation on reaching goals and remains unaware of the program goals.

Ideally, the evaluator suspends judgment concerning what the program is intended to accomplish and focuses on what actually happens. However, Popham (1988) sees this approach as oriented toward the output of the program and as a judgmental approach, since the evaluator is required to present a judgment regarding the program to the decision makers.

The techniques that the evaluator uses include examining preintervention test results, reading expert reviews, visiting program sites, reviewing the literature, examining similar programs, interviewing staff and clients, and examining materials. The techniques are generally qualitative methods, but quantitative methods can also be used.

The goal-free approach is not often used in evaluation. It is difficult for evaluators to determine what to evaluate when program objectives are not to be used. One concern is that evaluators will substitute their own goals, since there is a lack of clear methodology as to how to proceed. The goal-free evaluation approach may be most useful in combination with other approaches.

On the other hand, this approach has certain advantages. One is that it avoids classifying side effects and unanticipated effects as being of secondary interest, since these may be crucial to setting new priorities in a program. A classic example of this model was an evaluation of an educational program for coronary care patients. The results of the evaluation indicated no increase in knowledge, which was the program goal. However, an unanticipated side effect was reduction in patients' anxiety during exercise. Without the use of goal-free evaluation, this benefit of the program might not have been discovered.

The main differences between the goal-attainment and goal-free approaches are presented in Table 14.1. The types of questions asked in each approach reflect the difference in focus of the evaluation.

Framework for Program Evaluation

Once evaluators have selected the approach or approaches that will be used in the evaluation, they are ready to apply an evaluation framework. In 1999, the Centers for Disease Control and Prevention (CDC) (1999c) published an evaluation framework to be used with public health activities. Since the framework is applicable to all health promotion programs, an overview of it is provided here. The framework was developed by a working group that included evaluation experts, public health program managers and directors, state and local public health officials, teachers, researchers, U.S. Public Health Service agency representatives, and CDC staff.

The framework (see Figure 14.1) is comprised of six steps that must be completed in any evaluation, regardless of the setting. They are not a prescription; rather, they are starting points for tailoring the evaluation. The early steps provide the foundation, and all steps should be finalized before moving to the next step:

- *Step 1—Engaging stakeholders:* This step begins the evaluation cycle. Stakeholders must be engaged to insure that their perspectives are understood. The three primary groups of stakeholders are (1) those involved in the program operations, (2) those served or affected by the program, and (3) the primary users of the evaluation results. The scope and level of stakeholder involvement will vary with each program being evaluated.
- *Step 2—Describing the program:* This step sets the frame of reference for all subsequent decisions in the evaluation process. At a minimum, the program should be described in enough detail that the mission, goals, and objectives

TABLE 14.1 *Comparison of the Goal-Attainment and Goal-Free Approaches*

Goal-Attainment Approach	*Goal-Free Approach*
Have the objectives been reached?	What is the outcome of the program?
Has the program met the needs of the target population?	Who has been reached by the program?
How can the objectives be reached?	How is the program operating?
Are the needs of the program administrators and funding source being met?	What has been provided?

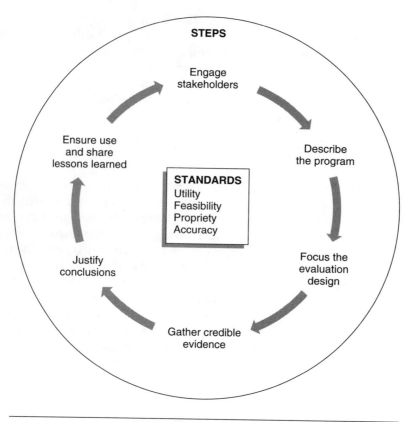

FIGURE 14.1   *Framework for Program Evaluation*

Source: Centers for Disease Control and Prevention (CDC) (1999c), p. 4.

are known. Also, the program's capacity to effect change, its stage of development, and how it fits into the larger organization and community should be known.

- *Step 3—Focusing the evaluation design:* This step entails making sure that the interests of the stakeholders are addressed while using time and resources efficiently. Among the items to consider at this step are articulating the purpose of the evaluation (i.e., gain insight, change practice, assess effects, affect participants), determining the users and uses of the evaluation results, formulating the questions to be asked, determining which specific design type will be used, and finalizing any agreements about the process.
- *Step 4—Gathering credible evidence:* This step includes many of the items mentioned in Chapter 5 of this text. At this step, evaluators need to decide on the measurement indicators, sources of evidence, quality and quantity of evidence, and logistics for collecting the evidence.

- *Step 5—Justifying conclusions:* This step includes the comparison of the evidence against the standards of acceptability; interpreting those comparisons; judging the worth, merit, or significance of the program; and creating recommendations for actions based upon the results of the evaluation.
- *Step 6—Ensuring use and sharing lessons learned:* This step focuses on the use and dissemination of the evaluation results. When carrying out this final step, concern must be given to each group of stakeholders.

In addition to the six steps of the framework, there are four standards of evaluation. These standards are noted in the box at the center of Figure 14.1. The standards provide practical guidelines for the evaluators to follow when having to decide among evaluation options. For example, these standards help evaluators avoid evaluations that may be "accurate and feasible but not useful or one that would be useful and accurate but is infeasible" (CDC, 1999c, p. 27). The four standards are:

- "Utility standards ensure that information needs of evaluation users are satisfied" (CDC, 1999c, p. 27).
- "Feasibility standards ensure that the evaluation is viable and pragmatic" (CDC, 1999c, p. 27).
- "Propriety standards ensure that the evaluation is ethical (i.e., conducted with regard for the rights and interests of those involved and effected)" (CDC, 1999c, p. 27).
- "Accuracy standards ensure that the evaluation produces findings that are considered correct" (CDC, 1999c, p. 29).

Selecting an Evaluation Design

As noted in the section above evaluators must give careful consideration to the evaluation design, since the design is critical to the outcome of the program.

There are few perfect evaluation designs, because no situation is ideal, and there are always constraining factors, such as limited resources. The challenge is to devise an *optimal* evaluation—as opposed to an *ideal* evaluation (CDC, 1999c). Planners should give much thought to selecting the best design for each situation. The following questions may be helpful in the selection of a design:

- How much time do you have to conduct the evaluation?
- What financial resources are available?
- How many participants can be included in the evaluation?
- Are you more interested in qualitative or quantitative data?
- Do you have data analysis skills or access to computers and statistical consultants?
- In what ways can validity be increased?

- Is it important to be able to generalize your findings to other populations?
- Are the stakeholders concerned with validity and reliability?
- Do you have the ability to randomize participants into experimental and control groups?
- Do you have access to a comparison group?

Dignan (1995) presents four steps in choosing an evaluation design. These four steps are outlined in Figure 14.2. The first step is to orient oneself to the situation. The evaluator must identify resources (time, personnel), constraints, and hidden agendas (unspoken goals). During this step, the evaluator must determine what is to be expected from the program and what can be observed.

The second step involves defining the problem—determining what is to be evaluated. During this step, definitions are needed for independent variables (what the sponsors think makes the difference), dependent variables (what will show the difference), and confounding variables (what the evaluator thinks could explain additional differences).

The third step involves making a decision about the design—that is, whether to use qualitative or quantitative methods of data collection or both. The **quantitative method** is **deductive** in nature (applying a generally accepted principle to an

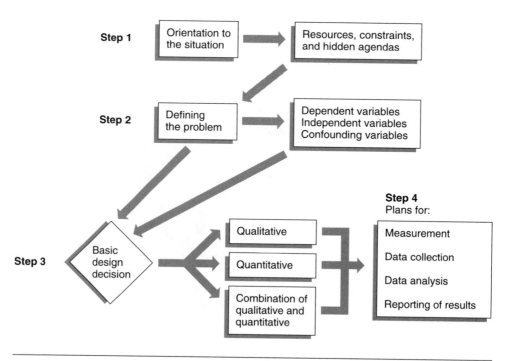

FIGURE 14.2 *Steps in Selecting an Evaluation Design*

Source: From M. B. Dignan, *Measurement and Evaluation of Health Education,* 3rd ed., 1995 (p. 151). Courtesy of Charles C Thomas, Publisher, Ltd., Springfield, Illinois.

individual case), so that the evaluation produces numeric (hard) data, such as counts, ratings, scores, or classifications. Examples of quantitative data would be the number of participants in a stress-management program, the ratings on a participant satisfaction survey, and the pretest scores on a nutrition knowledge test. This approach is suited to programs that are well defined and compares outcomes of programs with those of other groups or the general population. It is the method most often used in evaluation designs.

The **qualitative method** is an **inductive** method (individual cases are studied to formulate a general principle) and produces narrative (soft) data, such as descriptions. This is a good method to use for programs that emphasize individual outcomes or in cases where other descriptive information from participants is needed. Figure 14.3 provides a summary of the various qualitative methods presented by McDermott and Sarvela (1999).

FIGURE 14.3 *Methods Used in Evaluation*

Case studies: In-depth examinations of a social unit, such as an individual, family, household, worksite, community, or any type of institution as a whole

Content analysis: A systematic review identifying specific characteristics of messages

Delphi techniques: See Chapter 4 for an in-depth discussion of the Delphi technique

Elite interviewing: Interviewing that focuses on a certain type ("elite") of respondent

Ethnographic studies: A variety of techniques (participant-observer, observation, interviewing, and other interactions with people) used to study an individual or group

Films, photographs, and videotape recording (film ethnography): Includes the data collection and study of visual images

Focus group interviewing: See Chapter 4 for an in-depth discussion of focus group interviewing

Historical analysis: A review of historical accounts that may include an interpretation of the impact on current events

In-depth interviewing: A less structured, deeper interview in which the interviewees share their view of the world

Kinesics: "The study of body communication" (p. 233)

Nominal group process: See Chapter 4 for an in-depth discussion of the nominal group process

Participant-observer studies: Those in which the observers (evaluators) also participate in what they are observing

Quality circle: "A group of people who meet at regular intervals to discuss problems and to identify possible solutions" (p. 236)

Unobtrusive techniques: "Data collection techniques that do not require the direct participation or cooperation of human subjects" (p. 236) and include such things as unobtrusive observation, review of archival data, and study of physical traces

Source: Adapted from McDermott and Sarvela (1999).

Patton (1988) offers a checklist to determine whether qualitative data might be appropriate in a particular program evaluation. Collecting qualitative data may be a good strategy if there is a need to describe individual outcomes, to understand the dynamics and process of the programs, to obtain in-depth information on certain clients or sites, to focus on the diversity of program clients or sites; or to gather information to improve the program during formative evaluation.

Rather than choose one method, it may be advantageous to combine quantitative and qualitative methods. Steckler and colleagues (1992) have discussed integrating qualitative and quantitative methods, since, to a certain extent, the weaknesses of one method is compensated for by the strengths of the other. Figure 14.4 illustrates four ways that the qualitative and quantitative methods might be integrated. In Model 1, qualitative methods are used to help develop quantitative methods and instruments. For example, evaluators could use a focus group with stakeholders to determine what type of questions should be included on a data collection instrument. With Model 2, qualitative results are used to help interpret and explain findings from a quantitative evaluation. For example, evaluators could collect quantitative data from a large sample of people and more in-depth qualitative data from a few in the sample. Supplementing the hard data with anecdotal information further describes the findings. Model 3 is just the reverse of Model 2. In this model, quantitative results are used to help interpret predominately qualitative findings. For example, after observing a group of people for a period of time, evaluators may want to conduct a survey of the group. In the last model, Model 4, qualitative and quantitative are used equally and parallel to cross-validate the findings.

The fourth step in selecting an evaluation design includes choosing how to measure the dependent variable, deciding how to collect the data (these components were discussed in Chapter 5) and how the data will be analyzed, and determining how the results will be reported. (These components are discussed in Chapter 15.)

Experimental and Control Groups

As in other types of research studies, the group of individuals participating in the program that is to be evaluated is known as the **experimental group.** The evaluation is designed to determine what effects the program has on these individuals. To make sure that the effects are caused by the program and not by some other factor, a **control group** should be used. The control group should be as similar to the experimental group as possible, but the members of this group do not receive the program (intervention or treatment) that is to be evaluated.

Without the use of a properly selected control group, the apparent effect of the program could actually be due to a variety of factors, such as differences in participants' educational background, environment, or experience. By using a control group, the evaluator can show that the results or outcomes are due to the program and not to those other variables. In an ideal situation, participants should be randomly selected, then randomly assigned to one of two groups, and finally it should

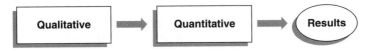

Model 1
Qualitative methods are used to help develop
quantitative measures and instruments.

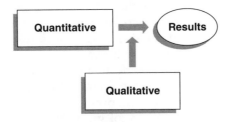

Model 2
Qualitative methods are used to help explain quantitative findings.

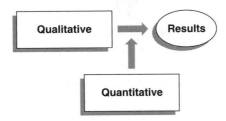

Model 3
Quantitative methods are used to embellish a primarily qualitative study.

Model 4
Qualitative and quantitative methods are used equally and parallel.

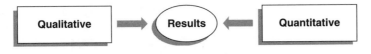

FIGURE 14.4 *Four Possible Ways That Qualitative and*
Quantitative Methods Might Be Integrated

Source: A. Steckler, K. R. McLeroy, R. M. Goodman, S. T. Bird, & L. McCormick, "Toward Integrating Qualitative and Quantitative Methods: An Introduction," *Heath Education Quarterly, 19*(1), p. 5. Copyright © 1992 by Sage Publications, Inc. Reprinted by permission of Sage Publications, Inc.

be randomly determined which group would become the experimental group and which the control group. Theoretically, this would evenly distribute the characteristics (independent variables) of the participants. This technique increases the credibility of the evaluation by controlling for extraneous events and factors.

It is not always possible or ethical to assign participants to a control group, especially if doing so would mean that they would be denied a necessary program or service. For example, a health promotion program could be designed for individuals with hypertension. Individuals diagnosed with hypertension could be referred by a physician into a health promotion class focused on reducing the risk factors associated with this disease. Denying some individuals access to the program in order to form a control group would clearly be unethical.

One way to deal with this problem is to provide the control group with an alternative program or to offer the regular program to the group at a later time (if a delay is not potentially harmful). Another alternative is to compare two programs: Offer an innovative program to some participants and continue the conventional program for others. Wagner and Guild (1989) see the advantage of this strategy as providing service to all participants (which fulfills a moral obligation) and still providing a comparison to assess the effectiveness of the innovative program.

Since the main purpose of social programs is to help clients, the client's viewpoint should be the primary one. It is important to keep this in mind when considering ethical issues in the use of control groups. Conner (1980) identifies four underlying premises for the use of control groups in social program evaluation:

1. All individuals have a right to status quo services.
2. All individuals involved in the evaluation are informed about the purpose of the study and the use of a control group.
3. Individuals have a right to new services, and random selection gives everyone a chance to participate.
4. Individuals should not be subjected to ineffective or harmful programs.

The ethical issues that must be considered involve the potential denial of a service and allocation of scarce resources. When randomization is not feasible, planners should consider an equitable process of providing services for individuals while maintaining control over the evaluation design.

When participants cannot be randomly assigned to an experimental or control group, a nonequivalent control group may be selected. This is known as a **comparison group.** It is important to find a group that is as similar as possible to the experimental group, such as two classrooms of students with similar characteristics or a group of residents in two comparable cities. Factors to consider include participants' age, gender, education, location, socioeconomic status, and experience, as well as any other variable that might have an impact on program results.

Evaluation Designs

Measurements used in evaluation designs can be collected at three different times: after the program; both before and after the program; and several times before, during, and after the program. **Measurement** is defined by Green and Lewis (1986) as the method or procedure of assigning numbers to objects, events, and people. How such information is obtained has been discussed in Chapter 5.

Figure 14.5 presents evaluation designs commonly used in health promotion. In the figure, the letter *O* refers to measurement (or data collection), such as surveys, tests, interviews, observations, or other methods of gaining information. Measurement before the program begins is known as the **pretest,** and measurement after the completion of the program is known as the **posttest.** The letter *X* represents the program (or intervention); the relative positions of the two letters in the table indicate when measurements are made in relation to when the program is provided. The figure also shows which groups receive the program and when participants are randomly assigned to groups [*(R)*].

Windsor and colleagues (1994) differentiate among three types of evaluation designs: experimental, quasi-experimental, and nonexperimental. **Experimental design** offers the greatest control over the various factors that may influence the results. It involves random assignment to experimental and control groups with

FIGURE 14.5 *Evaluation Designs*

I. Experimental design

1. Pretest-posttest design

—Experimental group	(R)	O	X	O			
—Control group	(R)	O		O			

2. Posttest-only design

—Experimental group	(R)		X	O			
—Control group	(R)			O			

3. Time series design

—Experimental group	(R)	O	O	O	X	O	O	O
—Control group	(R)	O	O	O		O	O	O

II. Quasi-experimental design

1. Pretest-posttest design

—Experimental group	O	X	O				
—Comparison group	O		O				

2. Time series design

—Experimental group	O	O	O	X	O	O	O
—Comparison group	O	O	O		O	O	O

III. Nonexperimental design

1. Pretest-posttest design

—Experimental group	O	X	O				

2. Time series design

—Experimental group	O	O	O	X	O	O	O

Key: (R) = Random assignment
 O = Measurement/Observation
 X = Program/Intervention

measurement of both groups. This evaluation design produces the most interpretable and defensible evidence of effectiveness. **Quasi-experimental design** results in interpretable and supportive evidence of program effectiveness, but usually cannot control for all factors that affect the validity of the results. There is no random assignment to the groups, and comparisons are made on experimental and comparison groups. **Nonexperimental design,** without the use of a comparison or control group, has little control over the factors that affect the validity of the results.

The most powerful design is the experimental design, in which participants are randomly assigned to the experimental and control groups. The difference between I.1 and I.2 in Figure 14.5 is the use of a pretest to measure the participants before the program begins. Use of a pretest would help assure that the groups are similar. Random assignment should equally distribute any of the variables (such as age, gender, and race) between the different groups. Potential disadvantages of the experimental design are that it requires a relatively large group of participants and that the intervention may be delayed for those in the control group.

A design more commonly found in evaluations of health promotion programs is the quasi-experimental pretest-posttest design using a comparison group (II.1 in Figure 14.5). This design is often used when a control group cannot be formed by random assignment. In such a case, a comparison group (a nonequivalent control group) is identified, and both groups are measured before and after the program. For example, a program on fire safety for two fifth-grade classrooms could be evaluated by using pre- and postknowledge test. Two other fifth-grade classrooms not receiving the program could serve as the comparison group. Similar pretest scores between the comparison and experimental groups would indicate that the groups were equal at the beginning of the program. However, without random assignment, it would be impossible to be sure that other variables (a unit on fire safety in a 4-H group, distribution of smoke detectors, information from parents) did not influence the results.

Sometimes participants cannot be assigned to a control group and no comparison group can be identified. In such cases, a nonexperimental pretest-posttest design (III.1 in Figure 14.5) can be used, but the results are of limited significance, since changes could be due to the program or to some other event. An example of this type of nonexperimental design would be the incidence of safety belt use after a community program on that topic. An increase in use might mean that the program successfully motivated individuals to use safety belts; however, it could also reveal the impact of increased enforcement of the mandatory safety belt law, of a traffic fatality in the community, or a safety article in the local newspaper.

A time series evaluation design (I.3, II.2, III.2 in Figure 14.5) can be used to examine differences in program effects over time. Random assignment to groups (I.3) offers the most control over factors influencing the validity of the results. The use of a comparison group (II.2) offers some control; without a control group or comparison group (III.2), it is possible to determine changes in the participants over time, but one cannot be sure that the changes were due only to the program.

In the time series design, several measurements are taken over time both before and after the program is implemented. This process helps to identify other factors that may account for a change between the pretest and posttest measurements and is especially appropriate for measuring delayed effects of a program. A time series design could be used in a weight loss program to indicate the amount of weight loss over time and the ability to maintain a desired weight.

When more than one experimental group is part of the evaluation, they can be included in the designs we have discussed. These designs could be used to evaluate several types of programs—for example, to compare the effect of lectures, workshop, and self-study. Measurements could be collected from all groups at the same points in time, and programs could occur simultaneously.

Another design that may be used is the staggered treatment design (Figure 14.6), which is used to determine the effects of a program over time by including several measurements after the end of the program. It also indicates the effects of testing, since not all groups in this design receive a pretest. The staggered treatment design can also be used in quasi-experimental and nonexperimental designs, although with the limitations of not using a control group or comparison group.

Internal Validity

The **internal validity** of evaluation is the degree to which the program caused the change that was measured. Many factors can threaten internal validity, either singly or in combination, making it difficult to determine if the outcome was brought about by the program or some other cause. Cook and Campbell (1979) have identified some of the threats to internal validity, summarized as follows:

- *History* occurs when an event happens between the pretest and posttest that is not part of the health promotion program. An example of history as a threat to internal validity is having a national antismoking campaign coincide with a local smoking cessation program.
- *Maturation* occurs when the participants in the program show pretest-to-posttest differences due to growing older, wiser, or stronger. For example, in tests of muscular strength in an exercise program for junior high students, an increase in strength could be the result of muscular development and not the effect of the program.

FIGURE 14.6 *Staggered Treatment Design*

Experimental group 1	(R)	X	O			O		O		O
Experimental group 2	(R)		O	X		O		O		O
Experimental group 3	(R)					O	X	O		O
Experimental group 4	(R)								X	O

Key: (R) = Random assignment
O = Measurement/Observation
X = Program

- *Testing* occurs when the participants become familiar with the test format due to repeated testing. This is why it is helpful to use a different form of the same test for pretest and posttest comparisons.
- *Instrumentation* occurs when there is a change in the measuring between pretest and posttest, such as the observers becoming more familiar with or skilled in the use of the testing format over time.
- *Statistical regression* is when extremely high or low scores (which are not necessarily accurate) on the pretest are closer to the mean or average scores on the posttest.
- *Selection* reflects differences in the experimental and comparison groups, generally due to lack of randomization. Selection can also interact with other threats to validity, such as history, maturation, or instrumentation, which may appear to be program effects.
- *Mortality* refers to participants who drop out of the program between the pretest and posttest. For example, if most of the participants who drop out of a weight loss program are those with the least (or the most) weight to lose, the group composition is different at the posttest.
- *Diffusion or imitation of treatments* results when participants in the control group interact and learn from the experimental group. Students randomly assigned to an innovative drug prevention program in their school (experimental group) may discuss the program with students who are not in the program (control group), biasing the results.
- *Compensatory equalization of treatments* occurs when the program or services are not available to the control group and there is an unwillingness to tolerate the inequality. For instance, the control group from the previous example (students not enrolled in the innovative drug prevention program) may complain, since they are not able to participate.
- *Compensatory rivalry* is when the control group is seen as the underdog and is motivated to work harder.
- *Resentful demoralization of respondents receiving less desirable treatments* occurs among participants receiving the less desirable treatments compared to other groups, and the resentment may affect the outcome. For example, an evaluation to compare two different smoking cessation programs may assign one group (control) to the regular smoking cessation program and another group (experimental) to the regular program plus an exercise class. If the participants in the control group become aware that they are not receiving the additional exercise class, they may resent the omission, and this may be reflected in their smoking behavior and attitude toward the regular program.

The major way in which threats to internal validity can be controlled is through randomization. By random selection of participants, random assignment to groups, and random assignment of types of treatment or no treatment to groups, any differences between pretest and posttest can be interpreted as a result of the program. When random assignment to groups is not possible and quasi-experimental designs are used, the evaluator must make all threats to internal validity explicit and then rule them out one by one.

External Validity

The other type of validity that should be considered is **external validity,** or the extent to which the program can be expected to produce similar effects in other populations. This is also known as **generalizability.** The more a program is tailored to a particular population, the greater the threat to external validity, and the less likely it is that the program can be generalized to another group.

As with internal validity, several factors can threaten external validity. They are sometimes known as *reactive effects,* since they cause individuals to react in a certain way. The following are several types of threats to external validity:

- *Social desirability* occurs when the individual gives a particular response to try to please or impress the evaluator. An example would be a child who tells the teacher she brushes her teeth every day, regardless of her actual behavior.
- *Expectancy effect* is when attitudes projected onto individuals cause them to act in a certain way. For example, in a drug abuse treatment program, the facilitator may feel that a certain individual will not benefit from the treatment; projecting this attitude may cause the individual to behave in self-defeating ways.
- *Hawthorne effect* refers to a behavior change because of the special status of those being tested. This effect was first identified in an evaluation of lighting conditions at an electric plant; workers increased their productivity when the level of lighting was raised as well as when it was lowered. The change in behavior seemed to be due to the attention given to them during the evaluation process.
- *Placebo effect* causes a change in behavior due to the participants' belief in the treatment.

Cook and Campbell (1979) discuss the threats to external validity in terms of statistical interaction effects. These include interaction of selection and treatment (the findings from a program requiring a large time commitment may not be generalizable to individuals who do not have much free time); interaction of setting and treatment (evaluation results from a program conducted on campus may not be generalizable to the worksite); and interaction of history and treatment (results from a program conducted on a historically significant day may not be generalizable to other days).

Conducting the program several times in a variety of settings, with a variety of participants, can reduce the threats to external validity. Threats to external validity can also be counteracted by making a greater effort to treat all subjects identically. In a **blind** study, the participants do not know what group (control or type of experimental group) they are in. In a **double blind** study, the type of group participants are in is not known by either the participants or the program planners. In a **triple blind** study, this information is not available to the participants, planners, or evaluators.

It is important to select an evaluation design that provides both internal and external validity. This may be difficult, since lowering the threat to one type of validity may increase the threat to the other. For example, tighter evaluation controls make it more difficult to generalize the results to other situations. There must be enough control over the evaluation to allow evaluators to interpret the findings while sufficient flexibility in the program is maintained to permit the results to be generalized to similar settings.

Summary

This chapter focused on evaluation approaches, an evaluation framework, and evaluation designs. House's (1980) taxonomy of eight evaluation approaches was presented. No one approach is useful in all situations; therefore, evaluators should select an approach or parts of approaches to structure the evaluation based on the needs of the stakeholders involved with each program. The Framework for Program Evaluation in Public Health (CDC, 1999c) presents a process that is adaptable to all health promotion programs, yet is not prescriptive in nature.

The steps for selecting an evaluation design were also presented with a discussion about quantitative and qualitative methods. Evaluation design should be considered early in the planning process. Planners/evaluators need to identify what measurements will be taken as well as when and how. In doing so, a design should be selected that controls for both internal and external validity.

Questions

1. List the eight major evaluation approaches in the taxonomy by House (1980). Discuss the major audiences and some of the evaluation questions that could be answered.

2. What are the major features of the behavioral objective, goal-free, decision-making, and systems analysis approaches? What are the strengths and limitations of each of these approaches?

3. What is the difference between cost-benefit analysis and cost-effectiveness analysis? Which is more appropriate for use in health promotion programs?

4. What are the six steps and four standards of the framework for program evaluation presented in this chapter? Why are the standards important?

5. What is the difference between quantitative and qualitative evaluation? When would one method be more appropriate than the other? How could they be combined in an evaluation design?

6. Name at least five different qualitative methods of evaluation and describe each.

7. What are the advantages of using a control group? What types of evaluation design do not use control groups? What is the difference between a control group and a comparison group?

8. What are the strengths and weaknesses of the various evaluation designs?

9. What is the difference between internal validity and external validity?

10. What are some considerations in the selection of an evaluation design presented in this chapter? What considerations can you add to this list?

Activities

1. Identify which approach or approaches you would use in developing an evaluation for a program you are planning. Provide a rationale for your decision.

2. Look at an evaluation of a health promotion program that has been conducted in your community. Identify the evaluation approach that it most closely follows. Discuss your view with the program evaluator.

3. Talk with a program administrator or other decision makers about their view of evaluation; discuss the advantages and disadvantages of the major approaches from their perspective. For example, who should make the decision about how the evaluation results are used? What are the questions they would like answered? Conduct the same activity using program partici-

pants instead of administrators. How does the view of the participants differ from the view of administrators?

4. Develop an evaluation design for a program you are planning. Explain why you chose this design, and list the strengths and weaknesses of the design.

5. If you were hired to evaluated a safety belt program in a community, what evaluation design would you use and why? Assume you have all the resources you need to conduct the evaluation.

6. Explain what evaluation design you would use in evaluating the difference between two teaching techniques. Why would you choose this design?

Activities on the Web

1. The Community Tool Box website from the University of Kansas has many resources for health educators. Visit the program evaluation page of the site **<http://ctb.lsi. ukans.edu/tools/c30/progeval.html>**. This site presents an adapted version of the Framework for Program Evaluation presented in this chapter. Read the information at the site and then write a two-page paper summarizing the "new" information that you learned from the site that was not in this chapter.

2. Visit the website of ERIC (Educational Resources Information Center) Clearinghouse on assessment and evaluation **<http:// www.ericae.net>**. This site offers a variety of resources for evaluation. Search the site

for links to other sites that could be useful in program evaluation. After you have visited a number of sites, create a list of five sites that you feel would be helpful in program evaluation. Print out a copy of the home page from each of the five sites and attach them to your list.

3. Visit the website for the National Science Foundation's site for User-Friendly Handbook for Mixed Method Evaluations **<www. ehr.nsf.gov/EHR/REC/pubs/NSF97-153/start. htm>**. Read Chapter 1 of the handbook, "Introduction to Mixed Method Evaluations." Then write a one-page summary of the value of mixed method evaluations. Print out a copy of the chapter and attach it to your list.

15

Data Analysis and Reporting

After reading this chapter and answering the questions at the end, you should be able to:

- List examples of univariate, bivariate, and multivariate analysis and explain how they could be used in evaluation.
- Differentiate between descriptive and inferential statistics.
- Explain the difference between the null hypothesis and the alternative hypothesis in significance testing.
- Define *level of significance, Type I error,* and *Type II error.*
- Define *independent variable* and *dependent variable.*
- Describe how statistical results can be interpreted.
- Describe the format for the evaluation report, guidelines for presenting data, and ways to enhance the report.
- Discuss ways to increase the utilization of the evaluation findings.

Key Terms

alpha level	inferential data analyses	multivariate data analysis
alternative hypothesis	level of significance	null hypothesis
analysis of variance (ANOVA)	mean	practical significance
bivariate data analysis	measures of central tendency	program significance
chi-square	measures of spread	statistical significance
correlation	or variation	Type I error
dependent variable	median	Type II error
descriptive data analysis	mode	univariate data analysis
independent variable	multiple regression	variables

Like all other aspects of evaluation, the types of data analysis to be used in the evaluation should be determined in the program-planning stage. Basically, the analysis determines whether the outcome was different from what was expected. The evaluator then draws conclusions and prepares reports and/or presentations. The types of analysis to be used and how the information is presented are determined by the evaluation questions and the needs of the stakeholders.

This chapter describes different types of analyses commonly used in evaluating health promotion programs. To present them in detail or to include all possible techniques is beyond the scope of this text. If you need more information, refer to statistics textbooks, research methods and statistics courses, or statistical consultants.

Evaluations that suffer from major methodological problems are not likely to inspire confidence. A common problem is inadequate documentation of methods, results, and data analysis. The evaluation itself should be well designed; the report should contain a complete description of the program, objective interpretation of facts, information about the evaluation design and statistical analysis, and a discussion of features of the study that may have influenced the findings. In order to add accurate findings to the knowledge base of the profession, appropriate evaluation standards should be adopted to serve as guidelines for reporting and reviewing evaluation research (Moskowitz, 1989).

Organization of Data

Once evaluators have collected the data, they must compile and analyze the information collected in order to interpret the findings. The data must be cleaned, reduced, coded, and pulled into a usable form. Information from surveys and observation sheets, for example, must be coded and entered into the computer to be compiled and analyzed. This is done with both quantitative and qualitative data.

Types of Analyses

Statistical analysis techniques can be used to describe data, generate hypotheses, or test hypotheses. Techniques that summarize and describe characteristics of a group or make comparisons of characteristics between groups are known as *descriptive statistics.* Inferential statistics are used to make generalizations or inferences about a population based on findings from a sample.

Variables are characteristics, such as age, level of knowledge, or type of educational program. **Independent variables** are controlled by the evaluator; an example is the type of fitness program chosen (high-impact aerobics or stretching and toning). This choice results in an outcome, known as the **dependent variable.** Examples of dependent variables include scores on an alcohol knowledge test, fitness level, or attitude toward safety. When one variable is analyzed, this is called **univariate data analysis.** Analysis of two or more variables is called **bivariate** and **multivariate data analysis,** respectfully.

The choice of a type of analysis is based on the evaluation questions, the type of data collected, and the audience who will receive the results (Newcomer, 1994). For some types of evaluation, descriptive data are all that is needed, and techniques are chosen to determine frequencies or relationships between variables. Other evaluation questions focus on testing a hypothesis about relationships between variables; in such cases, more elaborate statistical techniques are needed. Table 15.1 lists the types of evaluation questions that can be answered by using different types of data analyses.

The level of measurement (i.e., nominal, ordinal, interval, or ratio, discussed in Chapter 5) is an important factor in selecting the type of data analysis. For the most part, analytical techniques have been developed for use with selected levels of measurement. In other words, not all analytical techniques can be used with all levels of measurement. For example, multiple regression analysis is a technique that has been reserved for use with interval and ratio data. Newcomer (1994) has created a very useful summary (see Table 15.2) to assist evaluators in selecting appropriate statistical techniques.

The issue of who will be the recipients of the final evaluation report should also be considered when selecting the type of analysis. Evaluators want to be able to present the evaluation results in a form that can be understood by the stakeholders. With regard to this issue, it is probably best to err on the side of too simple an analysis rather than one that is too complex.

Finally, regardless of the type of analysis selected for an evaluation, the method should be chosen early in the evaluation process and should be in place before the data are collected.

TABLE 15.1   *Examples of Evaluation Questions Answered Using Univariate, Bivariate, and Multivariate Data Analysis*

Univariate Analysis	Bivariate Analysis	Multivariate Analysis
What was the average score on the cholesterol knowledge test?	Is there a difference in smoking behavior between the individuals in the experimental and control groups after the healthy lifestyle program?	Can the risk of heart disease be predicted using smoking, exercise, diet, and heredity?
How many participants at the worksite attended the healthy lifestyle presentation?	Is peer education or classroom instruction more effective in increasing knowledge about the effects of drug abuse?	Can mortality risk among motorcycle drivers be predicted from helmet use, time of day, weather conditions, and speed?
What percentage of the participants in the corporate fitness program met their target goal?	Do students' attitudes about bicycle helmets differ in rural and urban settings?	

TABLE 15.2 *Selecting Statistical Techniques*

Purpose of the Analysis	How the Variables Are Measured	Appropriate Technique	Appropriate Test for Statistical Significance	Appropriate Measure of Magnitude
To compare a sample distribution to a population distribution	Nominal/ordinal	Frequency counts	Chi-square	NA*
	Interval	Means/medians Standard deviations/ Interquartile range	Chi-square	NA
To analyze a relationship between two variables	Nominal/ordinal	Contingency tables	Chi-square	Percentage difference
	Interval	Contingency tables/test of differences of means	Chi-square or t	Difference in means
To reduce data through identifying factors that explain variation in a set of measures	Nominal/ordinal	NA	NA	NA
	Interval	Factor analysis	t	Pearson's correlations
To sort units into similar clusters or groupings	Nominal/ordinal	NA	NA	NA
	Interval	Cluster or discriminant analysis	t	Equivalent of R-square
To predict or estimate program impact	Nominal/ordinal	Loglinear regression	t and F	R-square, beta weights
	Interval	Regression	t and F	R-square, beta weights
To describe or predict a trend in a series of data collected over time	Nominal/ordinal	Regression	t and F	R-square, beta weights
	Interval	Regression	t and F	Same as above

Note: *NA = not applicable

Source: K. E. Newcomer, "Using Statistics Appropriately," in J. S. Wholey, H. P. Hatry, & K. E. Newcomer (Eds.), *Handbook of Practical Program Evaluation* (San Francisco: Jossey-Bass, 1994), p. 397. Copyright 1994 by Jossey-Bass, Inc., Publishers. Used by permission.

Univariate Data Analyses

Univariate data analysis examines one variable at a time. It is common for univariate analysis to be descriptive in nature. **Descriptive data analyses** are used to describe, classify, and summarize data. Summary counts (frequencies) are totals, and they are the easiest type of data to collect and report. Summary counts could be used in formative evaluation—for example, to count the number of participants in blood pressure screening programs at various sites. The information would assist the program planners in publicizing sites with low attendance or adding additional personnel to busy sites. Other examples of frequencies, or summary counts, are, for instance, the number of participants in a workshop, those who scored over 80% on a knowledge posttest, or the number of individuals wearing a safety belt.

   Measures of central tendency are other forms of univariate data analyses. The **mean** is the arithmetic average of all the scores. The **median** is the midpoint of all the scores, dividing scores ranked by size into equal halves. The **mode** is the score that occurs most frequently. These are all useful in describing the results, and reporting all three measures of central tendency will be especially helpful if extreme scores are found.

   Measure of spread or variation refers to how spread out the scores are. *Range* is the difference between the highest and lowest scores. For example, if the high score is 100 and the low score is 60, the range is 40. **Measures of spread or variation**—such as range, standard deviation, or variance—can be used to determine whether scores from groups are similar or spread apart.

Bivariate Data Analyses

Bivariate data analyses analyze the relationship between two variables. Measures of relationship, or **correlation,** are used to establish a relationship between two variables. Correlation is expressed as a value between +1 (positive correlation) and –1 (negative correlation), with 0 indicating no relationship between the variables. Correlation between variables only indicates a relationship; this technique does not establish cause and effect. An example of the use of correlation would be to determine the relationship between safety belt use and age of the driver. If older people were found to wear their safety belts more often than younger people, that would constitute a positive correlation between age and belt use. If younger people wore their safety belts more often, it would be a negative correlation. If age made no difference in who wore the belts more often, the correlation would be 0.

   Analysis of variance (ANOVA) is a statistical test used to compare the difference in means of two or more groups. It does not prove that there is a difference between groups; it only allows the evaluator to reject or retain the null hypothesis, then make inferences about the population.

   Chi square is a statistical technique to test hypotheses about frequencies in various categories. This technique uses categories that can be distinguished from one another but are not hierarchical. This type of analysis could be used to analyze attitudes toward the use of bicycle helmets (strongly agree, agree, neutral, disagree, and strongly disagree) between children in three different grade levels.

Inferential data analyses use statistical tests to draw tentative conclusions about the relationship between variables; conclusions are drawn in the form of probability statements, not absolute proof. The evaluation question is stated in the form of hypotheses. The **null hypothesis** holds that there is no observed difference between the variables. The **alternative hypothesis** says that there is a difference between the variables. For example, a null hypothesis states that there is no difference between the experimental and control groups in knowledge about cancer risk factors. The alternative hypothesis states that there is a difference.

Statistical tests are used to determine whether the null hypothesis can be rejected (meaning that a relationship between the variables probably does exist) or whether it should be retained (indicating that any apparent relationship between variables is due to chance). There is the possibility that the null hypothesis can be rejected when it is, in fact, true; this is known as a **Type I error.** There is also the possibility of failing to reject the null hypothesis when it is, in fact, not true; this is a **Type II error.** The probability of making a Type I error is reflected in the alpha level. The **alpha level,** or **level of significance,** is established before the statistical tests are run and is generally set at .05 or .01. This indicates that the decision to reject the null hypothesis is incorrect 5% (or 1%) of the time; that is, there is a 5% probability (or 1% probability) that the outcome occurred by chance alone.

When a smaller alpha level is used (.01 or .001), the possibility of making a Type I error is reduced; at the same time, however, the possibility of a Type II error increases. An example of a Type I error is the adoption of a new program due to higher scores on a knowledge test, when, in reality, increases in knowledge occurred by chance and the new program is not more effective than the existing program. An example of a Type II error is not adopting the new program when it is, in reality, more effective.

Multivariate Data Analyses

Multivariate data analyses are used to determine the relationships between more than two variables. One type of multivariate statistic is **multiple regression.** It is used to make a prediction from several variables. For example, the risk of heart disease may be predicted from the following variables: smoking, exercise, diet, and family history.

Applications of Data Analyses

Many evaluation concepts have been presented—so many, in fact, that you might find it difficult to keep them all clear in your mind or to apply them. Therefore, a few examples here will help you see how to move from a program goal to an intervention to an evaluation design to data analysis. To illustrate these concepts, a couple of statistics have been selected that are commonly used with health promotion programs: chi square and *t*-tests.

Case #1

Program goal: Reduce the prevalence of smoking in the target population
Target population: The seventy smoking employees of Company XYZ
Intervention (independent variable): Two different smoking cessation programs
Variable of interest (dependent variable): Smoking cessation after one year
Evaluation design: R   A X_1 O_1
                          R   B X_2 O_1

where:

R = random assignment
A = group A
B = group B
X_1 = method 1
X_2 = method 2
O_1 = self-reported smoking behavior

Data collected: Nominal data; quit yes or no

Smoking Employees

	Group A Method 1	Group B Method 2
Quit	24%	33%
Did not quit	76%	67%

Data analysis: A chi-square test of statistical significance can be used to test the null hypothesis that there is no difference in the success of the two groups.

Case #2

Program goal: Increase the AIDS knowledge of the target population
Target population: The 1,200 new freshmen at ABC University
Intervention (independent variable): A two-hour lecture-discussion program given during the freshmen orientation program
Variable of interest (dependent variable): AIDS knowledge
Evaluation design: O_1 X O_2

where:

O_1 = pretest scores
X = two-hour program at freshman orientation
O_2 = posttest scores

Data collection: Ratio data; scores on 100-point-scale test

Test Results

	Pretest	Posttest
Number of students	1,200	1,200
Mean score	69.0	78.5

Data analysis: A dependent *t*-test of statistical significance can be used to test the null hypothesis that there is no difference between the pre- and post-test means on the knowledge test.

Case #3

Program goal: To improve the testicular self-examination skills of the target population

Target population: All boys enrolled in the eighth grade at Jones Junior High School

Intervention (independent variable): Two-week unit on testicular cancer

Variable of interest (dependent variable): Score on testicular self-exam skills test

Evaluation design:

$$
\begin{array}{lccc}
A & O_1 & X & O_2 \\
B & O_1 & & O_2
\end{array}
$$

where:

$$
\begin{array}{ll}
A & = \text{eighth-grade boys at Jones Junior High School} \\
B & = \text{eighth-grade boys at Hastings Junior High School} \\
O_1 & = \text{pretest scores} \\
X & = \text{two-week unit on testicular cancer} \\
O_2 & = \text{posttest scores}
\end{array}
$$

Data collected: Ratio data; scores on 100-point skills test

Test Results

	Jones Junior High ($n = 142$)	Hastings Junior High ($n = 131$)
Pre	62	63
Post	79	65

Data analysis: An independent *t*-test of statistical significance can be used to (1) test the null hypothesis that there is no difference in the pretest scores of the two groups, since the groups were not randomly assigned, and (2) test the null hypothesis that there is no differences in the posttest scores of the two groups.

Interpreting the Results

After the results of the analyses are available, evaluators must interpret them to answer the evaluation questions. Utilization-focused evaluation suggests having a preevaluation session with the stakeholders to simulate interpreting the results of the data. The purpose of this session is to check on the evaluation design, train the stakeholders to interpret data, help stakeholders set realistic expectations, and build a commitment to use the findings, or else reveal the lack of commitment (Patton, 1986).

Evaluators should also seek input from the leaders of the group affected by the program to assist in the interpretation of the results and to develop recommendations. They should present the facts in a logical order, allowing for questions about the possible relationships among the findings. Various courses of action can then be discussed (Solomon, 1987).

Standards of acceptability should be established in the program-planning stage. These standards can be modified after a session with stakeholders, during instrument development, or before data collection. The role of evaluators as decision makers may vary in the different evaluation models. Even if evaluators are responsible for making decisions and recommendations, they should still seek input from stakeholders.

The interpretation of the results must distinguish between **program significance (practical significance)** and **statistical significance.** Programmatic significance measures the meaningfulness of a program regardless of statistical significance. Statistical significance is determined by statistical testing. It is possible—especially when a large number of people are included in the data collection—to have statistically significant results that indicate gains in performance but are not meaningful in terms of program goals. Statistical significance is similar to reliability in that they are both measures of precision. It is important to consider whether statistical significance justifies the development, implementation, and costs of a program (Fink & Kosecoff, 1978).

Evaluation Reporting

The results and interpretation of the data analyses, as well as a description of the evaluation process, are incorporated into the final report to be presented to the stakeholders. The report itself generally follows the format of a research report, including an introduction, methodology, results, conclusions, and discussion.

The number and type of reports needed are determined at the beginning of the evaluation based on the needs of the stakeholders. For a formative evaluation, reports are needed early and may be provided on a weekly or monthly basis. The formative evaluations may be formal or informal, ranging from scheduled presentations to informal telephone calls. They must be submitted on time in order to provide immediate feedback so that program modifications can be made. Generally, a report is submitted at the end of an evaluation and may be written and/or oral.

Evaluators must be able to communicate to all audiences when presenting the results of the evaluation. The reaction of each audience—participants, media, administrators, funding source—must be anticipated in order to prepare the necessary information. In some cases, technical information must be included; in other cases, anecdotal information may be appropriate. The evaluator must fit the report to the audience as well as prepare for a negative response if the results of the evaluation are not favorable. This involves looking critically at the results and developing responses to anticipated reactions.

The format for communicating the evaluation results may include several methods, such as a technical report, journal article, news release, meeting, presentation, press conference, letter, or workshop. Generally, more than one method is selected in order to meet the needs of all stakeholders. For example, following an innovative worksite health promotion program, the evaluator might prepare a news release for the community, a letter to all staff who participated, a technical report for the funding source, and an executive summary for the administrators.

Designing the Written Report

As previously mentioned, the evaluation report follows a similar format to that used in a research report. The evaluation report generally includes the following sections:

- *Abstract or executive summary:* This is a summary of the total evaluation, including goals and objectives, methods, results, conclusions, and recommendations. It is a concise presentation of the evaluation, since it may be the only portion of the report that some of the stakeholders may read. Most abstracts/executive summaries range in length from 150 to 600 words.
- *Introduction:* This section of the report includes a complete description of the program and the evaluation. Goals and objectives of the program are listed, as are the evaluation questions to be answered.
- *Methods/procedures:* The methods/procedures section of the report includes information on the evaluation design, the target groups, the instruments used, and how the data were collected and analyzed.
- *Results:* This section is the main part of the report. It includes the findings from the evaluation, summarizing and simplifying the data and presenting them in a clear, concise format. Data are presented for every evaluation question.
- *Conclusions/recommendations:* This section uses the findings (presented in the previous section) to answer the evaluation questions. The results are interpreted to determine significance and explanations. Judgments and recommendations are included in this section; they may have been made by the evaluator and/or the administrator, depending on the evaluation model used.

Figure 15.1 summarizes what is included in the evaluation report.

Presenting Data

The data that have been collected and analyzed are presented in the evaluation report. The presentation of the data should be simple and straightforward. Graphic displays and tables may be used to illustrate certain findings; in fact, they are often a central part of the report. They also often make it easier for the readers of a

FIGURE 15.1 *What to Include in the Evaluation Report*

Abstract/executive summary	Overview of the program and evaluation
	General results, conclusions, and recommendations
Introduction	Purpose of the evaluation
	Program and participant description (including staff, materials, activities, procedures, etc.)
	Goals and objectives
	Evaluation questions
Methods/procedures	Design of the evaluation
	Target population
	Instrument
	Sampling procedures
	Data collection procedures
	Pilot study results
	Validity and reliability
	Limitations
	Data analyses procedures
Results	Description of findings from data analyses
	Answers to evaluation questions
	Addresses any special concerns
	Explanation of findings
	Charts and graphs of findings
Conclusions/recommendations	Interpretation of results
	Conclusions about program effectiveness
	Program recommendations
	Determining if additional information is needed

written report or the audience for an oral report to understand the findings of an evaluation. When presenting the data in graphic form, it is often helpful to include a frame of reference—such as a comparison with national, state, local, or other data—and explain any limitations of the data. If graphic displays are used in a report, it is recommended (USDHHS, CDC, no date) that such displays are appropriate for the results:

1. Use horizontal bar charts to focus attention on how one category differs from another.
2. Use vertical bar charts to focus attention on a change in a variable over time.

3. Use cluster bar charts to contrast one variable among multiple subgroups.
4. Use line graphs to plot data for several periods and show a trend over time.
5. Use pie charts to show the distribution of a set of events or a total quantity.

If many tables are included, the main ones can be placed in the text of the report and the rest relegated to an appendix. Figure 15.2 lists guidelines to follow when presenting data in the evaluation report and/or presentation.

FIGURE 15.2 *Guidelines for Presenting Data*

1. Use graphic methods of presenting numerical data whenever possible.
2. Build the results and discussion section of the evaluation report—and perhaps other sections as well—around tables and figures. Prepare the tables and graphs first; then write text to explain them.
3. Make each table and figure self-explanatory. Use a clear, complete title, a key, label, footnotes, and so forth.
4. Discuss in the text the major information to be found in each table and figure.
5. Play with, and consider using, as many graphs as you have the time and ingenuity to prepare. Not only do they communicate clearly to your audiences, they also help you to see what is happening.
6. Since graphs tend to convey fewer details than numerical tables, consider providing both tables and graphs for the same data, where appropriate.
7. If you have used a mixed evaluation design with both quantitative and qualitative data collection procedures, use the direct quotations and descriptions from the qualitative results to add depth and clarity to information reported graphically.
8. When presenting complicated graphs to a live audience, give some instruction about how to read the graph and a few sample interpretations of simpler versions, then present the real data.
9. When a complete draft of the report has been completed, ask yourself the following questions:
   a. Do the figure titles give a comprehensive description of the figures? Could someone leafing through the report understand the graphs?
   b. Are both axes of every graph clearly labeled with a name?
   c. Is the interval size marked on all axes of graphs?
   d. Is the number of cases on which each summary statistic has been based indicated in each table or on each graph?
   e. Are the tables and figures labeled and numbered throughout the report?
   f. If the report is a lengthy one, does it include a list of tables and figures at the front following the table of contents?

Source: L. L. Morris, C. T. Fitz-Gibbon, and M. E. Freeman, *How to Communicate Evaluation Findings* (pp. 75–76). Copyright © 1987 by Sage Publications, Inc. Reprinted by permission of Sage Publications, Inc.

How and When to Present the Report

Evaluators must consider carefully the logistics of presenting the evaluation findings. They should discuss this with the decision makers involved in the evaluation. An evaluator may be in the position of presenting negative results, encountering distrust among staff members, or submitting a report that will never be read. Following are several suggestions for enhancing the evaluation report:

- Give key decision makers advance information on the findings; this increases the likelihood that the information will actually be used and prevents the decision makers from learning about the results from the media or another source.
- Maintain anonymity of individuals, institutions, and organizations; use sensitivity to avoid judging or labeling people in negative ways; maintain confidentiality of the final report according to the wishes of the administrators; maintain objectivity throughout the report (Windsor et al., 1994).
- Choose ways to report the evaluation findings so as to meet the needs of the stakeholders, and include information that is relevant to each group.

Increasing Utilization of the Results

Far too often, an evaluation will be conducted and a report submitted to the decision makers, but the recommendations will not be implemented. This occurs for a variety of reasons. Decision makers may not use findings because they are conducting the evaluation only to fulfill the requirements of the funding source, to serve their own self-interest, or to gain recognition for a successful program. Even decision makers who plan to use the evaluation results in their health promotion program may find that they are unable to state the evaluation question or that the final report contains language and concepts that are unfamiliar to them. Weiss (1984) sees the need to improve the quality both of evaluation research and of modes of disseminating the findings. Weiss developed the following guidelines to increase the chances that evaluation results will actually be used:

1. Plan the study with program stakeholders in mind and involve them in the planning process.
2. Continue to gather information about the program after the planning stage; a change in the program should result in a change in the evaluation.
3. Focus the evaluation on conditions about the program that the decision makers can change.
4. Write reports in a clear, simple manner and submit them on time. Use graphs and charts within the text, and include complicated statistical information in an appendix.

5. Base the decision on whether to make recommendations on how specific and clear the data are, how much is known about the program, and whether differences between programs are obvious. A joint interpretation between evaluator and decision maker may be best.
6. Disseminate the results to all stakeholders, using a variety of methods.
7. Integrate evaluation findings with other research and evaluation about the program area.
8. Provide high-quality research.

Summary

Evaluation questions developed in the early program-planning stages can be answered once the data have been analyzed. Descriptive statistics can be used to summarize or describe the data, and inferential statistics can be used to generate or test hypotheses. Evaluators then interpret the findings and present the results to the stakeholders, via a formal or informal report.

Questions

1. What are some common problems with evaluations, and how can these problems be reduced or overcome?

2. What are some types of univariate data analyses used in evaluation? When would these be used?

3. How are bivariate and multivariate data analyses used in evaluation?

4. Explain the concepts of hypothesis testing, level of significance, Type I error, and Type II error.

5. What is the role of evaluators and decision makers in interpreting the results and making recommendations?

6. What is the difference between statistical significance and program significance?

7. What information is included in the written evaluation report? How is the information modified for various audiences?

8. What are some guidelines for presenting data in an evaluation report?

9. How can the evaluation report be enhanced?

10. How can the evaluator increase the likelihood of utilization of the evaluation findings?

Activities

1. Obtain an actual report from a program evaluation. Look for the type of statistical test used, the level of significance, the independent and dependent variables, the interpretation of the findings, recommendations, and format for the report.

2. Discuss evaluation with a decision maker from a health agency. Find out what types of evaluation have been conducted, who has conducted them, what the findings have been, whether the findings were implemented, and how the information was reported.

3. Compare an evaluation report with a research report. What are the similarities and differences? How could you improve the report?

4. Using data that you have generated or data presented by your instructor, create one table and one graph.

Activities on the Web

1. Visit the website for the Association of State and Territorial Health Officials that link to the state/territorial page **<http://www.astho.org/state.html>**. Select the state or territory of your choice. Once you are on the state health department's home page, select the health data and statistics link. Locate data from a statewide survey (e.g., BRFSS). Then find at least three different ways (i.e., graphs, charts, tables) data are presented. Critique each of the presentations with a written response to these questions:
   a. Is the presentation easy to understand? Why or why not?
   b. Do you think that the data are presented in an appropriate manner? Why or why not?
   c. How could you change the format of the presentation to make it easier to understand?

   Print out the three data presentations and attach them to your critique.

2. Visit the website for at least one of the following voluntary health organizations:

   American Cancer Society **<http://www.cancer.org/>**

   American Diabetes Association **<http://www.diabetes.org/>**

   American Heart Association **<http://www.americanheart.org/>**

   American Lung Association **<http://www.lungusa.org/>**

   Search the site for the presentation of data in a chart, graph, or table. Critique the presentation by providing a written response to the following questions:
   a. What did you like and dislike about the presentation?
   b. How would you change it to make it more easily understood?

   Print out the home page of the organization and the data presentation and attach them to your critique.

Appendixes

Appendix A

Examples of a News Release and Copy for a Newspaper Column

NEWS RELEASE

Delaware City-County Health Department

For Immediate Release   **Contact: Susan Sutherland**
                                             Phone: (740) 368-1700

Food Safety: A Health Department Priority at Fair

Health Inspectors are busy this week checking every food concession stand at the fair for food safety. Health Department staff are looking for proper food temperatures, concession stand cleanliness, a safe water supply, and proper control of insects.

"The Health Department provides this service to ensure that our community and guests to our county are protected from food borne illnesses such a E. coli and Salmonella," said Susan Sutherland, Food Protection Program Manager. Sutherland and her staff will be reminding all food handlers to wash their hands before they touch foods, thoroughly cook food and test for temperature by using a reliable food thermometer. "It's as simple as keeping hot foods hot and cold foods cold," advised Sutherland.

Should you have any questions about food safety, please contact Ms. Sutherland at the Health Department.

The Delaware City-County Health Department promotes good health and improved quality of life in Delaware County. For more information contact the Delaware City-County Health Department at (740)368-1700 or (740)548-7055. You may e-mail Susan Sutherland at ssutherland@iwaynet.net or you may visit the Health Department's home page at www.health.co.delaware.oh.us

–end–

Source: Reprinted by permission of Delaware City-County Health Department.

Delaware Gazette Bi-monthly Column
Roger Wren, Health Educator
February 24, 2000

WHICH AILMENT: COLD OR FLU?

Delaware City-County Health Department

Much to the displeasure of a great many people, winter is still alive and well. Colds and influenza are still around too, and it looks like they will be for awhile. When you catch one of these bugs, how do you know one from the other?

People associate sneezing, stuffy nose, and sore throat with both ailments, but they are more common with the cold than with the flu. People can have the flu and have none of these symptoms.

Chest congestion and coughing are common in both illnesses, but can be more severe with the flu. Being less severe, a cold's symptoms are usually limited to sneezing, runny nose, sore throat, coughing, and chest congestion, with the occasional complications of sinus infection and earache.

The flu has much more to offer! Sudden onset of high fever, headaches, muscle aches, and fatigue are in store with influenza. Fever is characteristic of the flu and usually ranges between 102 and 104 degrees Fahrenheit and lasts three to four days. Headaches are prominent, and fatigue, usually not much of a problem with a cold, hits early and hard and tends to last from two to three weeks.

Although sinus infections and earaches are annoying complications of a cold, flu can give you a nasty dose of bronchitis or even pneumonia as an encore. Suffice it to say that the flu is usually much more severe than your common cold.

The only thing preferable about the flu over a cold is that there are preventative measures and treatment for influenza but not for a cold. You have to ride out a cold, getting only temporary relief of the symptoms. An annual flu vaccination is a good start from a prevention standpoint, but if you are unfortunate enough to get the flu anyway, your doctor may be able to prescribe antiviral drugs. Both illnesses are caused by a virus, so anti*biotic* drugs will not work.

This year, the influenza season started late and is expected to last a little longer than usual. The yearly flu vaccine lasts roughly four months, so people who got theirs early, in September or early October, may be at risk of contracting the flu, since the immunity may wear off. However, the Centers for Disease Control and the Ohio Department of Health are not recommending that people get an additional flu shot.

Remember, with or without the flu shot, there are still steps you can take to increase your chances of staying well! You can still affect your good health by doing the things that tend toward wellness—keep eating right, get enough rest, exercise, and wash your hands often to prevent the spread of germs. By staying fit, you can keep your immune system working effectively so it will fight off those scourges of winter—colds and flu.

The Delaware City-County Health Department promotes good health and improved quality of life in Delaware County. For more information, contact the Health Department at (740)368-1700 or (740) 548-7055. You can also e-mail the health education staff at **<healthed@rrcol.com>** *or go to* **<www.health.co.delaware.oh.us>** *and visit the Health Department's home page.*

–30–

Appendix B

Examples of PSAs for Radio and Television

30-SECOND PUBLIC SERVICE ANNOUNCEMENT

Delaware City-Council Health Department

For Immediate Release   Contact: Roger Wren
                                                             (740) 368-1700 or (740) 548-7055

Concern for the environment begins at home. Proper waste disposal has increasingly become a critical environmental concern, both globally and locally.

Recycling is an important part of the solution to this dilemma since it saves valuable landfill space and conserves natural resources.

Let's keep our home—Delaware County—an environmentally conscientious community.

Recycle. Because it's important.

Keep Delaware County beautiful.

Source: Reprinted by permission of Delaware City-County Health Department.

CABLE TELEVISION—PUBLIC SERVICE ANNOUNCEMENT

Delaware City-County Health Department

For Immediate Release

Contact: Melissa Sever
Delaware Health Dept.
(740) 368-1700

Cable Television

Most car seats aren't
installed safely!
Free car seat check up
at Nourse Chevrolet
1101 Columbus Pike
Saturday, Feb. 20th from 9 to 12 A.M.
Delaware Health Department
(740) 368-1700

Source: Reprinted by permission of Delaware City-County Health Department.

Appendix C

McSmeltzer Corporation Smoking Policy

McSMELTZER CORPORATION

Health Policy H-48
Effective January 1, 2000
Approved by the Board on August 4, 2000

Smoking Policy
It is the policy of the McSmeltzer Corporation that smoking will not be permitted on Corporation property (this includes the physical plant, the surrounding Corporation-owned grounds, and parking lots) and in Corporation vehicles (this includes vehicles owned by the Corporation and those leased vehicles that are being operated at Corporation expense). The policy applies to all employees, full- and part-time, and guests of the Corporation.

Violations of this policy will be dealt with according to the progressive discipline policy of the Corporation (see Policy A-5).

Appendix D

Model Ordinance Eliminating Smoking in Workplaces and Enclosed Public Places (100% Smokefree)

Sec. 1000. Title

This article shall be known as the Smoking Pollution Control Ordinance.

Sec. 1001. Findings and Purpose

The City Council [or Board of Supervisors] does hereby find that:

> Numerous studies have found that tobacco smoke is a major contributor to indoor air pollution, and that breathing secondhand smoke is a cause of disease, including lung cancer, in nonsmokers. At special risk are children, elderly people, individuals with cardiovascular disease, and individuals with impaired respiratory function, including asthmatics and those with obstructive airway disease; and

> Health hazards induced by breathing secondhand smoke include lung cancer, heart disease, respiratory infection, and decreased respiratory function, including bronchoconstriction and broncho-spasm.

Accordingly, the City Council [or Board of Supervisors] finds and declares that the purposes of this ordinance are (1) to protect the public health and welfare by prohibiting smoking in public places and places of employment; and (2) to guarantee the right of nonsmokers to breathe smoke- free air, and to recognize that the need to breathe smoke-free air shall have priority over the desire to smoke.

Sec. 1002. Definitions

The following words and phrases, whenever used in this article, shall be construed as defined in this section:

1. "Bar" means an area which is devoted to the serving of alcoholic beverages for consumption by guests on the premises and in which the serving of food is only incidental to the consumption of such beverages. A "bar" for the purpose of this definition does not include any establishment where tobacco smoke can filter into any area where smoking is prohibited through a passageway, ventilation system, or any other means. A "bar" for the purposes of this ordinance shall not include any area where full meals are served, but may include the service of appetizers and snacks.

2. "Business" means any sole proprietorship, partnership, joint venture, corporation or other business entity formed for profit-making purposes,

Source: Americans for Nonsmokers' Rights, 2530 San Pablo Avenue, Suite J, Berkeley, CA 94702, October 15, 1998. Reprinted by permission.

including retail establishments where goods or services are sold as well as professional corporations and other entities where legal, medical, dental, engineering, architectural or other professional services are delivered.

3. "Employee" means any person who is employed by any employer in the consideration for direct or indirect monetary wages or profit, and any person who volunteers his or her services for a non-profit entity.

4. "Employer" means any person, partnership, corporation, including a municipal corporation, or non-profit entity, who employs the services of one or more individual persons.

5. "Enclosed Area" means all space between a floor and ceiling which is enclosed on all sides by solid walls or windows (exclusive of door or passage ways) which extend from the floor to the ceiling, including all space therein screened by partitions which do not extend to the ceiling or are not solid, "office landscaping" or similar structures.

6. "Place of Employment" means any enclosed area under the control of a public or private employer which employees normally frequent during the course of employment, including, but not limited to, work areas, employee lounges and restrooms, conference and class rooms, employee cafeterias and hallways. A private residence is not a "place of employment" unless it is used as a child care, adult day care or health care facility.

7. "Public Place" means any enclosed area to which the public is invited or in which the public is permitted, including but not limited to, banks, educational facilities, health facilities, laundromats, public transportation facilities, reception areas, restaurants, retail food production and marketing establishments, retail service establishments, retail stores, theaters and waiting rooms. A private residence is not a "public place."

8. "Restaurant" means any coffee shop, cafeteria, sandwich stand, private and public school cafeteria, and any other eating establishment which gives or offers for sale food to the public, guests, or employees, as well as kitchens in which food is prepared on the premises for serving elsewhere, including catering facilities, except that the term "restaurant" shall not include a cocktail lounge or tavern if said cocktail lounge or tavern is a "bar" as defined in Section 1002 (1).

9. "Retail Tobacco Store" means a retail store utilized primarily for the sale of tobacco products and accessories and in which the sale of other products is merely incidental.

10. "Service Line" means any indoor line at which one (1) or more persons are waiting for or receiving service of any kind, whether or not such service involves the exchange of money.

11. "Smoking" means inhaling, exhaling, burning or carrying any lighted cigar, cigarette, pipe, weed, plant or other combustible substance in any manner or in any form.

12. "Sports Arena" means sports pavilions, gymnasiums, health spas, boxing arenas, swimming pools, roller and ice rinks, bowling alleys and other similar places where members of the general public assemble either to engage in physical exercise, participate in athletic competition, or witness sports events.

Sec. 1003. Application of Article to City-Owned [County-Owned] Facilities

All enclosed facilities owned by the City [County] of _____ shall be subject to the provisions of this article.

Sec. 1004. Prohibition of Smoking in Public Places

A. Smoking shall be prohibited in all enclosed public places within the City [County] of _____, including, but not limited to, the following places:
1. Elevators.
2. Restrooms, lobbies, reception areas, hallways and any other common-use areas.
3. Buses, taxicabs, and other means of public transit under the authority of the City [County] of _____, and ticket, boarding, and waiting areas of public transit depots.
4. Service lines.
5. Retail stores.
6. All areas available to and customarily used by the general public in all businesses and non-profit entities patronized by the public, including but not limited to, attorneys' offices and other offices, banks, laundromats, hotels and motels.
7. Restaurants.
8. Public areas of aquariums, galleries, libraries and museums when open to the public.
9. Any facility which is primarily used for exhibiting any motion picture, stage, drama, lecture, musical recital or other

similar performance, except *perfomers* when smoking is part of a stage production.

10. Sports arenas and convention halls, including bowling facilities.
11. Every room, chamber, place of meeting or public assembly, including school buildings under the control of any board, council, commission, committee, including joint committees, or agencies of the City [County] or any political subdivision of the State during such time as a public meeting is in progress, to the extent such place is subject to the jurisdiction of the City [County].
12. Waiting rooms, hallways, wards and semiprivate rooms of health facilities, including, but not limited to, hospitals, clinics, physical therapy facilities, doctors' offices, and dentists' offices.
13. Lobbies, hallways, and other common areas in apartment buildings, condominiums, trailer parks, retirement facilities, nursing homes, and other multiple-unit residential facilities.
14. Polling places.
15. Bingo games.

B. Notwithstanding any other provision of this section, any owner, operator, manager or other person who controls any establishment or facility may declare that entire establishment or facility as a nonsmoking establishment.

Sec. 1005. Prohibition of Smoking in Places of Employment

A. It shall be the responsibility of employers to provide a smoke-free workplace for all employees, but employers are not required to incur any expense to make structural or other physical modifications.
B. Within 90 days of the effective date of this article, each employer having an enclosed place of employment located within the City [County] shall adopt, implement, make known and maintain a written smoking policy which shall contain the following requirements:

Smoking shall be prohibited in all enclosed facilities within a place of employment without exception. This includes common work areas, auditoriums, classrooms, conference and meeting rooms, private offices, elevators, hallways, medical facilities, cafeterias, employee lounges, stairs, restrooms, vehicles, and all other enclosed facilities.

C. The smoking policy shall be communicated to all employees within three (3) weeks of its adoption.
D. All employers shall supply a written copy of the smoking policy upon request to any existing or prospective employee.

Sec. 1006. Reasonable Distance

Smoking shall occur at a reasonable distance outside any enclosed area where smoking is prohibited to insure that tobacco smoke does not enter the area through entrances, windows, ventilation systems or any other means.

Sec. 1007. Where Smoking Not Regulated

A. Notwithstanding any other provision of this article to the contrary, the following areas shall not be subject to the smoking restrictions of this article:
   1. Bars which meet the requirements of Section 1002 (1) of this article.
   2. Private residences, except when used as a child care, adult day care or health care facility.
   3. Twenty-five percent (25%) of hotel and motel rooms rented to guests.
   4. Retail tobacco stores.
   5. Restaurants, hotel and motel conference or meeting rooms and public and private assembly rooms while these places are being used for private functions.
B. Notwithstanding any other provision of this section, any owner, operator, manager or other person who controls any establishment described in this section may declare that entire establishment as a nonsmoking establishment.

Sec. 1008. Posting of Signs

A. "No Smoking" signs or the international "No Smoking" symbol (consisting of a pictorial representation of a burning cigarette enclosed in a red circle with a red bar across it) shall be clearly, sufficiently and conspicuously posted in every building or other area where smoking is prohibited by this article, by the owner, operator, manager or other person having control of such building or other area.
B. Every public place where smoking is prohibited by this Article shall have posted at every entrance a conspicuous sign clearly stating that smoking is prohibited.

C. All ashtrays and other smoking paraphernalia shall be removed from any area where smoking is prohibited by this article by the owner, operator, manager or other person having control of such area.

Sec. 1009. Enforcement

A. Enforcement of this article shall be implemented by the Department of Health [or City Manager], or his or her designee.

B. Notice of the provisions set forth in this article shall be given to all applicants for a business license in the City [County] of _____.

C. Any citizen who desires to register a complaint under this chapter may initiate enforcement with the Department of Health for City Manager].

D. The Health Department or the Fire Department shall require, while an establishment is undergoing otherwise mandated inspections, a "self-certification" from the owner, manager, operator or other person having control of such establishment that all requirements of this article have been complied with.

E. Any owner, manager, operator or employee of any establishment regulated by this article may inform persons violating this article of the appropriate provisions thereof.

F. Notwithstanding any other provision of this article, a private citizen may bring legal action to enforce this article.

Sec. 1010. Nonretaliation

No person or employer shall discharge, refuse to hire or in any manner retaliate against any employee, applicant for employment, or customer because such employee, applicant, or customer exercises any right to a smokefree environment afforded by this article.

Sec. 1011. Violations and Penalties

A. It shall be unlawful for any person who owns, manages, operates or otherwise controls the use of any premises subject to regulation under this article to fail to comply with any of its provisions.

B. It shall be unlawful for any person to smoke in any area where smoking is prohibited by the provisions of this article.

C. Any person who violates any provision of this article shall be guilty of an infraction, punishable by:

1. A fine not exceeding one hundred dollars ($100) for a first violation.
2. A fine not exceeding two hundred dollars ($200) for a second violation of this article within one (1) year.
3. A fine not exceeding five hundred dollars ($500) for each additional violation of this article within one (1) year.

D. Notwithstanding any other provision of this article, an employee or private citizen may bring legal action to enforce this article.

Sec. 1012. Public Education

The Department of Health [or City Manager] shall engage in a continuing program to explain and clarify the purposes and requirements of this ordinance to citizens affected by it, and to guide owners, operators and managers in their compliance with it. Such program may include publication of a brochure for affected businesses and individuals explaining the provisions of this ordinance.

Sec. 1013. Other Applicable Laws

This article shall not be interpreted or construed to permit smoking where it is otherwise restricted by other applicable laws.

Sec. 1014. Severability

If any provision, clause, sentence or paragraph of this article or the application thereof to any person or circumstances shall be held invalid, such invalidity shall not affect the other provisions of this article which can be given effect without the invalid provision or application, and to this end the provisions of this article are declared to be severable.

Sec. 1015. Effective Date

This article shall be effective thirty (30) days from and after the date of its adoption.

Appendix E

How to Select the Right Vendor for Your Company's Health Promotion Program

The development of interest by employers in health promotion programs for their employees has been paralleled by a growth of vendors interested in selling health promotion services to these employers. A checklist indicating the particular services offered and the methods by which they will be provided and at what costs can help the employer make the decision for the most suitable and efficient service.

There has been a tremendous growth during the past 15 years in the number of corporate employers who have begun offering employee health promotion programs (EHPPs) (1). Many of the early programs were begun because of the intuitive projection that improved employee lifestyle would not only improve the health of the individual employees but also have an impact on the health care programs of the company. However, much of the recent growth has come about because of the relatively recent empirical data indicating that EHPPs can be cost-effective and can have a significant effect on employee health, absenteeism, morale, and productivity. Additionally, the data have indicated that EHPPs may help a company increase its own image and its ability to recruit new personnel and decrease employee turnover (2–9).

With the growth of EHPPs in the business community there has come a parallel growth in the number of organizations (vendors) who are inter-ested in selling health promotion services (products) to the companies. It is not uncommon to find hospitals, health clubs, YMCAs/YWCAs, voluntary health agencies (i.e., American Lung Association, American Red Cross, etc.), health departments, other community organizations, and for-profit health promotion companies trying to market their services. Just as with any service, some of what these vendors are marketing is good, while some is not. Unless your company employs trained health promotion professionals who can identify the difference in these services, a good salesperson can make the poor services appear comparable to, if not better than, the good ones. Because of the newness of the EHPPs, there are few guidelines (10) to help companies select appropriate vendors. Thus, in order to help those companies who do not employ trained health promotion professionals and those who have hired one with limited experience, a checklist for evaluating health promotion vendors has been developed.

The Instrument

The checklist comprises 50 yes–no type questions. It includes several questions that are "common sense" or basic "good business" questions. However, it has been our experience that unless a company specifically asks the questions of the vendor, the vendor

Source: J. H. Harris, J. F. McKenzie, and W. B. Zuti, "How to Select the Right Vendor for Your Company's Health Promotion Program," by 1986, *Fitness in Business,* 1 (October 1986), pp. 53–56. Reprinted by permission.

may not provide information, and thus a company must make a decision to buy or not to buy based upon insufficient and/or perhaps inaccurate data.

The checklist is divided into six sections. The first section deals with the initial meeting with the vendor. Basically, this portion of the checklist presents questions which ask: "How well prepared was the vendor for the meeting?"

The second and third portions of the checklist pose questions that ask about the quality of the service being marketed. These include questions such as: "How effective is it?" "How does it compare to services being marketed by other vendors?" and "What are the qualifications of those who will actually provide the service?"

Section four of the checklist presents a series of questions that examine how the vendor will deliver and service the product. You want to work with a vendor who will provide excellent service when the agreement has been signed. The fifth section of the checklist provides questions that can be used in determining an appropriate cost for the product. The last portion of the checklist includes several general questions that deal with image, contracts, and legal concerns.

It should be noted that the checklist has been standardized and there is no set score that will assure that a vendor will be a good supplier of health promotion services. When using the checklist, those responsible for EHPPs should be very skeptical of those vendors who have a large number of checks in the "no" column of the instrument. At the same time, it will probably be difficult to find a vendor that will receive all "yes" responses. Although final decisions are usually made on a subjective basis, one should feel more confident when using the services of a vendor with a large number of "yes" responses. And finally, it should be pointed out that some areas of the country are better supplied with vendors than others, and thus all ratings would be relative to the geographic locations.

References

1. Fielding JE, Breslow L. Health promotion programs sponsored by California employees. *Am J Public Health* 73:538–542, 1983.
2. Erfurt JC, Foote A. Cost-effectiveness of worksite blood pressure control programs. *J Occup Med* 26:892–900, 1984.
3. Fielding JE. Effectiveness of employee health improvement programs. *J Occup Med* 24:907–916, 1982.
4. Fielding JE. Health promotion and disease prevention at the worksite. *Annu Rev Public Health* xx:237–265, 1984.
5. Gibbs JO, Mulvaney D, Henes C, Reed RW. Work-site health promotion: five-year trend in employee health care costs. *J Occup Med* 27:826–830, 1985.
6. Kristein MM. The economics of health promotion at the worksite. *Health Educ Q* 9 (special suppl):27–36, 1982.
7. Rogers PJ, Eaton EK, Bruhn JG. Is health promotion cost effective? *Prev Med* 10:324–339, 1981.
8. Schwartz RM, Rollins PL. Measuring the cost benefit of wellness strategies. *Business Health* 2(10):24–26, 1985.
9. Stason WG. Measuring the "payoff" of worksite health strategies. *Business Health* 1(4):19–22, 1984.
10. Zuti WB. Weighting–and minimizing–the risks of joint venturing. *Promoting Health* January–February, 4–5, 1986.
11. Kelly KE. Building a successful health promotion program. *Business Health* 3(March):44–45, 1986.
12. Opatz JP. *A Primer of Health Promotion: Creating Healthy Organizational Cultures.* Oryn Publications, Inc., Washington, DC, 1985.
13. Kelly KE. Separate yourself from the crowd. *Optimal Health* 2(March/April):30–32, 34, 1986.

Checklist for Selecting Health Promotion Vendors

Code: Yes—Yes, the vendor does/did this.   **NA**—Not applicable
No—No, the vendor does not/did not do this.   **NS**—Not sure

	Yes	No	NA/NS	Comments
1. Initial experience with vendor				
A. Did the vendor present a good professional image?				
B. Did the vendor do his/her homework on your company prior to the initial meeting?				
C. Is the vendor's philosophy of health promotion consistent with your company's philosophy (11)?				
D. Can the vendor explain why his/her product is appropriate for your company?				
E. Did the vendor appear responsive to your company's needs?				
F. Did the vendor explain how his/her product can meet the needs of your company (11)?				
G. Was the vendor willing to listen to you or was he/she too busy trying to sell his/her product?				
H. Is the vendor willing to make a presentation to your company's management?				
I. Did the vendor demonstrate his/her organization's expertise with regard to the product?				
J. Did the vendor provide you with a reference list of other customers (12)?				
K. Did the vendor leave written materials that summarize his/her product?				
2. Product quality				
A. Did the vendor provide an overview of the product content?				
B. Can the vendor provide careful documentation of product effectiveness?				
C. Does the vendor have evaluative data to back up the product?				
D. Does the vendor have data to compare success rates of the product to those of his/her competitors?				
E. Can the vendor provide data which show the adequacy of his/her products with a population similar to yours (12)?				
F. Can the vendor provide several different products (health promotion activities), or does he/she just specialize in one area?				

Continued

Checklist for Selecting Health Promotion Vendors

Code:	Yes—Yes, the vendor does/did this.			NA—Not applicable
	No—No, the vendor does not/did not do this.			NS—Not sure

	Yes	No	NA/NS	Comments
2. Product quality (continued)				
G. Did the vendor explain the types of interventions (behavior modification, aversive techniques, etc.) that are used with the product?				
H. Will the vendor "customize" the product to meet the needs of your company?				
I. Can the vendor offer a variety of interventions (i.e., different approaches to smoking cessation) from which you can choose to best meet the needs of your employees (13)?				
J. Can the vendor offer a product which can meet special needs of your employees (e.g., reading levels, various levels of health status, etc.) (13)?				
K. When appropriate, does the vendor provide written instructional materials to accompany the product?				
L. If written informational materials are provided, are they written clearly and presented in an attractive way?				
3. Individuals who provide the service				
A. What type of education and training do the staff and/or instructors have?				
B. Are the instructors certified by a professional and/or health organization?				
C. Are the instructors required to update their training periodically?				
D. Are the instructor-to-participant ratios reasonable?				
4. Product delivery and service				
A. Can the vendor put in writing the actual services that will be provided?				
B. If a written presentation of services is made, does it spell out the responsibilities of both parties?				
C. Is the vendor willing to market the product inside your company?				
D. Does purchase of the product include an evaluation?				
E. Can the vendor appropriately serve the size of your company's population?				

(continued)

Continued

Checklist for Selecting Health Promotion Vendors

Code: Yes—Yes, the vendor does/did this.   **NA**—Not applicable
         No—No, the vendor does not/did not do this.   **NS**—Not sure

	Yes	No	NA/NS	Comments
4. Product delivery and service (continued)				
F. Can the vendor provide the product at all sites desired?				
G. Can the vendor provide the product at the time desired?				
H. Are the length of the product sessions appropriate for your work day?				
I. Does the vendor provide you with the name of one of their employees who can act as a troubleshooter?				
J. Can the vendor also provide other products/services to other departments (units) (i.e., the safety division, health policy, etc.) in your company?				
K. Has the vendor been in business for at least five years (10)?				
L. Is the vendor's company well managed and financially sound (10)?				
M. Does the vendor enjoy a good repuation in the community (10)?				
5. Product cost				
A. Is the cost of the product competitive with the cost of other vendors?				
B. Does the vendor provide written bids for the product?				
C. Does the cost per unit go down when the number of participants increases?				
D. Does the cost per unit go down if additional products are purchased from the same vendor?				
E. Does the vendor offer corporate discounts?				
6. General concerns				
A. Does the vendor carry adequate liability insurance?				
B. Does the vendor put in writing a "statement of reasonable expectations" for the product (13)?				
C. Is the vendor willing to sign a contract?				
D. If you buy the product of this vendor, will it improve the image of your company in the community?				
E. If you buy the product of this vendor, will it improve the image of your company with the employees?				

Appendix F

Organizations/Agencies Offering Health Promotion Materials

Name	Address	Website	Topic
Alzheimer's Association	919 N. Michigan Ave. Suite 1000 Chicago, IL 60611-1676		Alzheimer's disease; aging
American Association of Retired Persons (AARP)	601 E. St., NW Washington, DC 20049	http://www.aarp.org/	Aging
American Cancer Society	Contact local affiliate	http://www.cancer.org/	Cancer; nutrition; smoking; smokeless tobacco; smoking cessation
American Diabetes Association	Contact local affiliate	http://www.diabetes.org/	Diabetes
American Dietetic Association	216 W. Jackson Blvd. Chicago, IL 60606-6995	http://www.eatright.org/	Nutrition
American Heart Association	Contact local affiliate	http://www.americanheart.org/	Cardiovascular disease; CPR; nutrition; food certification program; smoking; worksite wellness programs
American Hospital Association	One North Franklin Chicago, IL 60606	http://www.aha.org/	Variety of health areas
American Lung Association	Contact local affiliate	http://www.lungusa.org/	Lung diseases; smoking; smoking cessation

Continued

Name	Address	Website	Topic
American Red Cross	Contact local affiliate	http://www.redcross.org/	CPR; blood pressure; first aid; nutrition; safety; stress management; workplace HIV/AIDS education
CDC National Prevention Information Network	P.O. Box 6003 Rockville, MD 20849-6003	http://www.cdcnpin.org/	HIV/STD/TB prevention
Centers for Disease Control and Prevention	1600 Clifton Rd., NE Atlanta, GA 30333	http://www.cdc.gov/	Variety of health areas
Consumer Information Center	Pueblo, CO 81009		Variety of health areas
Health departments— local and state	Check local telephone directory		Variety of health areas
Johnson and Johnson	One Johnson & Johnson Plaza New Brunswick, NJ 08933	http://www.johnsonandjohnson.com/	SAFE KIDS campaign; general health promotion
Local colleges and universities	Check local telephone directory		Variety of health areas
Local public library	Check local telephone directory		Variety of health areas
March of Dimes	Contact local affiliate		Birth defects; pregnancy; worksite wellness
Metropolitan Life Insurance Company	One Madison Ave. New York, NY 10010	http://www.metlife.com	Health information
Mothers Against Drunk Driving	P.O. Box 541688 Dallas, TX 75345	http://www.madd.org/	Alcohol and driving
National Cancer Institute	Bldg. 31, Room 10A03 31 Center Dr. Bethesda, MD 20852	http://www.nci.nih.gov/	Cancer
National Center for Chronic Disease Prevention and Health Promotion	1600 Clifton Rd., NE Atlanta, GA 30333	http://www.cdc.gov/nccdphp/	Variety of health areas
National Dairy Council	Contact local affiliate	http://www.nationaldairycouncil.org/	Nutrition

Continued

Name	Address	Website	Topic
National Health Information Center	P.O. Box 1133 Washington, DC 20013-1133	http://www.nhic-nt. health.org/	Referral to health information
National Heart, Lung, and Blood Institute	Bethesda, MD 20892	http://www.nhlbi. nih.gov/	Cholesterol; heart/lung disease; high blood pressure; smoking
National Institute for Occupational Safety and Health	Hubert Humphrey Bldg. 200 Independence Ave., SW Room 715H Washington, DC 20201	http://www.cdc.gov. niosh/	Occupational safety and health
National Institutes of Health	Bethesda, MD 20892	http://www.nih.gov/	Consumer health; health information
National Kidney Foundation	Contact local affiliate	http://www.kidney. org/	Kidney disease; blood pressure control
National Rural Health Resource Center	600 E. Superior St. Suite 404 Duluth, MN 55802	http://www. ruralcenter.org/nrhrc/	Variety of rural health topics
National Safety Council	1121 Spring Lake Dr. Itasca, IL 60143-3201	http://www.nsc.org/	Safety; first aid
National Wellness Institute, Inc.	P.O. Box 827 Stevens Point, WI 54481	http://www. nationalwellness.org/	Variety of health areas
Office on Smoking and Health	Mail Stop K-50 Centers for Disease Control and Prevention 4770 Buford Highway, NE Atlanta, GA 30341-3724	http://www.cdc.gov/ nccdphp/divosh.htm	Smoking cessation
Planned Parenthood Federation of America	Contact local affiliate	http://www. plannedparenthood. org/	Contraception; pregnancy; STDs
U.S. Consumer Product Safety Commission	Washington, DC 20207	http://www.cpsc.gov/	Safety
U.S. Dept. of Agriculture (USDA)/ Cooperative Extension Service	Contact county extension office or state land-grant university	http://www.nal.usda. gov/fnic/	Nutrition

(continued)

Continued

Name	Address	Website	Topic
U.S. Dept. of Transportation—National Traffic and Highway Safety Administration	400 7th St., SW Washington, DC 20590	http://www.nhtsa.dot.gov/	Occupant safety; child safety seats; drunk driving prevention; injury prevention
United Way	Contact local affiliate	http://www.unitedway.org/	Variety of health areas
Wellness Councils of America	9802 Nicholas St. Suite 315 Omaha, NE 68114	http://www.welcoa.org/	Worksite wellness
YMCAs and YWCAs	Contact local YMCA or YWCA	http://www.ymca.com/	Exercise; safety; programs for children

Appendix G

Health Behavior Contract

Being of sound mind and in need of health behavior change, I (insert name of person wanting to make the change) do hereby commit myself to the following health behavior change for the next eight weeks. This contract with (insert the name of the other person who is entering into this contract) shall be in effect from (insert starting date) to (insert ending date). For completing this contract, I will be rewarded/reinforced with (insert reward or reinforcer). This reward/reinforcer will be received when I (insert desired behavior). If I do not successfully fulfill this contract, I will (insert what will happen if person is not successful).

A. The behavior I plan to change is:

_____

_____

B. The reason I want to change this behavior is because:

_____

_____

C. I have set the following objectives for myself (Reminder: objectives must be measurable so that you will know if you have reached them. For example, choose practicing relaxation techniques once a day, 5 times per week as an objective rather than indicating stress reduction as a goal.

1. _____

2. _____

3. _____

D. To meet these goals, I will (provide a description of your daily/weekly activity):

_____

_____

(continued)

Continued

E. To carry out my plan, I am going to solicit the help of (names of friends, family, room-mate, or significant others and how they will help):

_____

_____

F. I expect to receive the following benefits from this activity:

_____

_____

Your signature: _____   Date: _____

Facilitator's signature: _____   Date: _____

Appendix H

Example of an Informed Consent Form for a Cholesterol Screening Program

I hereby grant permission to the Institute for Health Promotion personnel to perform a cholesterol screening on me. I am engaging in this screening voluntarily. I have been told that this screening is an analysis of total blood cholesterol and that my blood will be taken from a fingerstick blood sample by a trained employee. I understand that the results of this screening are considered to be preliminary in nature and in no way conclusive. Results of a blood cholesterol screening like this can be affected by a number of factors including, but not limited to, smoking, stress level, amount of exercise, hormone levels, foods eaten, heredity, and pregnancy. I also understand that my physician can perform a more complete blood lipid (fat) analysis for me, if I so desire.

Further, I have been told that all information related to this screening is considered confidential.

I have read the above statement and understand what it means. I have also had an opportunity to ask questions about the screening, and all my questions have been answered to my satisfaction.

Participant's Signature	Date	Signature of Witness

To ensure it meets with all related local and state laws, this form, or any others like it, should be submitted to legal counsel before use.

Appendix I

Sample Medical Clearance Form

I hereby certify that (name of participant) has been examined and cleared by me to participate, with the noted restrictions, in the programs indicated below. This person should not be placed into any of the other programs until he/she has been cleared by me to do so.

❏ Vigorous exercise programs. This type of program would include all-out effort for the development of cardiovascular endurance, muscular strength, and flexibility.

Physician's comments: _____

_____

_____

❏ Moderate exercise program. This type of program is for those participants who would be unable to participate in the vigorous exercise program because of physical limitations. These programs should be modified as per my instructions.

Physician's comments: _____

_____

_____

❏ Mild exercise program. This type of program is for those participants who would be unable to participate in the moderate exercise program because of physical limitations. These programs should be modified as per my instructions.

Physician's comments: _____

_____

_____

_____

_____   _____
Physician's signature   Date

Appendix J

Code of Ethics for the Health Education Profession

Unabridged Version

Preamble

The Health Education profession is dedicated to excellence in the practice of promoting individual, family, organizational, and community health. Guided by common ideals, Health Educators are responsible for upholding the integrity and ethics of the profession as they face the daily challenges of making decisions. By acknowledging the value of diversity in society and embracing a cross-cultural approach, Health Educators support the worth, dignity, potential, and uniqueness of all people.

The Code of Ethics provides a framework of shared values within which Health Education is practiced. The Code of Ethics is grounded in fundamental ethical principles that underlie all health care services: respect for autonomy, promotion of social justice, active promotion of good, and avoidance of harm. The responsibility of each health educator is to aspire to the highest possible standards of conduct and to encourage the ethical behavior of all those with whom they work.

Regardless of job title, professional affiliation, work setting, or population served, Health Educators abide by these guidelines when making professional decisions.

Article I: Responsibility to the Public

A Health Educator's ultimate responsibility is to educate people for the purpose of promoting, maintaining, and improving individual, family, and community health. When a conflict of issues arises among individuals, groups, organizations, agencies, or institutions, health educators must consider all issues and give priority to those that promote wellness and quality of living through principles of self-determination and freedom of choice for the individual.

Section 1. Health Educators support the right of individuals to make informed decisions regarding health, as long as such decisions pose no threat to the health of others.

Section 2. Health Educators encourage actions and social policies that support and facilitate the best balance of benefits over harm for all affected parties.

Section 3. Health Educators accurately communicate the potential benefits and consequences of the services and programs with which they are associated.

Section 4. Health Educators accept the responsibility to act on issues that can adversely affect the health of individuals, families, and communities.

Section 5. Health Educators are truthful about their qualifications and the limitations of their expertise and provide services consistent with their competencies.

Section 6. Health Educators protect the privacy and dignity of individuals.

Section 7. Health Educators actively involve individuals, groups, and communities in the entire

Source: The Coalition of National Health Education Organizations, Ethics Task Force, November 9, 1999 <www.med.usf.ed/~kmbrown/CNHEO.htm>. Reprinted by permission.

educational process so that all aspects of the process are clearly understood by those who may be affected.

Section 8. Health Educators respect and acknowledge the rights of others to hold diverse values, attitudes, and opinions.

Section 9. Health Educators provide services equitably to all people.

Article II: Responsibility to the Profession

Health Educators are responsible for their professional behavior, for the reputation of their profession, and for promoting ethical conduct among their colleagues.

Section 1. Health Educators maintain, improve, and expand their professional competence through continued study and education; membership, participation, and leadership in professional organizations; and involvement in issues related to the health of the public.

Section 2. Health Educators model and encourage nondiscriminatory standards of behavior in their interactions with others.

Section 3. Health Educators encourage and accept responsible critical discourse to protect and enhance the profession.

Section 4. Health Educators contribute to the development of the profession by sharing the processes and outcomes of their work.

Section 5. Health Educators are aware of possible professional conflicts of interest, exercise integrity in conflict situations, and do not manipulate or violate the rights of others.

Section 6. Health Educators give appropriate recognition to others for their professional contributions and achievements

Article III: Responsibility to Employers

Health Educators recognize the boundaries of their professional competence and are accountable for their professional activities and actions.

Section 1. Health Educators accurately represent their qualifications and the qualifications of others whom they recommend.

Section 2. Health Educators use appropriate standards, theories, and guidelines as criteria when carrying out their professional responsibilities.

Section 3. Health Educators accurately represent potential service and program outcomes to employers.

Section 4. Health Educators anticipate and disclose competing commitments, conflicts of interest, and endorsement of products.

Section 5. Health Educators openly communicate to employers, expectations of job-related assignments that conflict with their professional ethics.

Section 6. Health Educators maintain competence in their areas of professional practice.

Article IV: Responsibility in the Delivery of Health Education

Health Educators promote integrity in the delivery of health education. They respect the rights, dignity, confidentiality, and worth of all people by adapting strategies and methods to meet the needs of diverse populations and communities.

Section 1. Health Educators are sensitive to social and cultural diversity and are in accord with the law, when planning and implementing programs.

Section 2. Health Educators are informed of the latest advances in theory, research, and practice, and use strategies and methods that are grounded in and contribute to development of professional standards, theories, guidelines, statistics, and experience.

Section 3. Health Educators are committed to rigorous evaluation of both program effectiveness and the methods used to achieve results.

Section 4. Health Educators empower individuals to adopt healthy lifestyles through informed choice rather than by coercion or intimidation.

Section 5. Health Educators communicate the potential outcomes of proposed services, strategies, and pending decisions to all individuals who will be affected.

Article V: Responsibility in Research and Evaluation

Health Educators contribute to the health of the population and to the profession through research and evaluation activities. When planning and conducting research or evaluation, health educators do so in accordance with federal and state laws and regulations, organizational and institutional policies, and professional standards.

Section 1. Health Educators support principles and practices of research and evaluation that do no harm to individuals, groups, society, or the environment.

Section 2. Health Educators ensure that participation in research is voluntary and is based upon the informed consent of the participants.

Section 3. Health Educators respect the privacy, rights, and dignity of research participants, and honor commitments made to those participants.

Section 4. Health Educators treat all information obtained from participants as confidential unless otherwise required by law.

Section 5. Health Educators take credit, including authorship, only for work they have actually performed and give credit to the contributions of others.

Section 6. Health Educators who serve as research or evaluation consultants discuss their results only with those to whom they are providing service, unless maintaining such confidentiality would jeopardize the health or safety of others.

Section 7. Health Educators report the results of their research and evaluation objectively, accurately, and in a timely fashion.

Article VI: Responsibility in Professional Preparation

Those involved in the preparation and training of Health Educators have an obligation to accord learners the same respect and treatment given other groups by providing quality education that benefits the profession and the public.

Section 1. Health Educators select students for professional preparation programs based upon equal opportunity for all, and the individual's academic performance, abilities, and potential contribution to the profession and the public's health.

Section 2. Health Educators strive to make the educational environment and culture conducive to the health of all involved, and free from sexual harassment and all forms of discrimination.

Section 3. Health Educators involved in professional preparation and professional development engage in careful preparation; present material that is accurate, up-to-date, and timely; provide reasonable and timely feedback; state clear and reasonable expectations; and conduct fair assessments and evaluations of learners.

Section 4. Health Educators provide objective and accurate counseling to learners about career opportunities, development, and advancement, and assist learners to secure professional employment.

Section 5. Health Educators provide adequate supervision and meaningful opportunities for the professional development of learners.

Abridged Version

Preamble

The Health Education profession is dedicated to excellence in the practice of promoting individual, family, organizational, and community health. The Code of Ethics provides a framework of shared values within which Health Education is practiced. The responsibility of each Health Educator is to aspire to the highest possible standards of conduct and to encourage the ethical behavior of all those with whom they work.

Article I: Responsibility to the Public

A Health Educator's ultimate responsibility is to educate people for the purpose of promoting, maintaining, and improving individual, family, and community health. When a conflict of issues arises among individuals, groups, organizations, agencies, or institutions, health educators must consider all issues and give priority to those that promote wellness and quality of living through principles of self-determination and freedom of choice for the individual.

Article II: Responsibility to the Profession

Health Educators are responsible for their professional behavior, for the reputation of their profession, and for promoting ethical conduct among their colleagues.

Article III: Responsibility to Employers

Health Educators recognize the boundaries of their professional competence and are accountable for their professional activities and actions.

Article IV: Responsibility in the Delivery of Health Education

Health Educators promote integrity in the delivery of health education. They respect the rights, dignity, confidentiality, and worth of all people by adapting strategies and methods to meet the needs of diverse populations and communities.

Article V: Responsibility in Research and Evaluation

Health Educators contribute to the health of the population and to the profession through research and evaluation activities. When planning and conducting research or evaluation, health educators do so in accordance with federal and state laws and regulations, organizational and institutional policies, and professional standards.

Article VI: Responsibility in Professional Preparation

Those involved in the preparation and training of Health Educators have an obligation to accord learners the same respect and treatment given other groups by providing quality education that benefits the profession and the public.

Appendix K

Cost-Benefit and Cost-Effectiveness as a Part of the Evaluation of Health Promotion Programs

Abstract

Economic evaluation should be a component of program evaluation. To encourage and help with this process, definitions of common economic terms, a review of the literature, steps for conducting an economic evaluation, and the use of economic evaluation, with health promotion program is presented.

Introduction

The idea of promoting good health practices is not new in the United States. However, it is only in recent years that the concept of health promotion has grown in popularity and that the number of health promotion programs has flourished. The growth has occurred because of the "...increasing evidence of an association between patterns of lifestyle and health status of individuals and population groups, and associations between environmental and workplace hazards and the health and well-being of communities and workers" (Work Group on Health Promotion/Disease Prevention, 1987).

Though the number of health promotion programs continues to increase, the evaluation of said programs lags behind. There are several reasons for this. First, many of the first generation health promotion programs were developed without regard to an appropriate plan of evaluation. Thus data were not and could not be collected. Second, the very nature of health promotion programs, that of being "in the field" and being geared toward the long-term outcome of "impovered health," makes them difficult to evaluate. Concerns such as evaluation expertise, confidentiality of participants, and resources of time, money, and personnel have proven to be stumbling blocks in collecting the needed data.

If health promotion programs are to prosper and grow, empirical evidence of their worth should be provided. This can be done only through appropriate evaluation of the programs; evaluation that pays considerable attention to problems of design and measurement, and that can be reproducible. Green (1979) stated that "Evaluation of a health promotion plan certifies its appropriateness and its effectiveness and ensures that the practitioner is accountable to the patient (consumer), the community, and the hospital administrator." Though Green's comments were directed toward hospital health promotion programs these same ideas can be transferred to any health promotion setting because

Source: J. F. McKenzie "Cost-Benefit and Cost-Effectiveness as a Part of the Evaluation of Health Promotion Programs," *The Eta Sigma Gamman,* 18(2) (1986): 10–16. Reprinted by permission from *Journal of Eta Sigma Gamma The Health Educator,* formerly *The Eta Sigma Gamman.*

all program planners need to be accountable to the consumer (Work Group on Health Promotion/Disease Prevention, 1987).

The question now is not whether or not health promotion programs should be evaluated but how should it be done? Green (1979) has defined three different levels of evaluation—process, impact, and outcome. Process evaluation deals with the professional practice of those presenting the health promotion program. Impact evaluation is concerned with the immediate difference that the health promotion program has on the knowledge, attitude, behavior, and environment. Outcome evaluation focuses on long-term concerns such as morbidity, morality, and years of survival following the health promotion program. There are many strategies for evaluating health promotion programs within each of these levels, and they have been thoroughly covered in the works of Windsor, Baranowski, Clark, and Cutter (1984) and Green and Lewis (1986). However, there is one evaluation strategy that these authors have addressed that merits further discussion because of the importance being placed on it in today's practice: the economic evaluation of health promotion programs. In the business world the economic evaluation of a program is often referred to as the "bottom line."

In writing about corporate health promotion programs, Fielding (1982, p. 85) has stated:

> Although current evidence suggests a very favorable return on investment for disease prevention and health promotion programs, much more information is needed to quantify costs and benefits and to suggest which models work best in different corporate settings. Therefore, it is imperative that all efforts include long-term evaluation of effects of programs on both direct and indirect costs.

The remaining portion of this paper will focus on the economic evaluation of health promotion programs. This refers to the cost-benefit and cost-effectiveness analysis (CBA and CEA, respectively) of the programs.

Definitions of CBA and CEA

Simply stated, CBA and CEA are formal analytical techniques used for comparing the negative and positive consequences of alternative uses of resources. They are not formulas for making decisions, but rather they are tools to help individuals make decisions (Warner & Luce, 1982). More specif-

ically, Green and Lewis (1986, p. 361) have defined cost-benefit as "a measure of the cost of an intervention relative to the benefits it yields, usually expressed as a ratio of dollars saved or gained for every dollar spent on the program," and cost-effectiveness as "a measure of the cost of an intervention relative to its impact, usually expressed in dollars per unit of effect." Common CEA measures may include years of life saved, days of morbidity and disability avoided, number of smokers who quit, and number of pounds lost.

When first reading these definitions, they appear to be very much alike. The basic technical distinction between CBA and CEA lies in the process of valuing the desirable consequences of health promotion programs (Warner & Luce, 1982). CBA requires that all desirable consequences be expressed in monetary (dollar) terms. For many of the consequences this is a manageable task, but there are some desirable consequences that researchers have found most difficult to quantify in dollars—the value of human life may be the most notable. Several researchers (Rice, 1966; Cooper and Rice, 1976; Acton, 1976) have offered means of dealing with the problem.

More recently the difference between CBA and CEA seems to be fading. Warner and Luce have pointed out that as they have reviewed the literature on CBA and CEA, the two techniques are becoming more alike in the way analysts are applying the concepts. They have indicated that "recent sophisticated health care CEAs are incorporating some dollar-valued benefits into the cost side of the equation (as negative costs), and increasing recognition of the meaning of CBA in health care is bringing it closer to CEA. The human capital approach to measuring indirect benefits in CBA values livelihood, not life itself; thus a CBA is really a net dollar benefit for some nonmonetized health outcomes. The newer more sophisticated CEA seems to be a significant step forward in that it combines the best of both CBA and CEA" (Warner & Luce, 1982, p. 213).

The Popularity of CBA and CEA

The evaluation techniques of CEA and CBA are by no means new concepts, for they can be traced back hundreds of years. However, there has been a tremendous growth in their use and interest in the health professions in the past fifteen years. Much of this growth has paralleled the increase of health care costs during the same period of time. Many feel that this burgeoning interest of CEA and CBA in the health professions has resulted from health professionals seeking to identify and convey the meaning of cost-beneficial and cost-effective health care interventions. It is now quite common to find CBA and CEA citations on most all health care topics.

Review of Literature

As Warner and Hutton (1980) have pointed out, the contributions to the health care CBA and CEA literature have grown exponentially in recent years. Over the years the majority of the literature has dealt with medical interventions. Since this paper is focused on nonmedical interventions—health promotion activities—the medical intervention CBA and CEA literature is not reviewed here. However, it is well presented in Warner and Luce (1982).

The references to the nonmedical CBA and CEA literature are much more limited. The nonmedical literature falls into three major areas—public health measures (i.e., water fluoridation, food inspection, etc.), identification of health risks via screenings (for hypertension, cancer and other diseases), and personal health lifestyle (i.e., exercise, smoking, nutrition, stress, etc.). Public health measures have generally not been considered a part of health promotion activities. And even though screenings have been a portion of a number of health promotion programs, it is the category of personal health lifestyle on which most health promotion programs are planned. It is this literature that is reviewed below.

A number of reviews of the CBA and CEA of health promotion type activities have been found in the literature (Fielding, 1982; Rogers, Eaton, & Bruhn, 1981; Scheffler & Paringer, 1980; and Warner, 1979). These reviews report on basically two types of studies. One group includes studies that have calculated a CBA or CEA on a specific health problem in terms of what the costs and benefits would be for the entire United States if a health promotion program were implemented. One such paper is presented by Kristein (1977). In his paper, Kristein examines several different health concerns such as hypertension, cancer of the colon, heavy cigarette smoking, alcohol abuse, and breast cancer. A summary of his heavy cigarette smoking calculations provides a good example of this approach. He calculated that the costs of heavy cigarette smoking were approximately $20.3 billion (in 1975 dollars). This includes the cost of hospital care, medical care, absenteeism, and premature deaths. If a smoking cessation program were implemented for the 22 million heavy smokers in the United States (a 1975 estimate) at $125 per person and there was a 25% success rate, Kristein estimated a cost-benefit ratio of 1.8 to 1.0. This means that for every dollar put into such a program a $1.80 could be saved. This type of CBA is useful in showing that smoking cessation programs can provide financial benefits, but the exactness of the figures must be put into perspective because of the lack of detail in the analysis.

The other major group of studies that appear in the reviews are those which report on the results of a CBA or CEA calculated on a specific health promotion activity offered by a specific organization. For example, Fielding (1982) has reviewed the results of a number of employee health promotion programs. His findings show that a number of different techniques have been used to calculate CBAs and CEAs, that calculations are based on a number of assumptions and thus the results are difficult to compare. In another paper, Fielding (1984) offers the following example:

> Campbell's analysis of the savings attributable to their colorectal cancer screening programs hinges on assumptions regarding the number of cases of colorectal cancer that would have occurred in the absence of screening, and the direct and indirect costs associated with each case. It also assumes that all cases prevented were due to on-site screening rather than screening that occurred in another setting (e.g., doctor's office or HMO) at the encouragement of an outside health professional. While these estimates of savings due to health promotion measures are useful in showing the value companies themselves have placed in the savings, it is difficult to know if their assertions can be applied to other companies. (p. 259)

Further indication of the inconsistency in the way CBA and CEA for health promotion activities have been calculated was noted by Rogers et al. (1981, p. 333)—"…carefully designed cost analyses have not been conducted so that various approaches can be compared as to the expense, as well as to short-term impact and long-term outcome." There is clearly a need for authors to describe in detail all the steps they follow in calculating their CBA or CEA so that other evaluators can use the same steps and thus be able to compare results.

The health promotion literature includes more reports of CBAs and CEAs on identification of health risks than in personal health lifestyle change, with the more reports dealing with hypertension screening programs than any other (Alderman, Madhavan, & Davis, 1983; Erfurt & Foote, 1984; Foote & Erfurt, 1977; Ruchlin & Alderman, 1980; and Ruchlin,

Melcher, & Alderman, 1984). Only two recent reports on personal health lifestyle change could be found. One dealt with weight loss (Seidman, Sevelius, & Ewald, 1984) and the other with smoking cessation (Weiss, Jurs, Lesage, & Iverson, 1984). Scheffler and Paringer (1980) have pointed out the need for empirical evidence of the economic soundness of other lifestyle change programs such as physical exercise and dietary changes.

Finally, there are many more reports using CEA than CBA in the health promotion literature. Only two reports of CBA (Alderman et al., 1983; and Weiss et al., 1984) could be found. All others were CEAs. The reasons for this will become clear from subsequent discussion.

Calculating CBAs and CEAs

As suggested in preceding portions of this paper, the calculation of CBAs and CEAs for health promotion activities is no easy task. In most cases they will be difficult and in some cases impossible to calculate. However, if evaluations of health promotion activities are going to be complete, they should be attempted.

Though there are certain processes that must be included in calculating CBAs and CEAs, the exact steps one could use may vary. The important point to remember is that whatever steps are used, they should be reported accurately and in detail so others can replicate and compare results. The steps presented below are a combination of techniques suggested by a governmental agency and several different individuals (OTA, 1978; OTA, 1980; Rogers et al., 1981; Shepard & Thompson, 1979; and Warner & Luce, 1982).

Step 1: Defining the Problem.   The initial step in calculating a CBA or CEA is defining the problem to be analyzed. The problem should be stated as clearly and explicitly as possible. Seemingly small differences in the definition of the problem could have a large impact on the calculated costs, benefits and effects. The statement of the problem should also clearly specify for whom the analysis is going to be calculated. For example, a cost-analysis of a health promotion program would differ greatly if it were being calculated from the employer's point of view as opposed to the costs, benefits, and effects experienced by the employee.

Commonly defined problems for which health promotion programs are usually designed deal with either a specific health concern or an economic issue. An example of a problem that deals with a health concern might be to reduce the risk of cardiovascular disease in white collar employees, while a problem revolving around an economic issue may be to reduce the amount of money the company spends on health insurance claims per year. Both of these problems would be appropriate for calculating a CBA or CEA; however, for the purposes of this paper, the cardiovascular disease problem will be used as an example through the remaining steps in the process.

Step 2: Specifying the Objectives.   Closely related to defining the problem is setting one or more objectives against which programmatic alternatives are to be evaluated. If the defined problem is not readily measurable, further specification may help qualify it. For example, the problem of reducing cardiovascular disease in white collar employees is too broad to be readily quantified.

A possible specification of an appropriate objective would be to reduce the risk of cardiovascular disease in this employee group by getting 50% of the high-risk employees in an appropriate exercise program. It is known that the high-risk group includes individuals who have hypertension and are overweight. These individuals cost a company more money in medical care, accidents, etc. than individuals without them. Exercise has been shown to help both of these health concerns.

Step 3: Identifying Alternatives.   To determine if a specific approach to a problem is cost-effective or cost-beneficial, it needs to be compared to other approaches that could also be used to achieve the stated objectives. Again using the problem of cardiovascular disease as an example, an alternative approach may be to reduce disease via a nutrition and weight control program as opposed to the exercise program.

When identifying alternatives for health promotion programs, it should be noted that the alternatives do not need to attack the problem using similar approaches. For example, if the problem is to reduce health costs due to cigarette smoking within an organization, one cost analysis may be completed on an educational smoking cessation approach. Another analysis of costs could be calculated on the alternative which mandates, via a company policy, that there be no smoking in the workplace.

It is helpful to keep the following concerns in mind when identifying appropriate alternatives: (1) select only alternatives that are believed to be potentially quite cost-effective, (2) select alternatives that offer variety in their approach, and (3) select alternatives that would be appropriate for comparison—do not select an alternative that is obviously an inappropriate approach for solving the problem (i.e., getting *every* employee to adopt a specific exercise program).

Step 4: Describing Production Relationships. The first three steps of this process set the conceptual framework for calculating a CBA or CEA. When one describes the production relationships, he/she is creating the technical framework for the quantitative assessment and comparison of costs and benefits of the alternatives. This may be the most important step in the CBA and CEA processes. To set up the technical framework, the evaluator must identify the resources necessary to carry out the alternative, explain how the resources are combined, and then predict the outcome(s). As Warner and Luce (1982) have pointed out, this can be completed in several different ways ranging from a simple flow chart to a sophisticated, multi-equation computer simulation.

In the cardiovascular disease problem, the resources would include personnel time—of both the high-risk employees participating in this program and the program leaders, educational materials (i.e., booklets, films, handouts, etc.), supplies (i.e., exercise clothing, laundry expenses, etc.), pre- and post-program exercise testings, pre-program medical examinations, fee for facility use, and any other pre-participant program expenses. The outcomes of the program may include 50% of the participants getting involved in a life-long exercise program, 50% reducing their weight, and 75% getting their blood pressure under control. These in turn may result in fewer health insurance claims because of reduced illness, less absenteeism, and fewer accidents, thus increasing productivity. In the long run it is hoped these programs will decrease both morbidity and premature mortality.

As one can see from this example, this step can become quite involved. One may need to examine previous programs—conducted either in house or in another setting—or obtain the services of a technical consultant to try to adequately identify all resources and outcomes. However, the evaluator of the health promotion programs should be aware that even this additional work may not ensure the identification of all health outcomes. It is because of this inability to identify specific health outcomes that the use of CBA with health promotion programs has been limited. If the health benefits of a program cannot be identified, then one cannot put a dollar value on them and thus the cost of the benefit cannot be analyzed. For example, what are the

health benefits of a nutrition education program? Unless these benefits can be identified,* CBA would be an inappropriate cost analysis technique to use with health promotion programs.

On the other hand, CEA can be applied very well to some health promotion programs. For the outcomes of concern are not benefits but effects, and with a CEA the evaluator is not required to put a dollar value on the effects. Thus when analyzing the nutrition education program, one can identify effects such as the reduction of calorie intake or the reduction of serum fat levels without trying to identify the health benefit of such. It should be noted that these effects are immediate (i.e., reduction in calories) or intermediate (i.e., decrease in serum fat levels) outcomes only and not long-term (i.e., decreased premature mortality) like some financiers of health promotion programs want to see.

Whether one is using CBA or CEA, the more completely the production relationships have been described, the easier it will be to complete steps 5 and 6 in the process—analyzing costs, benefits, and effectiveness.

Step 5: Analyzing the Costs. Costs should be defined as those resources that one must give up to gain some benefit or effect (Warner & Luce, 1982). This would include not only those direct controllable costs but also overhead uncontrollable costs.

The cost of some resources may be obvious. Using the cardiovascular disease example, it may be very easy to determine the cost of the educational materials because they can be purchased at a cost of Y per set. The cost of the group leader may be obvious, too, but how about the cost of the four volunteers who are helping conduct the program? Since the program could not be run without the four volunteers, this is a cost to the program. In this situation the economic concept of "opportunity cost" would be used. "The opportunity cost is its value in another use" (Warner & Luce, 1982, p. 77). So if these volunteers were not helping in this program, how much would they be worth in another setting? It may be found that they would be worth $7.50 per hour working in a similar capacity at a local health agency. Therefore, their cost could be determined with this figure.

Since one of the major reasons for calculating CBA and CEA is to be able to compare alternatives,

---

*See the related literature section of this paper for examples of where evaluators have been able to apply CBA to health promotion programs.

it is important that costs (and for that matter benefits and effects) of the different alternatives are calculated in a similar manner. For example, if one is comparing different cardiovascular exercise programs and both programs include the help of volunteers, the same opportunity costs should be used in determining the total cost of volunteers.

Step 6: Analyzing Benefits and Effectiveness.
There are usually numerous desired outcomes (benefits) that result from health promotion programs. Some are obvious while others are much more difficult to identify. For this reason, it may help the evaluator to try to categorize the different outcomes. Warner and Luce (1982) have identified the following classification scheme for outcomes associated with health care activities: (1) Personal health benefits—improvements in health such as increased life expectancy, decreased morbidity, and reduced disability; (2) Health care resource benefits—the saving of unused resources resulting from the implementation of an activity (for example, an exercise program could reduce the resources put into cardiac surgery); (3) Other economic benefits—desired outcomes that are not identified as either health or health care benefits, such as work productivity; (4) Other social benefits—desired outcomes that have positive social effects like increased access to health services or compassion; and (5) Intermediate outcomes—benefits that occur prior to a final outcome. Because it is sometimes difficult to measure final outcomes, one often must use the intermediate outcome. For example, the long-term impact of an exercise program on one's health would be difficult to determine, but one could measure the intermediate outcome of weight loss.

It should be noted that not all outcomes are benefits. The best example of this appears in screening programs when false positive outcomes appear. If such outcomes do exist, they need to be treated as costs.

The measurement of benefits and effectiveness is very much like the measurement of costs in that some aspects are straightforward while others are very difficult. For example, not all social benefits can be quantified, such as compassion. There is no standard unit of compassion on which one could attach a dollar value.

It is at this point in the calculations of CBA and CEA that the differences in the two analyses can be seen. The CEA ends with the measurement of effectiveness. No dollar value is placed on the outcomes. Thus, the number of lives saved, trips to the health clinic, or persons involved in the exercise program are all that are needed. However, in order to calculate

a CBA, monetary units must be attached to each outcome. This is not too difficult when market prices are available. But they are not always available, and the one area that has caused considerable discussion is trying to put a monetary label on the "value of life." Techniques that have been used include (1) human capital—value of being productively employed in the labor market plus direct benefit of health care resource savings, (2) willingness to pay—value that individuals place on reducing risks of death and illness, (3) court awards in civil cases—value of productive life and emotional costs, and (4) life insurance holdings—value of one's life insurance.

Step 7: Discounting. A necessary step in calculating an accurate CBA or CEA is that of discounting. Since the costs and benefits of some programs do not occur entirely in the present, for comparison purposes all future costs and monetary values of future benefits should be discounted to their present value. In other words, a dollar today is worth more to an individual than the promise of having the dollar tomorrow and more still than having the dollar the day after tomorrow. "The discount rate attempts to adjust for what a dollar invested today would earn in interest" (Collen & Goodman, 1985). "...Discounting is particularly important in the case of preventive activities since so many of the benefits occur well into the future. In addition, discounting helps to explain how 'postponing' illness costs can have the effect of 'containing them'" (Warner, 1979).

To carry out the discounting process, one must first decide on a discount rate. The discount rate expresses the degree to which tomorrow's dollar loses value relative to today's dollar. Since there is little consensus on what discount rate should be used and because the particular discount rate chosen can have a substantial impact on the outcome of the analysis [In relative terms, low discount rates tend to favor projects whose benefits occur in the distant future (OTA, 1980)], CBAs and CEAs are usually calculated using several different rates, usually ranging from 3–10%. This process of using several different rates is called sensitivity analysis.

For example, if one wanted to spend $1,000 today on an exercise program expecting to save $2,000 in medical costs in five years, there would be a need to discount the benefit ($2,000) to its estimated present value. For the sake of the example the discount rate will be set at 5%. The present discounted value today of the net benefit would be $567 ($1,567–1,000) and not $1,000 ($2,000–$1,000).

Both time (in years) and the discount rate have an impact on the discounted value. Tables 1

TABLE 1   *Effect of Time on Discounted Value*

Discount Rate	Time (in years)	Present Value of Cost	Present Value of Benefit	Present Value of Net Benefit
.05	0	$1,000	$2,000	$1,000
.05	1	1,000	1,905	905
.05	2	1,000	1,814	814
.05	5	1,000	1,567	567
.05	10	1,000	1,228	228
.05	20	1,000	754	−246

and 2 are presented to illustrate the effect of each. Table 1 shows how an expected $2,000 benefit decreases in value over time when the discount rate stays constant (5% in this example).

Table 2 illustrates how again a $2,000 benefit decreases in value as the discount rate increases and the time stays constant (5 years in this example).

It is obvious from these tables that given a large enough discount rate and/or a substantial number of years, the net benefit could be a negative number. Such a number would indicate that the costs would outweigh the benefits and the cost-benefits ratio would be less than one point zero (1.0) to 1.0. In other words, it would cost more than one dollar to get a dollar worth of benefit.

For those interested in other examples of the discounting process, see Collen and Goodman (1985) and Warner and Luce (1982).

Step 8: Analyzing Uncertainties. As has been demonstrated throughout this discussion of calculating a CBA or CEA, there will be times when the evaluator will be uncertain of some data that need to be included. In such cases there are several alternatives available to the evaluator. As with discounting, the evaluator could use a sensitivity analysis. For example, if the evaluator were figuring a CEA on a smoking cessation program and was not sure of the cost of an instructor for the program, he/she could make several different estimates of the cost. Each of these estimates could then be "plugged" into" the analysis to give the evaluator a range for the CEA.

Another approach to dealing with uncertainties would be to elicit the help of a group of experts in the field. Such a technique is called consensus development. With this technique a group of experts is brought together to listen to a presentation of uncertain areas. Following the presentation, the group is then isolated to discuss the presentation and to reach a consensus as to what should be used in place of the uncertain data.

TABLE 2   *Effect of Discount Rate on Discounted Value*

Discount Rate	Time (in years)	Present Value of Cost	Present Value of Benefit	Present Value of Net Benefit
0	5	$1,000	$2,000	$1,000
3	5	1,000	1,725	725
5	5	1,000	1,567	567
7	5	1,000	1,426	426
10	5	1,000	1,242	242
15	5	1,000	994	−6

Step 9: Interpreting the Results. Because of all the concerns noted in calculating a CBA or CEA, one needs to be careful in interpreting the results of an analysis. There are many assumptions and uncertainties that both the evaluator and/or the interpreter of the results could overlook. Thus, one needs to proceed with caution when reading the analysis reports.

Assuming all steps have been carried out properly and appropriate CBA and CEA data have been calculated, the decision maker must not forget that the economic evaluation is only one piece of the data needed to make decisions about programs. Most programs have important ethical, legal, and/or societal issues that must be identified and discussed before final program decisions can be made.

Using CBAs and CEAs with Health Promotion Programs. The need for incorporating an economic component in the evaluation of a health promotion program should be obvious. The question that remains is, what specific technique would be most appropriate? In most situations the answer would be CEA. The reasons for using CEA as opposed to CBA with health promotion programs are: (1) the inability to determine and then measure all the effects of a program, and (2) the inability to put a monetary value on the measured effect. These inabilities of not being able to identify the effects and then in turn being able to determine the value (in dollars) of these effects are critical steps in the CBA process. Without them an evaluator could not calculate an accurate CBA. It would probably be a rare situation in which a CBA would be an appropriate technique to use in an evaluation of a health promotion program. Even if an evaluator were able to determine these values, there are some (Fielding, 1979; Kristein, 1983) who believe the cost-benefit ratio would not favor the health promotion programs. These individuals have indicated that there are several cost issues that evaluators to date have not considered when calculating a CBA. One of these issues revolves around the additional costs of human longevity. When an individual lives longer, he/she is more likely to have incurred additional medical costs and an employee will have to pay pensions for a longer period of time.

Conclusion

Many of the early health promotion programs planned in this country were implemented on the premise that it was more economically sound to spend health care dollars on prevention activities than on curing disease. At the present time, there is little empirical data to prove such economic evaluation— even though CBA and CEA have been used in many other areas of the health care system. As one looks to the future, it seems reasonable that if health promotion program planners are going to convince policy makers that such programs are an effective means of improving health status, then economic evaluation must be a part of the total evaluation process.

References

Acton, J. (1976). Measuring the monetary value of lifesaving programs. *Law and Contemporary Problems, 40,* 46.

Alderman, M. H., Madhavan, S., & Davis, T. (1983). Reduction of cardiovascular disease events by worksite hypertension treatment. *Hypertension, 5* (supplement V). V138–V143.

Collen, M., & Goodman, C. (1985). Cost-effectiveness and cost-benefit analysis. In Institute of Medicine, *Assessing Medical Technologies* (pp. 136–144, 160–164). Washington, D.C.: National Medical Press.

Cooper, B., & Rice, D. (1976). The economic cost of illness revisited. *Social Security Bulletin, 39,* 21.

Erfurt, J. C., & Foote, A. (1984). Cost-effectiveness of work-site blood pressure control programs. *Journal of Occupational Medicine, 26,* 892–900.

Fielding, J. E. (1982). Effectiveness of employee health improvement programs. *Journal of Occupational Medicine, 24,* 907–916.

Fielding, J. E. (1984). Health promotion and disease prevention at the worksite. In L. Breslow (Ed.), *Annual review in public health* (pp. 237–265). Palo Alto, California: Annual Reviews, Inc.

Fielding, J. E. (1979). Preventive medicine and the bottom line. *Journal of Occupational Medicine, 21,* 79–88.

Foote, A., & Erfurt, J. C. (1977). Controlling hypertension: A cost-effective model. *Preventive Medicine, 6,* 319–343.

Green, L. W. (1979). How to evaluate health promotion. *Hospitals, 53,* 106–108.

Green, L. W., & Lewis, F. M. (1986). *Measurement and evaluation in health education and health promotion.* Palo Alto, California: Mayfield Publishing Company

Kristein, M. M. (1977). Economic issues in prevention. *Preventive Medicine, 6,* 252–264.

Kristein, M. M. (1983). How much can business expect to profit from smoking cessation? *Preventive Medicine, 12,* 358–381.

Office of Technology Assessment, U.S. Congress. (1978). *Assessing the efficacy and safety of medi-*

cal technologies. Washington, D.C.: U.S. Government Printing Office.

Office of Technology Assessment, U.S. Congress (1980). *The implications of cost-effectiveness analysis of medical technology/background paper #1: Methodological issues and literature review.* Washington, D.C.: U.S. Government Printing Office.

Rogers, P. J., Eaton, E. K., & Bruhn, J. G. (1981). Is health promotion cost effective? *Preventive Medicine, 10,* 324–339.

Rice, D. (1966). *Estimating the cost of illness.* U.S. Department of Health, Education and Welfare, PHS, Health Economic Series No. 6.

Ruchlin, H. S., & Alderman, M. H. (1980). Cost of hypertension control at the workplace. *Journal of Occupational Medicine, 22,* 795–800.

Ruchlin, H. S., Melcher, L. A., & Alderman, M. H. (1984). A comparative economic analysis of work-related hypertension care programs. *Journal of Occupational Medicine, 26,* 45–49.

Scheffler, R. M., & Paringer, L. (1980). A review of the economic evidence on prevention. *Medical Care, 18,* 473–484.

Schwartz, R. M., & Rollins, P. L. (1985). Measuring the cost benefit of wellness strategies. *Business and Health, 2,* 10, 24–26.

Seidman, L. S., Sevelius, G. G., & Ewald, P. (1984). A cost-effective weight loss program at the worksite. *Journal of Occupational Medicine, 26,* 725–730.

Shepard, D. S., & Thompson, M. S. (1979). First principles of cost-effectiveness analysis in health. *Public Health Reports, 94,* 535–543.

Warner, K. E., & Hutton, R. C. (1980). Cost-benefit and cost-effective analysis in health care. *Medical Care, 18,* 1069–1084.

Warner, K. E., & Luce, B. R. (1982). *Cost-benefit and cost-effectiveness in health care: Principles, practice, and potential.* Ann Arbor, Michigan: Health Administration Press.

Warner, K. E. (1979). The economic implications of preventive health care. *Social Science and Medicine, 13C,* 227–237.

Weiss, S. J., Jurs, S., Lesage, J. P., & Iverson, D. C. (1984). A cost-benefit analysis of a smoking cessation program. *Evaluation and Program Planning, 7,* 337–346.

Windsor, R. A., Baranowski, T., Clark, N., & Cutter, G. (1984). *Evaluation of health promotion and education programs.* Palo Alto, California: Mayfield Publishing Company.

Work Group on Health Promotion/Disease Prevention. (1987). Criteria for the development of health promotion and education programs. *American Journal of Public Health, 77,* 89–92.

References

Ad Hoc Work Group of the American Public Health Association. (1987). Criteria for the development of health promotion and education programs. *American Journal of Public Health, 77*(1), 89–92.

Agency for Health Care Policy and Research (AHCPR). (1996). *Smoking cessation: Clinical practice guideline no. 18.* (AHCPR Publication No. 96-0692). Rockville, MD: Author.

Ajzen, I. (1988). *Attitudes, personality, and behavior.* Chicago: Dorsey Press.

Alexander, G. (1999). Health risk appraisal. In G. C. Hyner, K. W. Peterson, J. W. Travis, J. E. Dewey, J. J. Foerster, & E. M. Framer (Eds.), *SPM handbook of health assessment tools* (pp. 5–8). Pittsburgh, PA: The Society of Prospective Medicine.

Albrecht, T. L. (1997). Defining social marketing: Twenty five years later. *Social Marketing Quarterly, 3,* 21–23.

Albrecht, T. L., & Bryant, C. (1996). Advances in segmentation modeling for health communication and social marketing campaigns. *Journal of Health Communication, 1,* 65–80.

Alexy, B. J. (1985). Health risk appraisal: Reliability demonstrated. In *Proceedings of the 20th Meeting of the Society of Prospective Medicine.* Bethesda, MD: Society of Prospective Medicine.

Alinsky, S. D. (1971). *Rules for radicals: A pragmatic primer for realistic radicals.* New York: Random House.

American Association for Health Education (AAHE), National Commission for Health Education Credentialing, Inc. (NCHEC), & Society for Public Health Education (SOPHE). (1999). *A competency-based framework for graduate-level health educators.* Reston, VA: Authors.

American Association of School Administrators (AASA). (1990). *Healthy kids for the year 2000: An action plan for schools.* Arlington, VA: Author.

American College Health Association (ACHA). (no date). *Healthy campus 2000: Making it happen.* Rockville, MD: Author.

American College of Sports Medicine (ACSM). (1998). *ACSM's resource manual for guidelines for exercise testing and prescription* (3rd ed.). Baltimore, MD: Williams & Wilkins.

American Indian Health Care Association (AIHCA). (no date). *Promoting health traditions workbook—A Guide to the healthy people 2000 campaign.* St. Paul, MN: Author.

American Public Health Association (1991). *Healthy communities 2000: Model standards—Guidelines for community attainment of the year 2000 national health objectives* (3rd ed.). Washington, DC: Author.

Anderson, D. M., & Portnoy, B. (1989). Diffusion of cancer education into the schools. *Journal of School Health, 59*(5), 214–217.

Anderson, D. R., & O'Donnell, M. P. (1994). Toward a health promotion research agenda: "State of the science" reviews. *American Journal of Health Promotion, 8*(6), 462–465.

Anderson, P., & Fenichel, E. (1989). *Serving culturally diverse families of infants and toddlers with disabilities.* Washington, DC: National Center for Clinical Infant Programs.

Andreasen, A. (1995). *Marketing sound change: Changing behavior to promote health, social development, and the environment.* San Francisco: Jossey-Bass.

Anspaugh, D. J., Hunter, S., & Savage, P. (1996). Enhancing employee participation in corporate health promotion programs. *American Journal of Health Behavior, 20*(3), 112–120.

Archer, S. E., & Fleshman, R. P. (1985). *Community health nursing.* Monterey, CA: Wadsworth Health Sciences.

Archer, S. E., Kelly, C. D., & Bisch, S. A. (1984). *Implementing change in communities: A collaborative process.* St. Louis: C. V. Mosby.

Arkin, E. B. (1990). Opportunities for improving the nation's health through collaboration with the mass media. *Public Health Reports, 105*(3), 219–223.

Association for the Advancement of Health Education (AAHE). (1994). *A cultural awareness and sensitivity: Guidelines for health educators.* Reston, VA: Author.

Auld, E. (1997). Practical tips for influencing public policy. *Health Education & Behavior, 24*(3), 272–274.

Bandura, A. (1977a). Self-efficacy: Toward a unifying theory of behavioral change. *Psychological Review, 84*(2), 191–215.

Bandura, A. (1977b). *Social learning theory.* Englewood Cliffs, NJ: Prentice-Hall.

Bandura, A. (1986). *Social foundations of thought and action.* Englewood Cliffs, NJ: Prentice-Hall.

Baranowski, T. (1985). Methodologic issues in self-report of health behavior. *Journal of School Health, 55*(5), 179–182.

Bartlett, E. E., Windsor, R. A., Lowe, J. B., & Nelson, G. (1986). Guidelines for conducting smoking cessation programs. *Health Education, 17*(1), 31–37.

Basch, C. (1984). Research on disseminating and implementing health education programs in schools. *Health Education, 15*(4), 57–66; *Journal of School Health, 54*(6), 57–66.

Basch, C. E., & Sliepcevich, E. M. (1983). Innovators, innovations, and implementation: A framework for curricular research in school health education. *Health Education, 14*(2), 20–24.

Bates, I. J., & Winder, A. E. (1984). *Introduction to health education.* Palo Alto, CA: Mayfield.

Baumgartner, T. A., & Strong, C. H. (1994). *Conducting and reading research on health and human performance.* Madison, WI: WCB Brown & Benchmark Publishers.

Becker, M. H. (Ed.). (1974). The health belief model and personal health behavior. *Health Education Monographs, 2* (entire issue).

Becker, M. H., Drachman, R. H., & Kirscht, J. P. (1974). A new approach to explaining sick-role behavior in low income populations. *American Journal of Public Health, 64*(March), 205–216.

Becker, M. H., & Green, L. W. (1975). A family approach to compliance with medical treatment, a selective review of the literature. *International Journal of Health Education, 18*(3), 2–11.

Becker, M. H., & Maiman, L. (1983). Models of health-related behavior. In D. Mechanic (Ed.), *Handbook of health, health care and the health professions* (pp. 539–568). New York: Free Press.

Beckwith, H. (1997). *Selling the invisible: A field guide to modern marketing* (p. 31). New York: Warner Books.

Behrens, R. (1983). *Work-site health promotion: Some questions and answers to help you get started.* Washington, DC: Office of Disease Prevention and Health Promotion.

Bellicha, T., & McGrath, J. (1990). Mass media approaches to reducing cardiovascular disease risk. *Public Health Reports, 105*(3), 245–252.

Bensley, L. B. (1989). A review of the use of mass media and marketing in health education: A look at theory and practice. *Eta Sigma Gamman, 21*(1), 18–23.

Bensley, L. B. (1991). Schoolsite health promotion: Ways of sustaining interest. *Journal of Health Education, 22*(2), 86–89.

Berkman, L. F., & Syme, S. L. (1979). Social networks, host resistance and mortality: A nine-year follow-up of Alameda County residents. *American Journal of Epidemiology, 109*(2), 186–204.

Best, J. A., & Milsum, J. H. (1978). HHA and the evaluation of lifestyle change programs: Methodological issues. In *Proceedings of the 13th Meeting of the Society of Prospective Medicine.* Bethesda, MD: Society of Prospective Medicine.

Black, D. R., Loftus, E. A., Chatterjee, R., Tiffany, S., & Babrow, A. S. (1993). Smoking cessation interventions for university students: Recruitment and program design considerations based on social marketing theory. *Preventive Medicine, 22,* 388–399.

Black, D. R., & Smith, M. A. (1994). Reducing alcohol consumption among university students: Recruitment and program design strategies based on social marketing theory. *Health Education Research, 9,* 375–384.

Blackburn, H. (1983). Research and demonstration projects in community cardiovascular disease prevention. *Journal of Public Health Policy, 4*(4), 398–421.

Bloomquist, K. (1981). Physical fitness programs in industry: Applications of social learning theory. *Occupational Health Nursing, 29*(7), 30–33.

Borg, W. R., & Gall, M. D. (1989). *Educational research: An introduction* (5th ed.). New York: Longman.

Bourque, L. B., & Fielder, E. P. (1995). *How to conduct self-administered and mail surveys.* Thousand Oaks, CA: Sage.

Bowling, A. (1997). *Measuring health: A review of quality of life measurement scales* (2nd ed.). Philadelphia, PA: Open University Press.

Brager, G., Specht, H., & Torczyner, J. L. (1987). *Community organizing.* New York: Columbia University Press.

Braithwaite, R. L., Murphy, F., Lythcott, N., & Blumenthal, D. S. (1989). Community organization and development for health promotion within an urban black community: A conceptual model. *Health Education, 20*(5), 56–60.

Breckon, D. J. (1997). *Managing health promotion programs: Leadership skills for the 21st century.* Gaithersburg, MD: Aspen.

Breckon, D. J., Harvey, J. R., & Lancaster, R. B. (1998). *Community health education: Settings, roles, and skills for the 21st century* (4th ed.). Gaithersburg, MD: Aspen.

Breen, M. (1999). Researching grants on the Internet. *Community Health Center Management,* March/April, p. 29.

Breslow, L. (1999). From disease prevention to health promotion. *Journal of the American Medical Association, 281*(11), 1030–1033.

Brownson, R. C., Koffman, D. M., Novotny, T. E., Hughes, R. G., & Eriksen, M. P. (1995). Environmental and policy interventions to control tobacco use and prevent cardiovascular disease. *Health Education Quarterly, 22*(4), 478–498.

Bryant, C. (1998, June). *Social marketing: a tool for excellence.* Eighth annual conference on social marketing in public health, Clearwater Beach, FL.

Bryant, C., Cole, S., Salazar, B., Lindenberger, J. H., Perrin, K., Sorrell, C., Flynn, M., Courtney, A., Dennis, C., Markesbery, B., & Gaskin, E. (1996). Breast cancer screening: A social marketing study. *Social Marketing Quarterly, 3,* 24–35.

Burdine, J. N., & McLeroy, K. R. (1992). Practitioners' use of theory: Examples from a workgroup. *Health Education Quarterly, 19*(3), 331–340.

Buxton, T. (1999). Effective ways to improve health education materials. *Journal of Health Education, 30*(1), 47–50.

Campbell, M. K., Devellis, B. M., Strecher,, V. J., Ammerman, A. S., Devillis, R. F., & Sandler, R. S. (1994). Improving dietary behavior: The effectiveness of tailored messages in primary care settings. *American Journal of Public Health, 84*(5), 783–787.

Campinha-Bacote, J. (1994). Cultural competence in psychiatric mental health nursing: A conceptual model. *Nursing Clinics of North America, 29,* 1–8.

Capwell, E. M., Butterfoss, F., & Francisco, V. T. (2000). Why evaluate? *Health Promotion Practice, 1*(1), 15–20.

Cardinal, B. J. (1995). The transtheoretical model of behavior change as applied to physical activity and exercise: A review. *Journal of Physical Education and Sport Science, 8,* 32–45.

Centers for Disease Control and Prevention (CDC), U.S. Department of Health and Human Services (USDHHS). (no date). *Planned approach to community health: Guide for local coordinator.* Atlanta, GA: Author.

Centers for Disease Control and Prevention (CDC), U.S. Department of Health and Human Services (USDHHS). (1999). *An ounce of prevention… What are the returns?* (2nd ed.). Atlanta, GA: Author.

Centers for Disease Control and Prevention (CDC), U.S. Department of Health and Human Services (USDHHS). (1999b). *CDCynergy CD-ROM.* Atlanta, GA: Author.

Centers for Disease Control and Prevention (CDC). (1999c). Framework for program evaluation in public health. *Morbidity and Mortality Weekly Report, 48* (RR-11), 1–40.

Centers for Disease Control and Prevention (CDC). (1999d). Ten great public health achievements—United States, 1900–1999. *Morbidity and Mortality Weekly Report, 48*(12), 241–243.

Centers for Disease Control and Prevention. (1999a). *CDCynergy Content and Framework Workbook.* Atlanta, GA: U.S. Department of Health and Human Services, Office of Communication, Office of the Director.

Chaplin, J. P., & Krawiec, T. S. (1979). *Systems and theories of psychology* (4th ed.). New York: Holt, Rinehart & Winston.

Chapman, L. S. (1997). Securing support from top management. *The Art of Health Promotion, 1*(2), 1–7.

Cheadle, A., Wagner, E., Koepsell, T., Kristal, A., & Patrick, D. (1992). Environmental indicators: A tool of evaluating community-based health promotion programs. *American Journal of Preventive Medicine, 8,* 345–350.

Checkoway, B. (1989). Community participation for health promotion: Prescription for public policy. *Wellness Perspectives: Research, Theory and Practice, 6*(1), 18–26.

Chenoweth, D. H. (1987). *Planning health promotion at the worksite.* Indianapolis: Benchmark Press.

Cinelli, B., Rose-Colley, M., & Hayes, D. M. (1988). Health promotion efforts in Pennsylvania schools. *American Journal of Health Promotion, 2*(4), 36–44.

Clapp, J. D., Packard, T. R., & Stanger, L. A. (1993). Community organizing in alcohol and other drug prevention coalition building: The role of strategic decisions. *Journal of Health Education, 24*(3), 157–161.

Clark, N. M., Janz, N. K., Dodge, J. A., & Sharpe, P. A. (1992). Self-regulation of health behavior: The "take PRIDE" program. *Health Education Quarterly, 19*(3), 341–354.

Cleary, M. J., & Neiger, B. L. (1998). *The certified health education specialist: A self-study guide for professional competency* (3rd ed.). Allentown, PA: The National Commission for Health Education Credentialing.

Clift, E., & Freimuth, V. (1995). Health communication: What is it and what can it do for you? *Journal of Health Education, 26*(2), 68–74.

Cohen, S., & Lichtenstein, E. (1990). Partner behaviors that support quitting smoking. *Jour-*

nal of Consulting and Clinical Psychology, 58, 304–309.

Colletti, G., & Brownell, K. (1982). *The physical and emotional benefits of social support: Application to obesity, smoking and alcoholism.* In M. Eisler et al. (Eds.), *Progress in behavior modification* (vol. 13). New York: Academic Press.

Conner, R. F. (1980). Ethical issues in the use of control groups. In R. Perloff & E. Perloff (Eds.), *New Directions for Program Evaluation* (pp. 63–75). San Francisco: Jossey-Bass.

Connor, D. M. (1968). *Strategies for development.* Ottawa: Development Press.

Cook, T. D., & Campbell, D. T. (1979). *Quasi-experimentation: Design and analysis issues for field settings.* Boston: Houghton Mifflin.

Cooper, K. H. (1982). *The aerobics program for total well-being.* Toronto: Bantam Books.

Cottrell, R. R., Girvan, J. T., & McKenzie, J. F. (1999). *Principles and foundations of health promotion and education.* Boston: Allyn and Bacon.

Cowdery, J. E., Wang, M. Q., Eddy, J. M., & Trucks, J. K. (1995). A theory driven health promotion program in a university setting. *Journal of Health Education, 26*(4), 248–250.

Cummings, C., Gordon, J. R., & Marlatt, G. A. (1980). Relapse: Prevention and prediction. In W. R. Miller (Ed.), *Addictive behaviors* (pp. 291–322). Oxford, U.K.: Pergamon Press.

Cummings, K., Becker, M. H., & Maile, M. (1980). Bringing the models together in an empirical approach to combining variables used to explain health actions. *Journal of Behavioral Medicine, 3*(2), 123–145.

Daniel, E. L., & Balog, J. E. (1997). Utilization of the world wide web in health education. *Journal of Health Education, 28*(5), 260–267.

Davis, J. (1990). Employee health newsletters: Analysis of characteristics. *AAOHN Journal, 38*(8), 360–367.

Davis, N. A., Lewis, M. J., Rimer, B. K., Harvey, C. M., & Koplan, J. P. (1997). Evaluation of a phone intervention to promote mammography in a managed care plan. *American Journal of Health Promotion, 11*(4), 247–249.

Davis, T. C., Mayeaux, E. J., Fredrickson, D., Bocchini, J. A., Jackson, R. H., & Murphy, P. W. (1994). Reading ability of parents compared with reading level of pediatric patient education materials. *Pediatrics, 93,* 460–468.

Deeds, S. G. (1992). *The health education specialist: Self- study for professional competence.* Los Alamitos, CA: Loose Canon.

DeJong, W. (1989). Condom promotion: The need for a social marketing program in Americas inner cities. *American Journal of Health Promotion, 3,* 5–10.

DiBlase, D. (1985). Small businesses lead into wellness. *Business Insurance,* (December 2), 16.

DiClemente, C. C., & Prochaska, J. O. (1982). Self-change and therapy change of smoking behavior: A comparison of processes of change in cessation and maintenance. *Addictive Behaviors, 7*(2), 133–142.

DiClemente, C. C., Prochaska, J. O., Fairhurst, S. K., Velicer, W. F., Velasquez, M. M., & Rossi, J. S. (1991). The process of smoking cessation: An analysis of precontemplation, contemplation, and preparation stages of change. *Journal of Consulting and Clinical Psychology, 59,* 259–304.

Dignan, M. B. (1995). *Measurement and evaluation of health education.* (3rd ed.) Springfield, IL: Charles C Thomas.

Dignan, M. B., & Carr, P. A. (1992). *Program planning for health education and health promotion.* Philadelphia: Lea & Febiger.

Dishman, R. K. (Ed.). (1988). *Exercise adherence: Its impact on public health.* Champaign, IL: Human Kinetics.

Dishman, R. K., Sallis, J. F., & Orenstein, D. R. (1985). The determinants of physical activity and exercise. *Public Health Reports, 100*(2), 158–171.

Division of Adolescent and School Health (DASH), National Center for Chronic Disease Prevention and Health Promotion. (1997). Youth risk behavior surveillance, national college health risk behavior survey—United States, 1995. *CDC Surveillance Summaries, November 14, 1997. MMWR, 46* (No. SS-6), pp. 1–56.

Dollahite, J., Thomson, C., & McNew, R. (1996). Readability of printed sources of diet and health information. *Patient Education and Counseling, 27*(2), 123–134.

D'Onofrio, C. N. (1992). Theory and the empowerment of health education practitioners. *Health Education Quarterly, 19*(3), 385–403.

Dunbar, J. M., Marshall, G. D., & Howell, M. F. (1979). Behavioral strategies for improving compliance. In R. B. Haynes, D. W. Taylor, & D. L. Sackett (Eds.), *Compliance in health care* (pp. 174–190). Baltimore: Johns Hopkins University Press.

Edington, D. W., & Yen, L. (1992). Is it possible to simultaneously reduce risk factors and excess health care costs? *American Journal of Health Promotion, 6*(6), 403–406, 409.

Edington, D. W., Yen, L., & Braunstein, A. (1999). The reliability and validity of HRAs. In G. C. Hyner, K. W. Peterson, J. W. Travis, J. E. Dewey, J. J.

Foerster, & E. M. Framer (Eds.), *SPM handbook of health assessment tools* (pp. 135–141). Pittsburgh, PA: The Society of Prospective Medicine.

Elias, W. S., & Dunton, S. (1981). Effect of reliability on risk factor estimation by a health hazard appraisal. In *Proceedings of the 16th Meeting of the Society of Prospective Medicine*. Bethesda, MD: Society of Prospective Medicine.

Emont, S. L., & Cummings, K. M. (1989). Adoption of smoking policies by automobile dealerships. *Public Health Reports, 104*(5), 509–514.

Emont, S. L., & Cummings, K. M. (1992). Using low-cost prize-drawing incentive to improve recruitment rate at a workshop smoking cessation clinic. *Journal of Occupational Medicine, 34*(8), 771–774.

Erfurt, J. C., Foote, A., Heirich, M. A., & Gregg, W. (1990). Improving participation in worksite wellness: Comparing health education classes, a menu approach, and follow-up counseling. *American Journal of Health Promotion, 4*(4), 270–278.

Erickson, A. C., McKenna, J. W., & Romano, R. M. (1990). Past lessons and new uses of the mass media in reducing tobacco consumption. *Public Health Reports, 105*(3), 239–244.

Faerber, M. (Ed.). (1999). *Gale directory of databases: Volume 1: Online databases*. Detroit, MI: Gale Group, Inc.

Feldman, R. H. L. (1983). Strategies for improving compliance with health promotion programs in industry. *Health Education, 14*(4), 21–25.

Fennell, R., & Beyrer, M. K. (1989). AIDS: Some ethical considerations for the health educator. *Journal of American College Health, 38*(November), 145–147.

Fink, A., & Kosecoff, J. (1978). *An evaluation primer*. Washington, DC: Capitol Publications.

Finkler, S. A. (1992). *Budgeting concepts for nurse managers* (2nd ed.). Philadelphia: W. B. Saunders.

Fishbein, M., & Ajzen, I. (1975). *Belief, attitude, intention and behavior: An introduction to theory and research*. Reading, MA: Addison-Wesley.

Fisher, D. S., Ryan, R., Esacove, A. W., Bishofsky, S., Wallis, J. M., & Roffman, R. A. (1996). The social marketing of Project ARIES: Overcoming challenges in recruiting gay and bisexual males for HIV prevention counseling. *Journal of Homosexuality, 37*, 177–203.

Forster, J., Jeffery, R., Sullivan, S., & Snell, M. (1985). A worksite weight control program using financial incentives collected through payroll deduction. *Journal of Occupational Medicine, 27*(11), 804–808.

Fowler, K., Celebuski, C., Edgar, T., Kroger, F., & Ratzan, S. C. (1999). An assessment of health communication job market across multiple types of organizations. *Journal of Health Communication, 4*, 327–342.

Frankish, C. J., Lovato, C. Y., & Shannon, W. J. (1998). Models, theories, and principles of health promotion with multicultural populations. In R. M. Huff & M. V. Kline (Eds.), *Promoting health in multicultural populations* (pp. 41–72). Thousand Oaks, CA: Sage.

Frederiksen, L. (1984). Using incentives in worksite wellness. *Corporate Commentary, 1*(2), 51–57.

Freimuth, V. S., & Mettger, W. (1990). Is there a hard-to-reach audience? *Public Health Reports, 105*(3), 232–238.

Freire, P. (1973). *Education: The practice of freedom*. London: Writer's and Reader's Publishing.

Freire, P. (1974). *Pedagogy of the oppressed*. New York: Seabury Press.

French, S. A., Jeffery, R. W., & Oliphant, J. A. (1994). Facility access and self-reward as methods to promote physical activity among healthy sedentary adults. *American Journal of Health Promotion, 8*(4), 257–259, 262.

French, S. A., Jeffery, R. W., Story, M., Hannan, P., & Snyder, M. P. (1997). A pricing strategy to promote low-fat snack choices through vending machines. *American Journal of Public Health, 87*(5), 849–851.

Gilbert, G., & Sawyer, R. (1995). *Health education: Creating strategies for school and community health*. Boston: Jones & Bartlett.

Gilmore, G. D., & Campbell, M. D. (1996). *Needs assessment strategies for health education and health promotion* (2nd ed.). Madison, WI: WCB Brown & Benchmark.

Gilmore, G. D., Campbell, M. D., & Becker, B. L. (1989). *Needs assessment strategies for health education and health promotion*. Indianapolis: Benchmark Press.

Glanz, K., Lewis, F. M., & Rimer, B. K. (Eds.). (1997). *Health behavior and health education: Theory, research, and practice*. San Francisco: Jossey-Bass.

Glanz, K., & Rimer, B. K. (1995). *Theory at a glance: A guide for health promotion practice* [NIH Pub. No. 95-3896]. Washington, DC: National Cancer Institute.

Glascoff, M. (1986). A social marketing approach to reducing salt intake. *Health Education, 3*, 11–14.

Glasgow, R. E., Vogt, T. M., & Boles, S. M. (1999). Evaluating the public health impact of health promotion interventions: The RE-AIM framework. *American Journal of Public Health, 89*(9), 1322–1327.

Godin, G., & Kok, G. (1996). The theory of planned behavior: A review of its applications to health-related behaviors. *American Journal of Health Promotion, 11*(2), 87–98.

Goetzel, R. Z., Anderson, D. R., Whitmer, R. W., Ozminkowski, R. J., Dunn, R. L., Wasserman, J., & The Health Enhancement Research Organization (HERO) Research Committee. (1998). The relationships between modifiable health risks and health care expenditures. *Journal of Occupational and Environmental Medicine, 40* (10), 843–854.

Golaszewski, T. J., Yen, L., Clearie, A., Lynch, W., & Vickery, D. (1989, September). Characteristics of employees reporting medical visits saved from use of the medical self-care text, Take care of yourself: The consumer's guide to medical care (pp. 152–161). In *Proceedings of the 25th Annual Meeting of the Society of Prospective Medicine*. Indianapolis, IN: Society of Prospective Medicine.

Gold, R. S. (1995). Application of technology to disease prevention and health promotion. In G. G. Gilbert & R. G Sawyer, *Health education: Creating strategies for school and community health* (pp. 79–81). Boston: Jones and Bartlett.

Goldman, K. D. (1994). Perceptions of innovations as predictors of implementation levels: The diffusion of nation-wide health education campaign. *Health Education and Behavior, 21*(4), 429–444.

Goldman, K. D. (1998). Promoting new ideas on the job: Practical theory-based strategies. *The Health Educator, 30*(1), 49–52.

Goldstein, M. G., DePue, J., Kazura, A, & Niaura, R. (1998). Models for provider-patient interaction: Applications to health behavior change. In S. A. Shumaker, E. B. Schron, J. K. Ockene, & W. L. McBee (Eds.), *The handbook of health behavior change* (2nd ed., pp. 85–113). New York: Springer.

Goldstein, S. M. (1997). Community coalitions: A self-assessment tool. *American Journal of Health Promotion, 11*(6), 430–435.

Goodman, R. M., McLeroy, K. R., Steckler, A. B., & Hoyle, R. H. (1993). Development of level of institutionalization scales for health promotion programs. *Health Education Quarterly, 20*(2), 161–178.

Graber, M. A., Roller, C. M., & Kaeble, B. (1999). Readability levels of patient education material on the World Wide Web. *The Journal of Family Medicine, 48*(1), 58–61.

Granat, J. P. (1994). *Persuasive advertising for entrepreneurs and small business owners: How to create more effective sales messages.* Binghamton, NY: Haworth Press.

Graves, E. J., & Owings, M. E. (1997). 1995 summary: National Hospital Discharge Survey. Advance data from *Vital and Health Statistics*, no. 291. Hyattsville, MD: National Center for Health Statistics.

Green, L. W. (1974). Toward cost-benefit evaluations of health education: Some concepts, methods, and examples. *Health Education Monographs, 2* (Suppl. 1), 34–64.

Green, L. W. (1975). Evaluation of patient education programs. Criteria and measurement techniques. In *Rx: Education for the patient: Proceedings of the Continuing Education Institution, Southern Illinois University* (pp. 89–98). Carbondale, IL: Southern Illinois University Press.

Green, L. W. (1976). Methods available to evaluate the health education components of preventive health programs. In *Preventive Medicine*, USA (pp. 162–171). New York: Prodist.

Green, L. W. (1979). National policy on the promotion of health. *International Journal of Health Education, 22, 161–168.*

Green, L. W. (1980). Healthy People: The Surgeon General's report and the prospects. In W. J. McNervey (Ed.), *Working for a healthier America* (pp. 95–110). Cambridge, MA: Ballinger.

Green, L. W. (1981a). Emerging federal perspectives on health promotion. In J. P. Allegrante (Ed.), *Health Promotion Monographs* (28 pp.). New York: Teachers College, Columbia University.

Green, L. W. (1981b). The objectives for the nation in disease prevention and health promotion: A challenge to health education training. *Proceedings of the National Conference for Institutions Preparing Health Educators,* (DHHS Publication No. 81–50171) (pp. 61–73). Washington, DC: U.S. Office of Health Information and Health Promotion.

Green, L. W. (1982). Reconciling policy in health education and primary care. *International Journal of Health Education, 24* (Suppl. 3), 1–11.

Green, L. W. (1983a). New policies in education for health. *World Health* (April—May), 13–17.

Green, L. W. (1983b). *New policies for health education in primary health care* (Background document for the technical discussions of the 36th World Health Assembly, May 1983). Geneva: World Health Organization.

Green, L. W. (1984a). A triage and stepped approach to self-care education. *Medical Times, 111,* 75–80.

Green, L. W. (1984b). Health education models. In J. D. Matarazzo, S. M. Weiss, & J. A. Herd (Eds.), *Behavioral health: A handbook of health enhancement and disease prevention* (pp. 181–198). New York: Wiley.

Green, L. W. (1984c). La educacion para la salud en el medio urbano. In *Conferencia InterAmericana de Educacion Para La Salud* (pp. 80–82). Mexico City: Sector Salud, SEP, and International Union for Health Education and World Health Organization.

Green, L. W. (1984d). Modifying and developing health behavior. *Annual Review of Public Health, 5,* 215–236.

Green, L. W. (1986a, October). *Applications and trials of the PRECEDE framework for planning and evaluation of health programs.* Paper presented at the meeting of the American Public Health Association, Las Vegas, NV.

Green, L. W. (1986b). Evaluation model: A framework for the design of rigorous evaluation of efforts in health promotion. *American Journal of Health Promotion, 1*(1), 77–79.

Green, L. W. (1986c). *New policies for health education in primary health care.* Geneva: World Health Organization.

Green, L. W. (1986d). Research agenda: Building a consensus on research questions. *American Journal of Health Promotion, 1*(2), 70–72.

Green, L. W. (1986e). The theory of participation: A qualitative analysis of its expression in national and international health policies. In W. B. Ward (Ed.), *Advances in Health Education and Promotion* (pp. 211–236). Greenwich, CT: JAI Press.

Green, L. W. (1987a). How physicians can improve patients' participation and maintenance in self-care. *Western Journal of Medicine, 147,* 346–349.

Green, L. W. (1987b). *Program planning and evaluation guide for Lung Associations.* New York: American Lung Association.

Green, L. W. (1989, March). *The health promotion program of the Henry J. Kaiser Family Foundation.* Paper presented at a public lecture at Mankato State University, Mankato, MN.

Green, L. W. (1990). The revival of community and the public obligation of academic health centers. In R. E. Bulger and S. J. Reiser (Eds.), *Integrity in institutions: Humane environments for teaching* (pp. 163–178). Iowa City: University of Iowa Press.

Green, L. W., (1999). Health education's contributions to public health in the twentieth century: A glimpse through health promotion's rearview mirror. In J. E. Fielding, L. B. Lave, & B. Starfield (Eds.). *Annual review of public health* (pp. 67–88). Palo Alto, CA: Annual Reviews.

Green, L. W., & Allen, J. (1980). *Toward a healthy community: Organizing events for community health promotion* (PHS Publication No. 80–50113). Washington, DC: USDHHS, Office of Disease Prevention and Health Promotion.

Green, L. W., Glanz, K., Hochbaum, G. M., Kok, G., Kreuter, M. W., Lewis, F. M., Lorig, K., Morisky, D., Rimer, B. K., & Rosenstock, I. M. (1994). Can we build on, or must we replace, the theories and models of health education? *Health Education Research, 9*(3), 397–404.

Green, L. W., Gold, R., Tan, J., & Kreuter, M. (1994). The EMPOWER/Canadian Health Expert System: The application of artificial intelligence and expert system technology to community health program planning and evaluation. *Canadian Medical Infamatics,* Nov./Dec., 20–23.

Green, L. W., & Kreuter, M. W. (1991). *Health promotion planning: An educational and environmental approach* (2nd ed.). Mountain View, CA: Mayfield.

Green, L. W., & Kreuter, M. W. (1992). CDC's planned approach to community health as an application of PRECEDE and an inspiration for PROCEED. *Journal of Health Education, 23*(3), 140–147.

Green, L. W., Kreuter, M. W. (1999). *Health promotion planning: An educational and ecological approach* (3rd ed.). Mountain View, CA: Mayfield.

Green, L. W., Kreuter, M. W., Deeds, S. G., & Partridge, K. B. (1980). *Health education planning: A diagnostic approach.* Palo Alto, CA: Mayfield.

Green, L. W., Levine, D. M., & Deeds, S. G. (1975). Clinical trials of health education for hypertensive outpatients: Design and baseline data. *Preventive Medicine, 4,* 417–425.

Green, L. W., & Lewis, F. M. (1986). *Measurement and evaluation in health education and health promotion.* Palo Alto, CA: Mayfield.

Green, L. W., & McAlister, A. L. (1984). Macro-intervention to support health behavior: Some theoretical perspectives and practical reflections. *Health Education Quarterly, 11,* 323–339.

Green, L. W., Mullen, P. D., & Friedman, R. (1986). An epidemiological approach to targeting drug information. *Patient Education and Counseling, 8,* 255–268.

Green, L. W., Wang, V. L., Deeds, S. G., Fisher, A. A., Windsor, R., & Rogers, C. (1978). Guidelines for health education in maternal and child health programs. *International Journal of Health Education, 21* (suppl.), 1–33.

Green, L. W., Wilson, A. L., & Lovato, C. Y. (1986). What changes can health promotion achieve and how long do these changes last? The tradeoffs between expediency and durability. *Preventive Medicine, 15,* 508–521.

Green, L. W., Wilson, R. W., & Bauer, K. G. (1983). Data required to measure progress on the objectives for the nation in disease prevention and health promotion. *American Journal of Public Health, 73,* 18–24.

Greenberg, J. (1978). Health education as freeing. *Health Education, 9*(2), 20–21.

Greene, G. W., Rossi, S. R., Reed, G. R., Willey, C., & Prochaska, J. O. (1994). Stages of change for reducing dietary fat to 30% of energy or less. *Journal of the American Dietetic Association, 94,* 1105–1110.

Greer, A. (1977). Advances in the study of diffusion of innovation in health care organizations. *Milbank Memorial Fund Quarterly, 55*(4) 505–532.

Grimley, D. M., Prochaska, J. O., Velicer, W. F., & Prochaska, G. E. (1995). Contraceptive and condom use adoption and maintenance: A stage paradigm approach. *Health Education Quarterly, 22*(1), 20–35.

Grimley, D. M., Riley, G. E., Bellis, J. M., & Prochaska, J. O. (1993). Assessing the stages of change and decision making for contraceptive use for the prevention of pregnancy, sexually transmitted diseases, and acquired immunodeficiency syndrome. *Health Education Quarterly, 20*(4), 455–470.

Grunbaum, J. A., Gingiss, P., Orpinas, P., Batey, L. S., Parcel, G. S. (1995). A comprehensive approach to school health program needs assessment. *Journal of School Health, 65*(2), 54–59.

Guyer, M. (1999). Grants: Finding a funding source. *Grant Source* (pp. 1–3). Columbus, OH: Office of the Auditor, State of Ohio.

Hall, C. L. (1943). *Principles of behavior.* New York: Appleton-Century-Crofts.

Hancock, T., & Minkler, M. (1997). Community health assessment of healthy community assessment. In M. Minkler (Ed.), *Community organizing and community building for health* (pp. 139–156). New Brunswick, NJ: Rutgers University Press.

Hanlon, J. J. (1974). *Administration of public health.* St. Louis: C. V. Mosby.

Harris, J. H., McKenzie, J. F., & Zuti, W. B. (1986). How to select the right vendor for your company's health promotion program. *Fitness in Business, 1*(October), pp. 53–56.

Harvey, P. D. (1994). The impact of condom prices on sales in social marketing programs. *Studies in Family Planning, 25,* 52–58.

Health Insurance Association of America. (1983). *Your guide to wellness at the worksite.* Pamphlet issued by the Public Relations Division of the Health Insurance Association of America, Washington, DC.

Healthy people: The Surgeon General's report on health promotion and disease prevention. (1979). (Publication No. 79–55071). Washington, DC: Department of Health, Education, and Welfare (Public Health Service).

Heiser, P. F., & Begay, M. E., (1997). The campaign to raise the tobacco tax in Massachusetts. *American Journal of Public Health, 87*(6), 968–973.

Hellerstedt, W. L., & Jeffery, R. W. (1997). The effects of a telephone-based intervention on weight loss. *American Journal of Health Promotion, 11*(3), 177–182.

Hertoz, J. K., Finnegan, J. R., Rooney, B., Viswanath, K., & Potter, J. (1993). *Health Communication, 5*(1), 21–40.

Hochbaum, G. M., Sorenson, J. R., & Lorig, K. (1992). Theory in health education practice. *Health Education Quarterly, 19*(3), 295–313.

Hopkins, K. D., Stanley, J. C., Hopkins, B. R. (1990). *Educational and psychological measurement and evaluation* (7th ed.). Englewood Cliffs, NJ: Prentice-Hall.

Horman, S. (1989). The role of social support on health throughout the lifestyle. *Health Education, 20*(4), 18–21.

Horne, W. M. (1975). Effects of a physical activity program on middle-aged, sedentary corporation executives. *American Industrial Hygiene Journal,* (March), 241–245.

Hosokawa, M. C. (1984). Insurance incentives for health promotion. *Health Education, 15*(6), 9–12.

House, E. R. (1980). *Evaluating with validity.* Beverly Hills, CA: Sage.

Houston, J. E. (Ed.). (1987). *Thesaurus of ERIC descriptors* (11th ed.). Phoenix, AZ: Oryx Press.

Hoyert, D. L., Kochanek, K. D., & Murphy, S. L., (1999). *Deaths: Final data for 1997.* Hyattsville, MD: U.S. Department of Health and Human Services, Public Health Service, CDC, National Center for Health Statistics.

Huff, R. M., & Kline, M. V. (1999). Health promotion in the context of culture. In R. M. Huff & M. V. Kline (Eds.), *Promoting health in multicultural populations* (pp. 3–22). Thousand Oaks, CA: Sage.

Hunt, W. A., Barnett, L. W., & Branch, L. G. (1971). Relapse rates in addiction programs. *Journal of Clinical Psychology, 27*(4), 455–456.

Hyner, G. C., Peterson, K. W., Travis, J. W., Dewey, J. E., Foerster, J. J., & Framer, E. M. (Eds.) (1999).

SPM handbook of health assessment tools. Pittsburgh, PA: The Society of Prospective Medicine.

Institute of Medicine (IOM). (1988). *The future of public health.* Washington, DC: National Academy Press.

IOX Assessment Associates. (1988). Program evaluation handbooks for health promotion and health education. Los Angeles: Author.

Israel, B. A., Checkoway, B., Schulz, A., & Zimmerman, M. (1994). Health education and community empowerment: Conceptualizing and measuring perceptions of individual, organizational, and community control. *Health Education Quarterly, 21*(2), 149–170.

Jacobsen, D., Eggen, P., & Kauchak, D. (1989). *Methods for teaching: A skills approach* (3rd ed.). Columbus, OH: Merrill, an imprint of Macmillan Publishing Company.

Jadad, A. R., & Gagliardi, A. (1998). Rating health information on the Internet. *Journal of the American Medical Association, 279,* 611–614.

Janz, N. K., & Becker, M. H. (1984). The health belief model: A decade later. *Health Education Quarterly, 11*(1), 1–47.

Jason, L. A., Jayaraj, S., Blitz, C. C., Michaels, M. H., & Klett, L. E. (1990). Incentives and competition in a worksite smoking cessation intervention. *American Journal of Public Health, 80*(2), 205–206.

Jeffery, R. W., Forster, J. L., Baxter, J. E., French, S. A., & Kelder, S. H. (1993). An empirical evaluation of the effectiveness of tangible incentives in increasing participation and behavior change in a worksite health promotion program. *American Journal of Health Promotion, 8*(2), 98–100.

Jessor, R., Graves, T. D., Hanson, R. C., & Jessor, S. L. (1968). *Society, personality, and deviant behavior: A study of tri ethnic community.* New York: Holt, Rinehart & Winston.

Jessor, R., & Jessor, S. L. (1977). *Problem behavior and psychosocial development: A longitudinal study of youth.* New York: Academic Press.

Joint Committee on Health Education Terminology. (1991). Report of the 1990 joint committee on health education terminology. *Journal of Health Education, 22*(2), 97–108.

Kaplan, B., & Cassel, J. (1977). Social support and health. *Medical Care, 15*(5), 47–58.

Kendall, R. (1984). Rewarding safety excellence. *Occupational Hazards,* (March), 45–50.

Kerlinger, F. N. (1986). *Foundations of behavioral research.* (3rd ed.). Austin, TX: Holt, Rinehart, & Winston.

Kim, S., McLeod, J. H., & Shantzis, C. (1992). Cultural competence for evaluators working with Asian American communities: Some practical considerations. In M. A. Orlandi, R. Weston, & L. G. Epstein (Eds.), *Cultural competence for evaluators.* Rockville, MD: Office of Substance Abuse Prevention.

Kittleson, M. J. (1995). Comparison of the response rate between e-mail and postcards. *Health Values, 19*(2), 27–29.

Kittleson, M. J. (1997). Determining effective follow-up of e-mail surveys. *American Journal of Health Behavior, 21*(3), 193–196.

Kline, M. V., & Huff, R. M., (1999). Tips for the practitioner. In R. M. Huff & M. V. Kline (Eds.), *Promoting health in multicultural populations* (pp. 103–111). Thousand Oaks, CA: Sage.

Koffman, D. M., Lee, J. W., Hopp, J. W., & Emont, S. L. (1998). The impact of including incentives and competition in a workplace smoking cessation program on quit rates. *American Journal of Health Promotion, 13*(2), 105–111.

Kolbe, L. J., & Iverson, D. C. (1981). Implementing comprehensive health education: Educational innovations and social change. *Health Education Quarterly, 8*(1), 57–80.

Kotler, P., & Andreasen, A. R. (1987). *Strategic marketing for nonprofit organizations* (3rd ed.). Englewood Cliffs, NJ: Prentice-Hall.

Kotler, P., & Andreasen, A. R. (1991). *Strategic marketing for nonprofit organizations* (4th ed.). Englewood Cliffs, NJ: Prentice-Hall.

Kotler, P., & Clarke, R. N. (1987). *Marketing for health care organizations.* Englewood Cliffs, NJ: Prentice-Hall.

Kotler, P., & Zaltman, G. (1971). Social marketing: An approach to planned social change. *Journal of Marketing, 35,* 3–12.

Kotecki, J. E., & Chamness, B. E. (1999). A valid tool for evaluating health-related WWW sites. *Journal of Health Education, 30*(1), 56–59.

Kotecki, J. E., & Siegel, D. (1997). Finding health information via the world wide web: An essential resource for the community health practitioner. *Journal of Health Education, 28*(2), 117–120.

Kreuter, M. W. (1992). PATCH: Its origin, basic concepts, and links to contemporary public health policy. *Journal of Health Education, 23*(3), 135–139.

Kreuter, M. W., Nelson, C. F., Stoddard, R. P., & Watkins, N. B. (1985). *Planned approach to community health.* Atlanta, GA: Centers for Disease Control.

Kreuter, M. W., Vehige, E., & McGuire, A. G. (1996). Using computer-tailored calendars to promote childhood immunization. *Public Health Reports, III* (March/April), 176–178.

Kumpfer, K., Turner, C., & Alvarado, R. (1991). A community change model for school health promotion. *Journal of Health Education, 22*(2), 94–96, 109–110.

Kviz, F. J., Crittenden, K. S., Madura, K. J., & Warnecke, R. B. (1994). Use and effectiveness of buddy support in a self-help smoking cessation program. *American Journal of Health Promotion, 8*(3), 191–201.

Laforge, R. G., Rossi, J. S., Prochaska, J. O., Velicer, W. F., Levesque, D. A., & McHorney, C. A. (1999). Stage of regular exercise and health-related quality of life. *Preventive Medicine, 28,* 349–360.

Lalonde, M. (1974). *A new perspective on the health of Canadians: A working document.* Ottawa, Canada: Minister of Health.

Langton, S. (Ed.). (1978). *Citizen participation in america.* Lexington, MA: Lexington Books.

Lefebvre, C. (1992). Social marketing and health promotion. In R. Burton & G. MacDonald (Eds.), *Health promotion: Disciplines and diversity* (pp. 153–181). London: Routledge.

Lefebvre, R. C., & Flora, J. A. (1988). Social marketing and public health intervention. *Health Education Quarterly, 15*(3), 299–315.

LeMaster, P. L., & Connell, C. M. (1994). Health education interventions among native Americans: A review and analysis. *Health Education Quarterly, 21*(4), 521–538.

Leventhal, H., & Cleary, P. D. (1980). The smoking problem: A review of the research and theory in behavioral risk modification. *Psychological Bulletin, 88*(2), 370–405.

Lewin, K. (1935). *A dynamic theory of personality.* New York: McGraw-Hill.

Lewin, K. (1936). *Principles of topological psychology.* New York: McGraw-Hill.

Lewin, K., Dembo, T., Festinger, L., & Sears, P. S. (1944). Level of aspiration. In J. Hunt (Ed.), *Personality and the behavior disorders* (pp. 333–378). New York: Ronald Press.

Lindberg, D. A. B. (Ed.). (1995). *Index Medicus* (NIH Publication No. 95–252). Washington, DC: U.S. Government Printing Office.

Lindsay, G. B., & Edwards, G. (1988). Creating effective health coalitions. *Health Education, 19*(4), 35–36.

Linkins, R. W., Dini, E. F., Watson, G., & Patriarca, P. A. (1994). A randomized trail of the effectiveness of computer-generated telephone messages in increasing immunization visits among preschool children. *Archives of Pediatric and Adolescent Medicine, 148*(9), 908–914.

Loughrey, K. A., Balch, G. I., Lefebvre, R. C., & Doner L. (1997). Bring five a day consumers into focus: Qualitative use of consensus research to guide strategic decision making. *Journal of Nutrition Education, 29,* 172–177.

Ludman, E. J., Curry, S. J., Meyer, D., & Taplin, S. H. (1999). Implementation of outreach telephone counseling to promote mammography participation. *Health Education & Behavior, 26*(5), 689–702.

Maccoby, N., & Solomon, D. S. (1981). Heart disease prevention: Community studies. In R. E. Rice, et al. (Eds.), *Public communication campaigns* (pp. 105–125). Beverly Hills, CA: Sage.

Maibach, E., & Holtgrave, D. R. (1995). Advances in public health communication. *Annual Review of Public Health, 16,* 219–238.

Maibach, E., Shenker, A., & Singer, S. (1997). Results of the Delphi survey. *Journal of Health Communication, 2,* 304–307.

Marcarin, S. (Ed.). (1995). *Cumulative index to nursing & allied health literature: CINAHL.* Volume 40, Part A. Glendale, CA.

Marcus, B. H., Banspach, S. W., Lefebvre, R. C., Rossi, J. S., Carleton, R. A., & Abrams, D. B. (1992). Using stages of change model to increase the adoption of physical activity among community participants. *American Journal of Health Promotion, 6,* 424–429.

Marcus, B. H., Emmons, K. M., Simkin-Silverman, L., Linnan, L. A., Taylor, E. R., Bock, B. C., Roberts, M. B., Rossi, J. S., & Abrams, D. B. (1998). Evaluation of motivationally-tailored versus standard self-help physical activity interventions at the workplace. *American Journal of Health Promotion, 12*(4), 246–253.

Marlatt, G. A. (1982). Relapse prevention: A self-control program for treatment of addictive behaviors. In R. B. Sturat (Ed.), *Adherence, compliance, and generalization in behavioral medicine* (pp. 329–377). New York: Brunner/Mazel.

Marlatt, G. A. (1985). Relapse prevention: Theoretical rationale and overview of the model. In G. A. Marlatt & J. R. Gordon (Eds.), *Relapse prevention* (pp. 3–70). New York: Guilford Press.

Marlatt, G. A., & George, W. H. (1998). Relapse prevention and the maintenance of optimal health. In S. A. Shumaker, E. B. Schron, J. K. Ockene, & W. L. McBee (Eds.), *The handbook of health behavior change* (2nd ed., pp. 33–58). New York: Springer.

Marlatt, G. A., & Gordon, J. R. (1980). Determinants of relapse: Implications for maintenance of behavior change. In P. O. Davidson & S. M. Davidson (Eds.), *Behavioral medicine: Changing health lifestyles* (pp. 410–452). New York: Brunner/Mazel.

Mason, J. O., & McGinnis, J. M. (1990). "Healthy people 2000": An overview of the national health promotion and disease prevention objectives. *Public Health Reports, 105*(5), 441–446.

Matson, D. M., Lee, J. W., & Hopp, J. W. (1993). The impact of incentives and competitions on participation and quit rates in worksite smoking cessation programs. *American Journal of Health Promotion, 7*(4), 270–280, 295.

McAlister, A. L., Puska, P., Salonen, J. T., Tuomilehot, J., & Koskelia, A. (1982). Theory and action for health promotion: Illustrations from the North Karelia project. *American Journal of Public Health, 72*(1), 43–50.

McCarthy, E. J. (1978). *Basic marketing: A managerial approach* (6th ed.). Homewood, IL: Richard D. Irwin.

McCaul, K. D., Bakdash, M. B., Geoboy, M. J., Gerbert, B., et al. (1990). Promoting self-protective health behaviors in dentistry. *Annuals of Behavioral Medicine, 12*, 156–160.

McCraig, L. F. (1997). National Hospital Ambulatory Medical Care Survey: 1995 outpatient department summary. Advance data from *Vital and Health Statistics*, no. 284. Hyattsville, MD: National Center for Health Statistics.

McDermott, R. J., & Sarvela, P. D. (1999). *Health education evaluation and measurement: A practitioner's perspective* (2nd ed.). New York: WCB/McGraw-Hill.

McDonald, T. L., Treser, C. D., & Hatlen, J. B. (1994). Development of an environmental health addendum to the assessment protocol for excellence in public health. *Journal of Public Health Policy, 15*(2), 203–217.

McDowell, I., Newell, C., & Rosser, W. (1989a). Computerized reminders for blood pressure screening in primary care. *Medical Care, 27*(3), 297–305.

McDowell, I., Newell, C., & Rosser, W. (1989b). Computerized reminders to encourage cervical screening in family practice. *Journal of Family Practice, 28*(4), 420–424.

McGuire, W. J. (1981). Behavioral medicine, public health and communication theories. *Health Education, 12*(3), 8–13.

McKenzie, J. F. (1986). Cost-benefit and cost-effectiveness as a part of the evaluation of health promotion programs. *The Eta Sigma Gamman, 18*(2), 10–16.

McKenzie, J. F. (1988). Twelve steps in developing a schoolsite health education/promotion program for faculty and staff. *The Journal of School Health, 58*(4), 149–153.

McKenzie, J. F., Luebke, J., & Romas, J. A. (1992). Incentives: A means of getting and keeping workers involved in health promotion programs. *Journal of Health Education, 23*(2), 70–73.

McKenzie, J. F., Pinger, R. R., & Kotecki, J. E. (1999). *An introduction to community health* (3rd ed.). Boston: Jones and Bartlett.

McKenzie, J. F., & Smeltzer, J. L. (1997). *Planning, implementing, and evaluating health promotion program: A primer* (2nd ed.). Boston: Allyn and Bacon.

McKenzie, J. F., Wood, M. L., Kotecki, J. E., Clark, J. K., & Brey, R. A. (1999). Establishing content validity: Using qualitative and quantitative steps. *American Journal of Health Behavior, 23*(4), 311–318.

McKnight, J. L., & Kretzmann, J. P. (1997). Mapping community capacity. In M. Minkler (Ed.), *Community organizing and community building for health.* (pp. 157–172). New Brunswick, NJ: Rutgers University Press.

McLeroy, K. R. (1993). Theory and practice in health education: Which practice, which theory? *American Public Health Association, Public Health Education and Health Promotion Section Newsletter,* Summer, 7–8.

McLeroy, K. R., Bibeau, D., Steckler, A., & Glanz, K. (1988). An ecological perspective on health promotion programs. *Health Education Quarterly, 15*, 351–377.

Meyer, J., & Rainey, J. (1994). Writing health education material for low-literacy populations. *Journal of Health Education, 25*(6), 372–374.

Mikanowicz, C. K., & Altman, N. H. (1995). Developing policies on smoking in the workplace. *Journal of Health Education, 26*(3), 183–185.

Miller, R. E. (1992). Health communication through workplace smoking discouragement posters. *Journal of Health Education, 23*(4), 250–252.

Miller, R. E., & Golaszewski, T. J. (1992). Analysis of commercial health newsletters by worksite decision makers. *American Journal of Health Promotion, 7*(1), 11–12, 75.

Minkler, M. (Ed.). (1997a). *Community organizing and community building for health.* New Brunswick, NJ: Rutgers University Press.

Minkler, M. (1997b). Introduction and overview. In M. Minkler (Ed.), *Community organizing and community building for health* (pp. 3–19). New Brunswick, NJ: Rutgers University Press.

Minkler, M., & Wallerstein, N. (1997). Improving health through community organization and community building: A health education perspective. In M. Minkler (Ed.), *Community organizing and community building for health* (pp. 30–52). New Brunswick, NJ: Rutgers University Press.

Monahan, J. L., & Scheirer, M. A. (1988). The role of linking agents in the diffusion of health promotion programs. *Health Education Quarterly, 15*(4), 417–433.

Mondros, J. B., & Wilson, S. M. (1994). *Organizing for power and empowerment.* New York: Columbia Press.

Morreale, M. (no date). Understanding public health research: A primer for youth workers. *Issue Brief.* Washington, DC: National Network for Youth.

Morris, L. L., Fitz-Gibbon, C. T., & Freeman, M. E. (1987). *How to communicate evaluation findings.* Newbury Park, CA: Sage.

Moskowitz, J. M. (1989). Preliminary guidelines for reporting outcome evaluation studies of health promotion and disease prevention programs. In M. Braverman (Ed.), *New directions for program evaluation* (pp. 59–74). San Francisco: Jossey-Bass.

National Association of County Health Officials (NACHO). (1991). *APEX/PH, Assessment protocol for excellence in public health.* Washington, DC: Author.

National Commission for Health Education Credentialing, Inc. (NCHEC). (1996). *A competency-based framework for professional development of certified health education specialists.* New York: Author.

National Dairy Council. (1992). *2000 and counting.* Rosemont, IL: Author.

National Task Force on the Preparation and Practice of Health Educators, Inc. (1985). *A framework for the development of competency-based curricula for entry-level health educators.* New York: Author.

Neiger, B. L., (1998). *Social marketing: Making public health sense.* Paper presented at the annual meeting of the Utah Public Health Association, Provo, UT.

Newcomer, K. E. (1994). Using statistics appropriately. In J. S. Wholey, H. P. Hatry, & K. E. Newcomer (Eds.), *Handbook of practical program evaluation* (pp. 389–416). San Francisco: Jossey-Bass.

Ngo, J. (1993). Social marketing and fat intake. *European Journal of Clinical Nutrition, 1,* 91–95.

Norcross, J. C., Prochaska, J. O., & Hambrecht, M. (1991). Treating ourselves vs. treating our clients: A replication with alcohol abuse. *Journal of Substance Abuse, 3,* 123–129.

Novelli, W. D. (1988). Marketing health and social issues: What works? In R. Dunmire (Ed.), *Social marketing: Accepting the challenge in public health.* Atlanta, GA: Centers for Disease Control.

Novelli, W. D., & Ziska, D. (1982). Health promotion in the workplace: An overview. *Health Education Quarterly, 9*(suppl.), 20–26.

Nye, R. D. (1979). *What is B. F. Skinner really saying?* Englewood Cliffs, NJ: Prentice-Hall.

Nye, R. D. (1992). *The legacy of B. F. Skinner: Concepts and perspectives, controversies, and misunderstandings.* Pacific Grove, CA: Brooks/Cole.

O'Donnell, M. (1992). Design of workplace health promotion programs (2nd ed.). Rochester Hills, MI: *American Journal of Health Promotion.*

O'Donnell, M. P. (1996). Editor's notes. *American Journal of Health Promotion, 10*(4), 244.

O'Donnell, M., & Ainsworth, T. (Eds.). (1984). *Health promotion in the workplace.* New York: John Wiley and Sons.

Office of Public Health and Science (OPHS), U.S. Department of Health and Human Services (USDHHS). (1998). *Healthy People 2010 objectives: Draft for public comment.* Washington, DC: Author.

Ogbu, J. (1987). Cultural influences on plasticity in human development. In J. L. Gallagher & C. T. Ramey (Eds.), *The malleability of children* (pp. 155–169). Baltimore, MD: Paul H. Brookes.

Olpin, M., & Gotthoffer, D. (2000). *Quick guide to the Internet for health.* Boston: Allyn and Bacon.

Orlaldi, M. A. (1986). The diffusion and adoption of worksite health promotion innovations: An analysis of barriers. *Preventive Medicine, 15*(5), 522–536.

Pahnos, M. L. (1992). The continuing challenge of multicultural health education. *Journal of School Health, 62*(1), 24–26.

Parcel, G. S. (1983). Theoretical models for application in school health education research. *Health Education, 15*(4), 39–49.

Parcel, G. S., & Baranowski, T. (1981). Social learning theory and health education. *Health Education, 12*(3), 14–18.

Parcel, G. S., Ericksen, M. P., Lovato, C. Y., Gottlieb, N. H., Brink, S. G., & Green, L. W. (1989). The diffusion of school-based tobacco-use prevention programs: Project description and baseline data. *Health Education Research, 4*(1), 111–124.

Parkinson, R. S., & Associates. (1982). *Managing health promotion in the workplace: Guidelines for implementation and evaluation.* Palo Alto. CA: Mayfield.

Pasick, R. J., D'Onofrio, C. N., & Otero-Sabogal, R. (1996). Similarities and differences across cultures: Questions to inform a third generation for health promotion research. *Health Education, 23* (Suppl.), S142–S161.

Patton, M. Q. (1986). *Utilization-focused evaluation.* Beverly Hills, CA: Sage.

Patton, M. Q. (1988). *How to use qualitative methods in evaluation.* Newbury Park, CA: Sage.

Patton, R. P., Corry, J. M., Gettman, L. R., & Graff, J. S. (1986). *Implementing health/fitness programs.* Champaign, IL: Human Kinetics.

Pavlov, I. (1927). *Conditional reflexes.* Oxford: Oxford University Press.

Pealer, L. N., & Dorman, S. M. (1997). Evaluating health-related web sites. *Journal of School Health, 67*(1), 232–235.

Penner, M. (1989). Economic incentives to reduce employee smoking: A health insurance surcharge for tobacco using state of Kansas employees. *American Journal of Health Promotion, 4*(1), 5–11.

Pentz, M. A., Johnson, C. A., Dwyer, J. H., MacKinnon, D. M., Hansen, W. B., & Flay, B. R. (1989). A comprehensive community approach to adolescent drug abuse prevention: Effects on cardiovascular disease risk behaviors. *Annals of Medicine, 21*(3), 382–388.

Perlman, J. (1978). Grassroots participation from neighborhood to nation. In S. Langton (Ed.), *Citizen participation in America* (pp. 65–79). Lexington, MA: Lexington Books.

Pickett, G. E., & Hanlon, J. J. (1990). *Public health: Administration and practice.* St. Louis: Mosby-Year Book, Inc.

Piniat, A. J. (1984). How to put spirit in an incentive program. *National Safety News,* (January), 46–49.

Pinto, B. M., & Marcus, B. H. (1995). A stages of change approach to understanding college students' physical activity. *Journal of American College Health, 44,* 27–31.

Pollock, M. L., Foster, C., Salisburg, R., & Smith, R. (1982). Effects of a YMCA starter fitness program. *The Physician and Sportsmedicine, 10*(1), 89–91, 95–99, 120.

Popham, W. J. (1988). *Educational evaluation.* Englewood Cliffs, NJ: Prentice-Hall.

Powell-Griner, E. J., Anderson, J. E., & Murphy, W. (1997). State- and sex-specific prevalence of selected characteristics—Behavioral risk factor surveillance system, 1994–1995. In *CDC Surveillance Summaries, August 1, 1997. MMWR, 46* (No. SS-3), pp. 1–31.

Price, J. H., Telljohann, S. K., Roberts, S. M., & Smit, D. (1992). Effects of incentives in an inner city junior high school smoking prevention program. *Journal of Health Education, 23* (7), 388–396.

Prochaska, J. O. (1979). *Systems of psychotherapy: A transtheoretical analysis.* Homewood, IL: Dorsey Press.

Prochaska, J. O., & DiClemente, C. C. (1983). Stages and processes of self-change of smoking: Toward an integrative model of change. *Journal of Consulting and Clinical Psychology, 51*(3), 390–395.

Prochaska, J. O., & DiClemente, C. C. (1985). Common processes of change for smoking, weight control, and psychological distress. In S. Shiffman & T. Wills (Eds.), *Coping and Substance Abuse* (pp. 345–363). New York: Academic Press.

Prochaska, J. O., DiClemente, C. C., & Norcross, J. C. (1992). In search of how people change: Applications to addictive behaviors. *American Psychologist, 47*(9), 1102–1114.

Prochaska, J. O., DiClemente, C. C., Velicer, W. F., Ginpil, S., & Norcross, J. C. (1985). Predicting change in smoking status for self-changers. *Addictive Behaviors, 10*(4), 395–406.

Prochaska, J. O., Harlow, L. L., Redding, C. A., Snow, M. G., Rossi, J. S., & Velicer, W. F. (1990). *Stages of charge, self-efficacy, and decisional balance of condom use in a high HIV risk sample.* Atlanta, GA: Technical Report for Centers for Disease Control Contract Grant 0–4115–002.

Prochaska, J. O., Johnson, S., & Lee, P. (1998). The transtheoretical model of behavior change. In S. A. Shumaker, E. B. Schron, J. K. Ockene, & W. L. McBee (Eds.), *The handbook of health behavior change* (2nd ed., pp. 59–84). New York: Springer.

Prochaska, J. O., Norcross, J. C., Fowler, J. L., Follick, M. J., & Abrams, D. B. (1992). Attendance and outcome in a worksite weight control program: Processes and stages of change as process and predictor variables. *Addictive Behaviors, 17,* 35–45.

Prochaska, J. O., Redding, C. A., Harlow, L. L., Rossi, J. S., & Velicer, W. F. (1994). The transtheoretical model of change and HIV prevention: A review. *Health Education Quarterly, 21*(4), 471–486.

Rakich, J. S., Longest, B. B., & O'Donovan, T. R. (1977). *Managing health care organizations.* Philadelphia: W. B. Saunders.

Ratzan, S. C. (1999a). Strategic health communication and social marketing on risk issues. *Journal of Health Communication, 4,* 1–6.

Ratzan, S. C. (1999b). Revolutionizing health: Communication can make a difference. *Journal of Health Communication, 4,* 255–257.

Redding, C. A., Rossi, J. S., Rossi, S. R., Velicer, W. F., & Prochaska, J. O. (1999). Health behavior models. In G. C. Hyner, K. W. Peterson, J. W.

Travis, J. E. Dewey, J. J. Foerster, & E. M. Framer (Eds.), *SPM handbook of health assessment tools* (pp. 83–93). Pittsburgh, PA: The Society of Prospective Medicine.

Rice, R. E., & Atkin, C. K. (1989). Trends in communication campaign research. In R. E. Rice & C. K. Atkin (Eds.), *Public communication campaigns* (2nd ed.). Newbury Park, CA: Sage.

Rich, R. F., & Sugrue, N. M. (1989). Health promotion, disease prevention, and public policy. *Wellness Perspectives: Research, Theory and Practice, 6*(1), 27–35.

Riedel, J. E. (1999). The cost-effectiveness of health promotion. In G. C. Hyner, K. W. Peterson, J. W. Travis, J. E. Dewey, J. J. Foerster, & E. M. Framer (Eds.), *SPM handbook of health assessment tools* (pp. 111–118). Pittsburgh, PA: The Society of Prospective Medicine.

Rifkin, S. B. (1986). Lessons from community participation in health programmes. *Health Policy and Planning, 1*(3), 240–249.

Robbins, L. C., & Hall, J. H. (1970). *How to practice prospective medicine.* Indianapolis, IN: Methodist Hospital of Indiana.

Rogers, E. M. (1962). *Diffusion of innovations.* New York: Free Press of Glencoe.

Rogers, E. M. (1983). *Diffusion of innovations* (3rd ed.). New York: Free Press.

Rogers, E. M., (1994). *Diffusion of innovations* (4th ed.). New York: Free Press.

Rogers, E. M. (1996). The field of health communication today: An up-to-date report. *Journal of Health Communication, 1,* 15–23.

Romer, D., & Kim, S. (1995). Health interventions for African American and Latino youth: The potential role of mass media. *Health Education Quarterly, 22*(2), 172–189.

Rosenstock, I. M. (1966). Why people use health services. *Milbank Memorial Fund Quarterly, 44,* 94–124.

Rosenstock, I. M., Strecher, V. J., & Becker, M. H. (1988). Social learning theory and the health belief model. *Health Education Quarterly, 15*(2), 175–183.

Ross, H. S., & Mico, P. R. (1980). *Theory and practice in health education.* Palo Alto, CA: Mayfield.

Ross, M. G. (1967). *Community organization: Theory, principles, and practice.* New York: Harper & Row.

Rothman, J., & Tropman, J. E. (1987). Models of community organization and macro practice perspectives: Their mixing and phasing. In F. M. Cox, J. L. Erlich, J. Rothman, & J. E. Tropman (Eds.), *Strategies of community organization: Macro practice* (pp. 3–26). Itasca, IL: F. E. Peacock.

Rotter, J. B. (1954). *Social learning and clinical psychology.* New York: Prentice-Hall.

Rotter, J. B. (1966). Generalized expectancies for internal versus external control of reinforcement. *Psychological Monographs, 80*(1).

Rubin, H. J., & Rubin, I. S. (1992). *Community organizing and development* (2nd ed.). New York: Macmillan.

Sachs, J. J., Krushat, W. M., & Newman, J. (1980). Reliability of the health hazard appraisal. *American Journal of Public Health, 70,* 730–732.

Samuels, S. E. (1993). Project LEAN: Lessons learned from a national social marketing campaign. *Public Health Reports, 108,* 45–53.

Scandrett, A. (1994). The black church as a participant in community interventions. *Journal of Health Education, 25*(3), 183–185.

Schechter, C., Vanchieri, C., & Crofton, C. (1990). Evaluating women's attitudes and perceptions in developing mammography promotion messages. *Public Health Reports, 105*(3), 253–257.

Schmid, T. L., Pratt, M., & Howze, E. (1995). Policy as intervention: Environmental and policy approaches to the prevention of cardiovascular disease. *American Journal of Public Health, 85,* 1207–1211.

Sciacca, J., Seehafer, R., Reed, R., & Mulvaney, D. (1993). The impact of participation in health promotion on medical costs: A reconsideration of the Blue Cross and Blue Shield of Indiana study. *American Journal of Health Promotion, 7*(5), 374–383, 395.

Scriven, M. (1973). Goal-free evaluation. In E. House (Ed.), *School evaluation: The politics and procedures* (pp. 319–328). Berkeley, CA: McCutchan.

Seffrin, J. R. (1994). America's interest in comprehensive school health education. *Journal of School Health, 64,* 397–399.

Shea, S., & Basch, C. E. (1990). A review of five major community-based cardiovascular disease prevention programs: Part I, rationale, design and theoretical framework. *American Journal of Health Promotion, 4*(3), 203–213.

Shepard, M. (1985). Motivation: The key to fitness compliance. *The Physician and Sportsmedicine, 13*(7), 88–101.

Shim, J. K., & Siegel, J. G. (1994). *Complete budgeting workbook and guide.* New York: New York Institute of Finance.

Silberg, W. M., Lundberg, G. D., & Musacchio, R. A. (1997). Assessing, controlling, and assuring the quality of medical information on the internet. *Journal of the American Medical Association, 277,* 1244–1245.

SilverPlatter. (1992, April). PsycLIT on SilverPlatter.

Simkin, L. R., & Gross, A. M. (1994). Assessment of coping with high-risk situations for exercise relapse among healthy women. *Health Psychology, 13*, 274–277.

Simmons, R. (1998). Quitting by phone. *Health Education & Behavior, 25*(6), 686–687.

Simons-Morton, B. G., Greene, W. H., & Gottlieb, N. H. (1995). *Introduction to health education and health promotion* (2nd ed.). Prospect Heights, IL: Waveland Press.

Simons-Morton, D. G., Simons-Morton, B. G., Parcel, G. S., & Bunker, J. F. (1988). Influencing personal and environmental conditions for community health: A multilevel intervention model. *Family and Community Health, 11*(2), 25–35.

Skinner, B. F. (1953). *Science and human behavior.* New York: Free Press.

Skinner, C. S., Strecher, V. J., & Hospers, H. (1994). Physicians' recommendations for mammography; Do tailored messages make a difference? *American Journal of Public Health, 84*(1), 43–49.

Sloan, R., Gruman, J., & Allegrante, J. (1987). *Investing in employee health.* San Francisco: Jossey-Bass.

Smith, K. W., McKinlay, S. M., & McKinlay, J. B. (1989). The reliability of health risk appraisals: A field trial of four instruments. *American Journal of Public Health, 79*(12), 1603–1606.

Snow, M. G., Prochaska, J. O., & Rossi, J. S. (1992). Stages of change for smoking cessation among former problem drinkers: A cross-sectional analysis. *Journal of Substance Abuse, 4*, 107–116.

Soet, J. E., & Basch, C. E. (1997). The telephone as a communication medium for health education. *Health Education & Behavior, 24*(6), 759–772.

Solomon, D. D. (1987). Evaluating community programs. In F. M. Cox, J. L. Erlich, J. Rolhman, & J. E. Tropman (Eds.), *Strategies of community organization: Macro practices* (pp. 366–368). Itasca, IL: F. E. Peacock.

Sorensen, G., Rigotti, N., Rosen, A., Pinney, J., and Prible, R. (1991). Effects of a worksite nonsmoking policy: Evidence for increased cessation. *American Journal of Public Health, 81*(2), 202–204.

Speers, M. (1992). Preface. *Journal of Health Education, 23*(3), 132–133.

SPM Board of Directors (SPMBoD). (1999). Ethics guidelines for the development and use of health assessments. In G. C. Hyner, K. W. Peterson, J. W. Travis, J. E. Dewey, J. J. Foerster, & E. M. Framer (Eds.), *SPM handbook of health assessment tools* (p. xxiii). Pittsburgh, PA: The Society of Prospective Medicine.

Stacy, R. D. (1987). Instrument evaluation guides for survey research in health education and health promotion. *Health Education, 18*(5), 65–67.

Steckler, A., Goodman, R. M., McLeroy, K. R., Davis, S., & Koch, G. (1992). Measuring the diffusion of innovative health promotion programs. *American Journal of Health Promotion, 6*(3), 214–224.

Steckler, A., McLeroy, K. R., Goodman, R. M., Bird, S. T., & McCormick, L. (1992). Toward integrating qualitative and quantitative methods: An introduction. *Health Education Quarterly, 19*(1), 1–8.

Strecher, V. J., DeVellis, B. M., Becker, M. H., & Rosenstock, I. M. (1986). The role of self-efficacy in achieving health behavior change. *Health Education Quarterly, 13*(1), 73–91.

Strecher, V. J., Kreuter, M. W., Den Boer, D. J., Kobrin, S., Hospers, H. J., & Skinner, C. S. (1994). The effects of computer-tailored smoking cessation messages in family practice. *Journal of Family Practice, 39*(3), 262–270.

Strecher, V. J., & Rosenstock, I. M. (1997). The health belief model. In K. Glanz, F. M. Lewis, & B. K. Rimer (Eds.), *Health behavior and health education: Theory, research, and practice* (pp. 41–59). San Francisco: Jossey-Bass.

Strycker, L. A., Foster, L. S., Pettigrew, L., Donnelly-Perry, J., Jordan, S., & Glasgow, R. E. (1997). Steering committee enhancements on health promotion program delivery. *American Journal of Health Promotion, 11*(6), 437–440.

Stufflebeam, D. L., & Members of the National Study Committee on Evaluation of Phi Delta Kappa (1971). *Educational evaluation and decision making.* Itasca, IL: F. E. Peacock.

Stunkard, A. J., & Braunwell, K. D. (1980). Worksite treatment for obesity. *American Journal of Psychiatry, 137*, 252–253.

Suchman, E. A. (1967). *Evaluative Research.* New York: Russell Sage Foundation.

Sullivan, D. (1973). Model for comprehensive, systematic program development in health education. *Health Education Report, 1*(1) (November–December), 4–5.

Sutherland, M. S., Harris, G. J., Kissinger, M., Barber, M., & Lewis, J. L. (1994). Creating awareness of drug prevention: Using beauty shops as information outlets. *Journal of Health Education, 25*(3), 186–187.

Syre, T. R., & Wilson, R. W. (1990). Health care marketing: Role evolution of the community health educator. *Health Education, 21*(1), 6–8.

Thompson, N. J., & McClintock, H. O. (1998). *Demonstrating your program's worth: A primer on eval-*

uation for programs to prevent unintentional injury. Atlanta, GA: National Center for Injury Prevention and Control, CDC.

Thorndike, E. L. (1898). Animal intelligence: An experimental study of the associative processes in animals. *Psychological Monographs, 2*(8).

Tillman, H. N. (1997). Evaluating quality on the web [Online]. Available: <http://tiac.net/users/hope/findqual.html>.

Timmreck, T. C. (1995). *Planning, program development, and evaluation: A handbook for health promotion, aging, and health services.* Boston: Jones and Bartlett.

Toufexis, A. (1985). Giving goodies to the good. *Time* (November 18), 98.

U.S. Bureau of Census (USBC). (1997). *Statistical abstract of the United States: 1997, 117th ed.* Washington, DC: U.S. Government Printing Office.

U.S. Department of Health and Human Services (USDHHS), Centers for Disease Control and Prevention (CDC). (no date). *Planned approach to community health: Guide for local coordinator.* Atlanta, GA: Author.

U.S. Department of Health and Human Services (USDHHS), Office of Disease Prevention and Health Promotion. (1997). *Developing objectives for healthy People 2010.* Washington, DC: U.S. Government Printing Office.

U.S. Department of Health and Human Services (USDHHS). (1995). *Healthy People 2000: Midcourse review and 1995 revisions.* Washington, DC: U.S. Government Printing Office.

U.S. Department of Health and Human Services. (1998). *Healthy People 2010 objectives: Draft for public comment.* Washington, DC: Office of Public Health and Science.

Udinsky, B. F., Osterlind, S. J., & Lynch, S. W. (1981). *Evaluation resource handbook: Gathering, analyzing, reporting data.* San Diego: EdITS.

U.S. Department of Health and Human Services (USDHHS). (1980). *Promoting health/preventing disease: Objectives for the nation.* Washington, DC: U.S. Government Printing Office.

U.S. Department of Health and Human Services (USDHHS). (1985). *No smoking: A decision maker's guide to reducing smoking at the worksite.* Washington, DC: U.S. Government Printing Office.

U.S. Department of Health and Human Services (USDHHS). (1986a). *Integration of risk factor interventions.* Washington, DC: U.S. Government Printing Office.

U.S. Department of Health and Human Services (USDHHS). (1986b). *The 1990 health objectives for the nation: A midcourse review.* Washington, DC: U.S. Government Printing Office.

U.S. Department of Health and Human Services (USDHHS). (1987). *Strategies for diffusing health information to minority populations: Executive summary.* Washington, DC: U.S. Government Printing Office.

U.S. Department of Health and Human Services (USDHHS). (1989). *Making health communication programs work: A planner's guide* (NIH Publication No. 89–1493). Washington, DC: U.S. Government Printing Office.

U.S. Department of Health and Human Services (USDHHS). (1990a). *Healthy people 2000: National health promotion disease prevention objectives* (DHHS Publication No. [PHS] 90–50212). Washington, DC: U.S. Government Printing Office.

U.S. Department of Health and Human Services (USDHHS). (1990b). *Prevention '89/'90.* Washington, DC: U.S. Government Printing Office.

U.S. Department of Health and Human Services (USDHHS). (1994). *Healthy People 2000 Review, 1993* (DHHS Publication No. [PHS] 94–1232–1). Washington, DC: U.S. Government Printing Office.

U.S. Department of Health and Human Services (USDHHS), Office of Substance Abuse Prevention (1991). *The fact is…you can prepare easy-to-read materials.* Rockville, MD: Author.

van Ryn, M., & Heaney, C. A. (1992). What's the use of theory? *Health Education Quarterly, 19*(3), 315–330.

Velicer, W. F., Fava, J. L., Prochaska, J. O., Abrams, D. B., Emmons, K. M., & Pierce, J. (1995). Distribution of smokers by stage in three representative samples. *Preventive Medicine, 24,* 401–411.

Velicer, W. F., Prochaska, J. O., Fava, J. L., Norman, G. J., & Redding, C. A. (1998). Smoking and stress: Applications of the transtheoretical model of behavior change. *Homeostasis, 38,* 216–233.

Venditto, G. (1997, January). Critic's choice: Six sites that rate the web. *Internet World,* pp. 82–96.

Wagner, E. H., & Guild, P. A. (1989). Choosing an evaluation strategy. *American Journal of Health Promotion, 4*(2), 134–139.

Walker, R. A., & Bibeau, D. (1985/1986). Health education as freeing—Part II. *Health Education, 16*(6), (December/January), 4–8.

Wallerstein, N. (1994). Empowerment education applied to youth. In A. C. Matiella (Ed.). *The multicultural challenge in health education* (pp. 153–176). Santa Cruz, CA: ETR Associates.

Wallerstein, N., & Bernstein, E. (1988). Empowerment education: Freier's ideas adapted to health education. *Health Education Quarterly, 15*(4), 379–394.

Wallerstein, N., Sanchez-Merki, V., & Dow, L. (1997). Freirian praxis in health education and community organizing: A case study of an adult prevention program. In M. Minkler (Ed.), *Community organizing and community building for health* (pp. 195–215). New Brunswick, NJ: Rutgers University Press.

Wallston, K. A. (1992). Hocus-pocus, the focus isn't strictly on locus: Rotter's social learning theory modified for health. *Cognitive Therapy and Research, 16,* 183–199.

Wallston, K. A. (1994). Theoretically based strategies for health behavior change. In M. P. O'Donnell, & J. S. Harris (Eds.). *Health promotion in the workplace* (2nd ed.). (pp. 185–203). Albany, NY: Delmar.

Wallston, K. A., Wallston, B. S., & DeVellis, R. (1978). Development of the multidimensional health locus of control (MHLC) scales. *Health Education Monographs, 6,* 160–170.

Walsh, D. C., Rudd, R. E., Moeykens, B. A., & Moloney, T. W. (1993). Social marketing for public health. *Health Affairs, 12,* 104–119.

Walter, C. L. (1997). Community building practice: A conceptual framework. In M. Minkler (Ed.), *Community organizing and community building for health* (pp. 68–83). New Brunswick, NJ: Rutgers University Press.

Warner, K. E. (1987). Selling health promotion to corporate America: Uses and abuses of the economic argument. *Health Education Quarterly, 14*(1), 39–55.

Warner, K. E., Wickizer, T., Wolfe, R., Schildroth, J., & Samuelson, M. (1988). Economic implications of workplace health promotion programs: Review of literature. *Journal of Occupational Medicine, 30*(2), 106–112.

Washington, R. (1987). Alternative frameworks for program evaluation. In F. M. Cox, J. L. Erlich, J. Rolhman, & J. E. Tropman (Eds.), *Strategies of community organization: Macro practices* (pp. 373–374). Itasca, IL: F. E. Peacock.

Watson, J. B. (1925). *Behaviorism.* New York: W. W. Norton.

Weinreich, N. K. (1999). What is social marketing [Online]. Available: <http://www.social-marketing.com.html>.

Weinstein, A. (1987). *Market segmentation.* Chicago: Probus.

Weiss, C. H. (1984). Increasing the likelihood of influencing decisions. In L. Rutman (Ed.), *Evaluation research methods: A basic guide* (2nd ed.) (pp. 159–190). Beverly Hills, CA: Sage.

Weiss, C. H. (1998). *Evaluation* (2nd ed.). Upper Saddle River, NJ: Prentice-Hall.

Wilbur, C. (1983). Live for life—The Johnson & Johnson program. *Preventive Medicine, 12*(5), 672–681.

Williams, B., & Suen, H. (1998). Formal vs. informal assessment methods. *American Journal of Health Behavior, 22*(4), 308–313.

Williams, J. E., & Flora, J. A. (1995). Health behavior segmentation and campaign planning to reduce cardiovascular disease risk among Hispanics. *Health Education Quarterly, 22*(1), 36–38.

Wilson, M. G. (1990). Factors associated with, issues related to, and suggestions for increasing participation in workplace health promotion programs. *Health Values, 14*(4), 29–36.

Wilson, M. G., and Olds, S. (1991). Application of the marketing mix to health promotion marketing. *Journal of Health Education, 22*(4), 254–259.

Windsor, R. A., Baranowski, T., Clark, N., & Cutter, G. (1984). *Evaluation of health promotion and education programs.* Palo Alto, CA: Mayfield.

Windsor, R., Baranowski, T., Clark, N., & Cutter, G. (1994). *Evaluation of health promotion, health education, and disease prevention programs* (2nd ed.). Mountain View, CA: Mayfield.

Wolfe, R., Slack, T., & Rose-Hearn, T. (1993). Factors influencing the adoption and maintenance of Canadian, facility-based worksite health promotion programs. *American Journal of Health Promotion, 7*(3), 189–198.

Woolf, H. B. (Ed.). (1979). *Webster's new collegiate dictionary.* Springfield, MA: G. & C. Merriam.

Wright, P. A. (Ed.). (1994). *Technical assistance bulletin: A key step in developing prevention materials is to obtain expert and gatekeepers' reviews.* Bethesda, MD: Center for Substance Abuse Prevention (CASP) Communications Team.

Wright, P. A. (Ed.). (1997). *Technical assistance bulletin: Identifying the target audience.* Bethesda, MD: Center for Substance Abuse Prevention (CASP) Communications Team.

Name Index

Subject Index